SMALLPOX,
SYPHILIS AND
SALVATION

SMALLPOX, SYPHILIS AND SALVATION

MEDICAL BREAKTHROUGHS

THAT CHANGED THE WORLD

SHERYL PERSSON

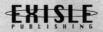

EXISLE
PUBLISHING

First published 2009

Exisle Publishing Limited
'Moonrising', Narone Creek Road, Wollombi, NSW 2325, Australia
P.O. Box 60–490, Titirangi, Auckland 0642, New Zealand
www.exislepublishing.com

National Library of Australia Cataloguing-in-Publication Data:

Persson, Sheryl Ann, 1952–

Smallpox, syphilis and salvation : medical breakthroughs
that changed the world / Sheryl Persson

ISBN 9781921497063 (pbk.)

Includes index.
Bibliography.

Discoveries in science.
Medicine – Biography.
Medicine – History.

509

Designed by saso content & design pty ltd
Typeset in Perpetua 12/15 by 1000 Monkeys Typesetting Services
Printed in China through Colorcraft Limited, Hong Kong

10 9 8 7 6 5 4 3 2 1

Two contrary laws seem to be wrestling with each other nowadays: the one, a law of blood and of death, ever imagining new means of destruction and forcing nations to be constantly ready for the battlefield — the other, a law of peace, work and health, ever evolving new means for delivering man from the scourges which beset him.

Louis Pasteur,
speech opening the Pasteur Institute,
Paris, 14 November 1888

CONTENTS

INTRODUCTION

It is a wonder that humans as a species have managed to survive and thrive. For thousands of years we have been bent on destroying our own kind and we continue to develop ever more sophisticated means of doing so. Apart from the wars we wage against each other we have also succeeded, particularly during the last century, in damaging our environment irreparably and destroying innumerable species that once shared Earth with us. But we are not our own worst enemy. It is the foe we cannot see that has from prehistoric times posed the greatest threat. Species of micro-organisms flourished before we did and they were the most determined killers of humankind long before we knew they existed. For millennia humans did not have the means with which to detect and identify these unseen disease-causing adversaries.

When I began the research for this book on world-changing cures and medical breakthroughs it soon became evident that I had to discard a number of preconceived notions. Firstly I had to examine my understanding of what constituted a 'cure'. My working definition was simple: you contract a disease, you are provided with some kind of medication, your symptoms disappear and they do not return. You are cured. What I came to realise is that until penicillin was discovered and used widely for the first time in the early 1940s, very few diseases actually had a cure.

Since ancient times the search for ways to prevent and cure the devastating scourges that have afflicted humankind has been ongoing but it is only within the last 200 years that significant advances have been possible. The age of monumental medical breakthroughs began as recently as 1796 with Edward Jenner's discovery of vaccination and his development of a vaccine for smallpox. Described as the 'Founding Father of Immunology', Jenner took the first of many protracted steps on the road to discovering the human immune system, how it works and how it can be manipulated to fight disease. In Jenner's day there were no cures as I understood them for the plethora of diseases that plagued all societies, often with cata-strophic consequences. If you were sick physicians could do little more than provide treatments that were often little more than comfort, an easing of symptoms perhaps, as you succumbed to your fate.

Although there was an accretion of medical knowledge over the centuries as human anatomy became more understood, it was necessary that advances in technology also take place, especially in the development of instruments vital for discoveries to be made. The invention of the microscope, for example, was critical. In the seventeenth century, Antonie van Leeuwenhoek, a Dutch merchant, developed a single lens microscope that was powerful enough to reveal a microscopic world where micro-organisms and human cells battled for dominance, a world that was still unknown to Jenner when he gave the world its first great 'cure'. As microscopes became more sophisticated, the microscopic realm of disease-causing organisms was slowly revealed.

Almost a century passed after Jenner's discovery until another effective vaccine was developed. It was Louis Pasteur who risked his reputation and roused the ire of the scientific elite of his day when he proposed Germ Theory and proved conclusively that microbes were the cause of human diseases. This knowledge facilitated the development of new vaccines. Pasteur discovered how to prepare and use attenuated disease-causing microbes as vaccines against anthrax and chicken cholera. In 1885 Pasteur developed the second human vaccine, a cure for the disease rabies even though at the time microscopes were still not powerful enough to enable him to see the rabies virus. The world applauded this momentous development and vaccination was established as an accepted and effective method of preventing disease.

Pasteur built on the work of Edward Jenner and established the science of microbiology. Other scientific superstars of the nineteenth century took up the challenge to identify and defeat the invisible viruses and bacteria that cause disease — diseases such as tuberculosis, bubonic plague, cholera, typhoid, tetanus and diphtheria. Many of the early significant medical advances were made in laboratories headed by Louis Pasteur in France and by his rival, Robert Koch in Berlin. Robert Koch furthered the understanding of the role of micro-organisms in causing disease. He was the first to demonstrate that a specific pathogen caused a specific disease.

Louis Pasteur and Robert Koch inspired a whole generation of 'microbe hunters', disciples who travelled the world in the search for the causes of disease and hopefully the cures. Producing a vaccine, however, often took years of painstaking work which could be fraught with both personal and professional difficulties for these early medical pioneers.

By 1900 the medical profession had an increasing understanding of health and disease. Pasteur's seminal work had revolutionised concepts of infection and the practice of surgery and obstetrics but still only a few 'cures' were to be found in the physician's little black bag: morphine and aspirin to ease pain; quinine to fight off malaria; digitalis from the foxglove plant for heart failure; and vaccines for smallpox, rabies, typhoid, cholera and bubonic plague. However, Germ Theory had shown scientists who the enemy was and 21 micro-organisms that were the cause of human disease had been identified. The war against them had begun in earnest and was gaining momentum. Once identified, the microbes that cause disease could be targeted with vaccines that were toxic only to those microbes and harmless to humans.

Although in the first decades of the twentieth century the number of vaccines being developed was increasing, there were at that time very few effective chemical treatments for disease. At the beginning of the century venereal syphilis was the most serious and dreaded of the sexually transmitted diseases. The micro-organism responsible for syphilis was isolated in 1905. The development of a chemical cure for the disease, a new 'magic bullet', took many years after that but the achievement was groundbreaking because it resulted in the establishment of the disciplines of chemotherapy and haematology.

A contemporaneous breakthrough was Blood Serum Therapy, which resulted from the discovery that antitoxins in blood could be used to make vaccines against diphtheria and tetanus. In 1921 a vaccine to prevent tuberculosis was developed in France and at the same time in Canada the discovery was made that diabetes could be treated with insulin therapy. Although not a cure for diabetes, insulin has saved the lives of countless diabetics.

During the 1930s and 1940s with the discovery and the introduction of penicillin and the subsequent development of other antibiotics a whole raft of cures became possible. Developed during World War II, the impact of penicillin on the war effort and the health of countless millions of people from that time on has been monumental. Since the introduction of antibiotics over 60 years ago the world has enjoyed an increasing mastery over microbial disease.

In the 1950s, summertime was a time of great anxiety for many parents as children by the thousands became infected with the crippling disease poliomyelitis, a disease that engendered fear worldwide. The development of a vaccine for polio was hailed as a miracle, but the long and tortuous race to find a cure led to bitter and acrimonious debate amongst the scientific elite in the United States.

New and astonishing cures resulted from the development of anti-viral drugs in the mid twentieth century. Using a process called rational drug design, scientists produced 'medical marvels' that worked against bacteria, protozoan parasites, malignant diseases and immune disorders. For the very first time acute childhood leukaemia could be cured.

About three-quarters of all human diseases involve the immune system in one way or another. The 1960s saw an exponential increase in immunological knowledge which has facilitated progress in the diagnosis and treatment of auto-immune and malignant diseases, immunodeficiency and allergies. Researchers established that the immune system is also responsible for the rejection of organ transplants, another burgeoning field of medical endeavour. The understanding and manipulation of immunological tolerance and rejection is what has made successful organ transplantation possible. If a diseased or failing organ could not be cured, then it could be

4

replaced. Following hard on the heels of this success was the introduction of bone marrow transplants.

What I came to realise as I investigated these milestones in medical progress was that the personal stories behind the great cures of the nineteenth and early twentieth centuries followed similar plot lines which were often characterised by rivalry, subterfuge, professional infighting and jealousy, public humiliation, deprivation and dedication, and great personal struggle and sacrifice. It was intriguing to examine too the personal motivation of those who had done so much for the good of humankind, to understand if they had been driven by altruism, by ambition and ego or by the thrill of scientific discovery for its own sake.

It was not only the pioneers of medical science who suffered or sacrificed as they dedicated themselves to the cause of combating disease. Many of the practices employed in medical experimentation in the past would be considered unethical today. As little as 50 years ago the ethics of a scientist trialling vaccines on prisoners, orphans or the scientist's own family may not have been questioned and some were certainly not averse to trying experimental vaccines on themselves. There are many examples of medical trailblazers who, driven by their desire to succeed, exercised poor judgment and took risks which at times resulted in tragic outcomes. They then had to deal with their own consciences.

Human trials were often preceded by many years of experimentation on animals and even today some vaccines have animal components. It would be impossible to estimate how many animals have been used in medical experiments since Edward Jenner's time. The practice of vivisection, experimentation with living animals, has always had its opponents and the debate continues today. There are those who espouse the view that human need is greater than the rights of animals while others believe that in this day and age vivisection is unnecessary and repugnant. As medical science progressed issues such as these have had to be faced, and as a result another discipline within the study of medicine has emerged: the field of medical ethics.

As my research brought me to the latter part of the twentieth century I found it more difficult to recognise a medical breakthrough, to pinpoint the exact moment when a cure was discovered and to identify an individual whose genius made it possible. There are singular moments however, such as the discovery of the DNA double helix in 1953 or the first cloning of a mammal, the creation of Dolly the sheep in 1997. Most scientific advances are now the result of accumulated knowledge resulting from research that has been undertaken by numerous people over the course of many years, dependent on progress and discoveries that have come before. The science behind medical breakthroughs has become more and more complex and specialised.

Edward Jenner gave the world vaccination and the means for those who followed to provide an armoury of 'cures' to fight humankind's major killers. How the doctor's black bag has expanded. There are now medicines and treatments for almost every illness. Today the medical profession draws upon a vast arsenal of drugs, vaccines, and diagnostic tools that could hardly have been dreamt of in 1900 let alone 1796. Scientists from every corner of the globe have contributed to the medical revolution that began ever so slowly centuries ago. We hear almost daily now of some new and astonishing medical breakthrough. Medicine has progressed through various stages: anatomy, physiology, microbiology, surgery, pharmacology and immunology and, in the 21st century, molecular biology and molecular medicine. During each stage scientists have made astonishing advances in treatment and cure.

Today, molecular biology, molecular medicine and genetic engineering are changing vaccine development by offering new and powerful ways of producing the antigens and attenuated materials necessary for vaccination. The manipulation of tolerance and the 'creation' of animals with cell-surface tissue antigens compatible with human self-recognition is also being pursued and extraordinary progress is being made in stem-cell research. All of this is nothing short of awe-inspiring. Even so, while cures for many diseases and conditions have been found, the causes of some diseases still elude the greatest scientific and medical minds.

Although many milestones have been reached in winning the war against bacterial and viral diseases, it is still two steps forward and one step back. Scientists are now sounding an ominous note of caution. The tide could be turning against us as some diseases are making a comeback. The overuse of antibiotics has resulted in the proliferation and resurgence of resistant strains of bacterial and viral diseases including outbreaks of multi-resistant tuberculosis and polio.

Today, when medicine has come so far and we are focused on new enemies such as terrorism and global warming, surely it is ironic that our oldest enemies are the most resilient and still present the greatest threat. They are tenacious foes, natural survivors, unseen and insidious, capable of engineering their own methods of making the weapons we use against them useless. With the emergence of bio-terrorism, humankind may yet face the threat of a disease like smallpox being brought back from the brink of extinction. The advances in medical science that have saved millions of lives are the very ones that could be used to bring about our destruction. The words of Louis Pasteur remain prescient: as a species we are capable of great good and inconceivable evil.

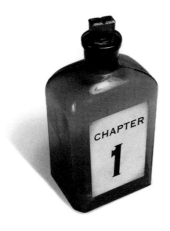

ERADICATING THE 'SPECKLED MONSTER'

EDWARD JENNER AND THE DISCOVERY OF VACCINATION

The joy I felt at the prospect before me of being the
instrument destined to take away from the world one
of its greatest calamities ... was so excessive that ...
I have sometimes found myself in a kind of reverie.[1]

Edward Jenner

In the late eighteenth century an English country doctor named Edward
Jenner set himself the herculean task of combating the most dreaded of diseases, smallpox. Without knowing its cause, however, the battle would
prove to be a very long one. Edward Jenner changed the course of medical
science and opened up a new and brighter future for humanity. A declaration on 8 May 1980 by the World Health Organization (WHO) that
smallpox had finally been eradicated was an acknowledgment that Edward
Jenner had been instrumental in removing from the world what had indeed
been one of its greatest calamities.

Smallpox, an ancient disease, was more vicious than any war ever
waged. Century after century this disease shaped human history in every

corner of the globe. It did not discriminate between kings and commoners or the rich and the poor, and countless millions were its victims. Contracting smallpox was an almost certain death sentence. Six out of every ten people who contracted the disease succumbed. In today's terms smallpox was deadlier and more feared than cancer. Around one quarter of the entire European population was killed, blinded or left permanently scarred by smallpox before the lid was closed on its own coffin. For those who managed to escape death the disfiguring scars that were left after the characteristic 'pox' had healed were a frightening reminder to all of the power of the disease. Smallpox was ever-present and omnipresent.

The ultimate victory against smallpox was achieved through inspired scientific discovery, technical innovation and international cooperation but this unparalleled triumph would not have been possible without the pioneering work, perseverance and great personal sacrifice of the 'simple' country doctor.[2] The breadth of Edward Jenner's work, his contribution to public health and the legacy he provided for humankind are extraordinary, even more so because in his own era he had to struggle against vociferous and jealous critics who were bent on destroying his idealism and his reputation. The hardships that Jenner faced and the personal sacrifices that he made are not uncommon amongst the stories of those who have given us salvation through monumental medical discoveries.

Edward Jenner's determination to develop a cure for smallpox brought about the discovery of vaccination, a procedure that has since saved an unimaginable number of lives and without which the world would not have advanced in the way it has. Taken for granted in the Western world today, vaccination remains the only method medicine has in its arsenal to prevent the onset and spread of rapacious and deadly infectious diseases. With Jenner's smallpox vaccination came the inception of one of the most important branches of modern medicine: immunology, the science of our body's defence against invading microbes and chemicals. In the long term, developments in immunology have led to an understanding of allergy, auto-immune diseases and transplantation. And it all started with Edward Jenner.

To appreciate how extraordinary Edward Jenner's achievement was it is necessary to understand the context in which he set out to defeat smallpox — we must visit his times and know his enemies. Born in the middle of the eighteenth century, Edward Jenner was a humanitarian who possessed a prodigious intellect and eclectic knowledge, and as a doctor he saw first-hand how smallpox afflicted those around him like no other disease. In Edward Jenner's eighteenth-century Europe, each year smallpox killed one-tenth of the population in rural areas, and in towns and cities where infection was rampant the losses were double that. It was a time when many children had little chance of living to adulthood and smallpox was responsible for 1 in 3 of their deaths. An even greater tragedy was the mortality rate among children younger than five years of age. In London where Jenner did his medical training, 80 per cent of children who were infected with smallpox died. Elsewhere in Europe the death toll was even worse. In Berlin, for example, a staggering 98 per cent of children under five did not survive the disease.[3]

Because of its indiscriminate killing power smallpox was universally feared, perhaps even more so than bubonic plague. Both diseases brought their own kind of terror but bubonic plague, which was known as the Black Death, was episodic, invading Europe in waves over the centuries while smallpox was a perennial enemy, a threat that never abated. Like bubonic plague, smallpox too had its own epithet. It was known as the 'speckled monster' because of the way it spotted its victims' bodies with pustules or pox that left deep, permanent scars when they healed. It is these pox which gave the disease its name. Around the end of the fifteenth century the term 'small pockes' was first used to distinguish this disease from syphilis — another dreaded disease. (Syphilis was called the 'great pockes' because the infected pustules that erupted on the skin of its victims were much larger.[4])

In 1800, the historian Thomas Macauley graphically described the horror that was smallpox, the fear that it engendered in individuals and the devastation it visited upon Edward Jenner's society:

> *Smallpox was always present, filling the churchyard with corpses,*
> *tormenting with constant fear all whom it had not yet stricken,*
> *leaving on those whose lives it spared the hideous traces of its power,*
> *turning the babe into a changeling at which the mother shuddered,*
> *and making the eyes and cheeks of the betrothed maiden objects of*
> *horror to the lover.*[5]

It was this formidable enemy that Edward Jenner challenged with his intellect but medical knowledge in Jenner's time was very limited in comparison to the 21st century. Although there were enormous changes in the way medicine was practised in the 1700s, there were crucial gaps in scientific knowledge which prevented progress, the most significant of which is something that seems so fundamental today — that micro-organisms cause disease. It was unlikely that a cure for infectious diseases such as smallpox and bubonic plague could be found if science was unable to provide an understanding of their cause.

The prevailing belief was that diseases could result from physiological dysfunction and so investigations into the chemical and material structure of the body through post-mortems became a way for doctors to expand their knowledge of anatomy and pathology. In the eighteenth century, for the first time, doctors were being formally educated and trained in hospitals and were acquiring certified qualifications in their profession.[6] But hospitals then were vastly different to the high-tech institutions they are today and procedures were carried out with no understanding of infection and its transmission.

When Edward Jenner developed the first vaccine he was unaware of the existence of micro-organisms and that smallpox, the highly contagious human disease, was caused by a virus one-millionth of a millimetre in size that can multiply only within human cells. To many intellectual minds in the eighteenth century, such an idea would have been both fanciful and preposterous. In keeping with the climate of enquiry prevalent in Jenner's era, however, the theory that smallpox arose from innate seeds that were present in all humans or was the result of unfavourable environmental conditions was questioned, and the view that smallpox was a specific disease that could be attributed to a specific material cause became current. Despite this step forward in medical knowledge identifying the real cause would be impossible until the end of the nineteenth century when Louis Pasteur proved his 'Germ Theory of Disease' and it became widely accepted that micro-organisms cause disease.

Today the smallpox virus is called the 'variola' virus, coming from the Latin word *varius*, meaning 'stained', or from *varus*, meaning 'mark on the skin', signifying the rash and disfiguring scars that are hallmarks of the disease. There are two strains of the virus: variola major, which has severe symptoms and a very high mortality rate (sometimes as high as 100 per cent); and variola minor, which as its name implies is much less severe, with a mortality rate of less than 2 per cent.

In the same way that there was uncertainty about the cause of smallpox, for many centuries there was also uncertainty about how people caught it. Smallpox is spread through droplet infection — in lay terms, coughs and sneezes. Breathing in just a few particles of the virus is all it takes to become infected. The virus enters the body through the lungs, passes through the respiratory tract and enters the bloodstream, eventually spreading to the internal organs and the skin. With variola major it takes twelve to fourteen days for symptoms (which are nothing short of gruesome) to appear. It begins with a fever and then a splitting headache and backache, an inability to stand and delirium. Nausea and vomiting are also common.

After two to four days, the fever eases and a rash appears. The rash is the result of the virus replicating in the skin. After several more days, pustules or pox form. The pustules contain a cloudy fluid and they cover the body, are excruciatingly painful and can spread to the throat, the eyes and the anus. In some cases the rash merges and can peel off the body in black sheets.[7] Although death usually occurs between day eleven and day fifteen of the rash, some people die before it has fully developed because of blood poisoning, secondary infections or internal bleeding. If a person survives, over a period of three to four weeks the pustules form crusts which actually contain the virus. The crusts then shrink, dry up and eventually fall off leaving deep scars.

A FAR-REACHING DISEASE WITH A LONG HISTORY

So how did a country doctor during a period in which medical knowledge and technological ability were limited, come to develop a vaccine for this horrifying disease without fully understanding the science behind his discovery?

The story begins with Edward Jenner's childhood. Born on 17 May 1749 in the small market town of Berkeley in Gloucestershire, Edward Jenner was the third of eight children born to the vicar of Berkeley, the Reverend James Stephen Jenner, and Sarah Jenner. When Edward was five years old his parents died and he was cared for by his eldest sister Mary until he was sent to boarding school. It was there, during a smallpox epidemic, that Edward was first confronted by the many horrors associated with smallpox that were part and parcel of life in the era in which he lived. His experience, however, would prove instrumental in providing both motivation and means in his later work.

Edward Jenner was only eight years old, away from home and family, when he was subjected to a medical procedure that was known as variolation. For him it was a horrendous experience, one he would never forget. Variolation provided the only hope of protection from smallpox. It involved deliberately infecting healthy people with smallpox in the hope that they would contract a less severe case and, as a result, would not catch it again. Healthy children and adults were exposed to various forms of material from people who had experienced fairly mild cases of smallpox.

Fluid from pustules or ground-up scabs were inserted into the nose or rubbed into a cut made in the skin. As only a small number of people who were variolated developed a fatal case of smallpox, for many the chance of salvation far outweighed the risk of death.

The ordeal that Edward went through when he was variolated we would now consider tantamount to abuse. First he had to be bled. Bleeding was a common but potentially dangerous medical treatment that involved cutting the veins or using leeches to suck out blood. Edward then had to fast and purge over a period of six weeks, which left him weak, emaciated and at his very young age utterly afraid. After this brutal ordeal Edward was variolated and locked in a stable with other boys who were desperately ill with smallpox, and left there until the disease had run its course.[8]

There are three things to be grateful for: Edward Jenner did not catch smallpox; he had witnessed at close quarters a disease that had visited its unique horror on many societies for thousands of years; and he had experienced variolation first-hand. The practice had reached England just some 30 years before this event. Until then, during smallpox epidemics very little could be done to stop the spread of the disease. Apart from individuals praying and fasting the only public measure available was to round up those who were symptomatic and isolate them in foul places called 'pest houses' or on derelict ships languishing in harbours. All in vain, of course. Once symptoms were in evidence it was too late.

Because there was no understanding of microbiology and hence the nature of infectious diseases, smallpox reigned unchecked for millennia. The theory is that it started as a rodent virus that jumped to humans in agricultural settlements in north-eastern Africa as long ago as 10,000 BC. There is evidence that smallpox was known in ancient Egypt. Mummies dated as belonging to the eighteenth to twentieth Dynasties, 1570 to 1085 BC, have marks that are consistent with smallpox scars and this includes the well-preserved mummy of the pharaoh, Ramses V, who died in 1157 BC.[9]

The first smallpox epidemic ever recorded occurred in 1350 BC during a war between the Egyptians and the Hittites. Egyptian prisoners were carriers of the disease which decimated the Hittite soldiers and citizens and killed their king, Suppiluliumas I, perhaps hastening the decline of the civilisation. Egyptian merchants also became unwitting carriers and smallpox began its slow but deadly journey to the rest of the world. Literary records place it in the Mediterranean area and in China in the third century AD.

Smallpox was the indomitable enemy of empires and a furtive assassin that changed the line of succession of ruling families in Europe and Asia. Around 180 AD smallpox attacked the Roman Empire. In the epidemic, called the Plague of Antonine, as many as 7 million people may have been killed, a massive number for ancient times. Roman legions returning from a military campaign against Parthia brought the disease with them from Armenia. The rate at which smallpox spread — 10,000 infections per day — gives some idea of its apocalyptic power.[10] The Roman population was decimated, and so great were the losses amongst the army that Emperor Marcus Aurelius, who soon succumbed to the disease himself, began relying on paid mercenaries to protect the empire from incursions by Goths and Vandals. The mercenaries began to exploit Rome's weakness and historians see this as marking the end of Rome's golden age, ushering in the beginning of the decline of the Roman Empire.

Smallpox took up residence in all corners of the globe. In Asia, the king of Burma died from smallpox in 1368 and the king and queen of Ceylon (modern-day Sri Lanka) and all of their sons succumbed in 1582. In Europe, smallpox had an exhaustive and impressive list of victims. It altered the succession of the British royal family. Queen Anne was the last monarch of the House of Stuart because in 1700 her heir, Prince William, died of smallpox at the age of eleven. In the 50 years before Edward Jenner's birth in 1749, the Japanese emperor Higashiyama, the Austrian emperor Joseph I, King Louis I of Spain, Tsar Peter II of Russia and Queen Ulrika Eleanora of Sweden all lost their lives to smallpox.[11]

Smallpox, the speckled monster, was carried to the Americas, the New World, during the voyages of discovery where it killed many more Aztecs and indigenous North Americans than were killed by invading colonisers.

Within 100 years of the Spanish conquistadors arriving in Mexico in 1518, the indigenous population of 25 million had contracted to 1.6 million, principally due to smallpox. In 1520 the Aztec emperor, Ciutláhuac, became one of the multitudes of victims.

The abhorrent slave trade also contributed to the introduction of smallpox in the Americas because many slaves came from regions of Africa where smallpox was endemic. On the eastern coast of what became the United States, smallpox had disastrous consequences for the original population. It was here that one of the first deplorable acts of biological warfare took place. In 1763 the leader of the British forces suggested grinding smallpox scabs into blankets that were to be distributed to Indian tribes, a practice that a century later was used by the American government in what could be interpreted as a deliberate act of genocide.[12]

It is ironic that the knowledge that smallpox material could be used to pass on the disease would eventually form part of the theoretical framework for its ultimate defeat. Also critical was the knowledge that those who survived smallpox did not succumb a second time. This view was present in many societies and was borne out by experience.

The Greek historian Thucydides made such an observation during a smallpox epidemic that hit Athens in 430 BC. Early in the tenth century AD, a Persian physician and philosopher, Abu Bakr Muhammad Ibn Zakariya al-Razi, known as Rhazes, wrote *De Variolis et Morbillis Commentaries*, a medical description of smallpox. In it he explained that smallpox survivors did not develop the disease again and also concluded that smallpox could be transmitted from person to person. In 1734, Voltaire in his *Philosophical Letters* noted that people known as the Circassians (Circassia is an historical region near the Black Sea) had observed that out of 1000 people 'hardly one was attacked twice by full-blown smallpox'. Three or four might experience a mild recurrence but 'one never truly has that illness twice in life'.[13]

Over time, the combined knowledge that smallpox material from one person could be used to infect another and that those who survived smallpox did not get the disease again brought about the practice of variolation.

For centuries before Edward Jenner experienced it, variolation had been practised without any sound medical evidence as to why it worked. In India where it had been used from around 1000 AD the most common method was to apply scabs or pus to the scratched skin of a healthy person. In China pox or scab material rubbed on a cotton pad was inserted into the nose or blown into the nostrils through a tube.[14] The Chinese also made pills from dried fleas taken from cows, an early hint that fleas played some part in the disease.

In the mid 1600s travelling merchants introduced variolation to the Ottoman Empire where it became frequently practised. Many women in the Turkish sultan's harem in Istanbul had been variolated during childhood on parts of their bodies where scars would not be seen.[15] Reports describing the method of variolation used in Turkey reached England in the early 1700s when smallpox was running rampant. Members of the Royal Society of London, the esteemed and prestigious national academy of science that had been founded in 1660, became aware of the practice but it was not immediately embraced by physicians.

It was an English aristocrat, a woman, Lady Mary Wortley Montague, who is credited with introducing variolation to England and western Europe where it was also called inoculation. Lady Mary had experienced the scourge first-hand in 1715. Once a reputed beauty, her face was ravaged by the speckled monster which had also robbed her of her brother. In 1717 Lady Mary's husband, Edward Wortley Montague was appointed as ambassador to Turkey and within two weeks of arriving, Lady Mary wrote to her friend Sarah Chiswell, describing how variolation, which she called 'ingrafting', was used at the Ottoman court.[16] Material from the pustules of people who had contracted a mild case of smallpox was introduced to the healthy through scratches or a puncture made on the arm.

Convinced that the method was a way to protect her children, in March 1718 Lady Montague instructed the embassy surgeon, Charles Maitland, to variolate her five-year-old son. When she returned to London in April 1721, Lady Montague had her four-year-old daughter variolated by Dr

Maitland in the presence of physicians appointed to the English royal court, including the king's physician, Sir Hans Sloane. Consequently members of the English royal family became interested in the possibility of saving their own children through variolation.

Charles Maitland was granted a Royal Licence to conduct a trial, which he carried out on six prisoners at Newgate Prison on 9 August 1721. The ethics of this may be questionable from a 21st-century perspective but the prisoners were promised a full pardon if they submitted. All six survived variolation and were released. One prisoner was then exposed directly to smallpox and proved to be immune. After the next successful trial, which Maitland carried out on six children from a charitable institution in London, the Princess of Wales allowed her two daughters to be treated.[17] The actions of Lady Mary had saved more children than her own but sadly her friend, Sarah, with whom she had shared her discovery, died from smallpox a few years later.

Not surprisingly, with a royal imprimatur, variolation soon gained general acceptance but it was not foolproof. Two to 3 per cent of people who were variolated died because success depended on physicians identifying a mild strain of smallpox and some people were inadvertently infected with other life-threatening illnesses such as tuberculosis or syphilis. An even greater risk was that those who were inoculated with a virulent strain, apart from losing their own lives, were potentially the source of new smallpox epidemics. However, mortality rates were ten times lower amongst those who caught smallpox from variolation than those who caught it naturally. In 1722 James Jurin, a physician and secretary to the Royal Society, conducted one of the first medical statistical surveys and found that the mortality rate in non-variolated children was 1 in 14 but for the inoculated, it was 1 in 91.[18]

In the Americas variolation found powerful supporters as well. Benjamin Franklin, whose son died of smallpox in 1736, also carried out a statistical study to assess the effectiveness of the procedure and promoted it enthusiastically. In 1766, during the War of Independence, American soldiers under George Washington were unable to wrest Quebec from the English because a smallpox epidemic halved their troop numbers. British troops on the other hand had been variolated and did not succumb. Being a witness to the success of variolation, George Washington made the practice mandatory for all his soldiers.

By the time Edward Jenner was born in 1749 variolation was widespread throughout England. As an indication of how enormous the social and economic repercussions of smallpox were, the London Smallpox and Inoculation Hospital, dedicated to the treatment and prevention of smallpox, had been established. In both England and Europe doctors began variolating on a large scale and many built up lucrative businesses. During the 1750s when the young Edward suffered his ordeal many of the nobility of Europe were ensuring that their children were given a chance to escape smallpox. Empress Marie-Therese of Austria and her children and grandchildren were variolated as was King Louis XVI of France and his children, and Catherine II of Russia and her son.[19] Variolation remained the only defence against smallpox until Jenner's vaccine became an accepted replacement in the mid nineteenth century.

Fortunately for us all, Edward Jenner recovered from the trauma of his experience with variolation and the road to salvation for generations of people began five years later, when at the age of thirteen he embarked on his long and exceptional medical career. It was common in those days for doctors to learn their craft by apprenticeship and Jenner went to work with Dr Daniel Ludlow, an eminent country surgeon who lived near Bristol. It soon became obvious that Jenner had a sharp and enquiring mind and he was a keen observer and listener, storing away many things that would later inform his research.

During his training, Jenner was reminded of another commonly held belief in regard to smallpox. He heard a dairymaid say, 'I shall never have smallpox for I have had cowpox. I shall never have an ugly pockmarked face.'[20] In rural areas of England and Europe it was well known that milkmaids became immune to smallpox after developing cowpox, which they caught because of their close contact with cows. Cowpox was not dangerous to humans and cows exhibited few symptoms other than pox or pustules on their udders accompanied by a slight decrease in milk production. This phenomenon had been noted by the medical profession and in 1765 a doctor from Gloucestershire reported to the Medical Society of London that people who had had cowpox had no reaction to variolation with smallpox material.

It was to be an odd marriage. Folklore was to become the foundation for the science that Edward Jenner would use to develop the first vaccine. As we understand it today, a vaccine which can be given by injection or orally consists of live, attenuated — meaning weakened in some way — or killed disease-causing micro-organisms, or in the case of some vaccines just a fragment of the organism's specific protein. Proteins are compounds that are essential constituents of all living organisms. A vaccine works by stimulating a person's immune system which then produces antibodies against that disease, thus killing or neutralising the infectious micro-organism.[21] Vaccines can be prophylactic, which means they prevent or ameliorate the effects of a future infection; or therapeutic, meaning they cure the disease after it has been contracted.

All that is now known about disease prevention by vaccination follows from Jenner's fundamental work, work that he did before medical science had an understanding of microbiology and immunology.

In 1770 Edward Jenner began further medical training at St George's Hospital in London under the tutelage of Dr John Hunter, a leading surgeon and a pioneer of medical practice. Hunter had a profound influence on Jenner's life. He became aware of Jenner's observational and investigational skills and taught his protégé not only surgical techniques but, more importantly, the use of scientific method, insisting that the young physician's medical practices and decisions be based on evidence. As a result Jenner developed a rigorous and methodical approach to scientific investigation. He would carefully make observations from his own experience, form a hypothesis, test it and modify it to make new predictions which in their turn were tested. His method provided the scaffolding for his own research and for future discoveries as well.

Hunter also fostered Jenner's great love of nature and natural science, encouraging him to assist the botanist Joseph Banks in classifying the botanical specimens he collected on Captain James Cook's expedition in search of Terra Australis Incognita.[22] Cook was the first European to explore the east coast of Australia, and Jenner was invited to join Cook's 1772 expedition as a botanist but turned the offer down. At the age of 23 Jenner returned home to Berkeley to take up the position of local doctor. The scene was set for a medical breakthrough that would change the world.

In his practice at Berkeley Jenner was frequently asked to variolate people against smallpox. He would insist that patients rest and maintain a strict diet for two weeks before the procedure. Jenner's method was to draw up a small quantity of fluid from a smallpox pustule with a lancet, and then, being careful not to draw blood, introduce it between the outer and inner layers of the skin of the upper arm of the patient. Ever the astute observer and listener, Jenner found that some of his patients were completely resistant to smallpox variolation and deduced that these patients had previously had cowpox.

It seems that by 1788, Jenner was convinced of the scientific truth of what was considered folklore. Jenner made a crucial connection: cowpox not only protected against smallpox but could be transferred from one human being to another to provide protection. At the time he drew sketches of cowpox marks on a milkmaid's hand and showed them to Hunter and other experts with whom he discussed the hypothesis he was forming, but the breakthrough would come a decade later after Jenner had embarked on marriage and family life.[23]

Edward Jenner may have been a country doctor but he was an extraordinarily talented and compassionate man with a universal outlook. As a response to the slave trade and the transportation of 18 million Africans he composed an anti-slavery song. He was fascinated by passenger-carrying hydrogen balloons so began building his own. He was an expert in natural history and wrote several scientific studies, the most outstanding of which, *Observations on the Natural History of the Cuckoo,* published in 1788, earned Jenner the honour, at the age of 35, of being named a Fellow of the Royal Society.

It was also in 1788 that Edward Jenner married Catherine Kingscote. Catherine, who with her introverted nature was the opposite of her outgoing husband, dedicated her life to her religion, to Jenner and his work and practice in Berkeley, and to their three children.

A confluence of circumstances in 1796 gave Jenner an opportunity to test his cowpox theory. In May, a milkmaid named Sarah Nelmes came to see her local doctor because she had a rash on her hand. Sarah was relieved when Jenner diagnosed not smallpox, as she had feared, but cowpox. She had caught it from one of her cows, Blossom, a name now as famous as Sarah's.[24] Wasting no time, on 14 May Jenner extracted fluid from the cowpox pustule on Sarah's hand and inoculated his gardener's son, James Phipps. James was eight, the same age Jenner had been when he was variolated. Jenner made two half-inch incisions on James' arm, rubbed the fluid in and then anxiously watched and waited. After a few days James became mildly ill with cowpox, developed a few pustules and a mild fever but was well again a week later.

This was the first step. Jenner had confirmed that cowpox could pass from person to person as well as from cow to person. But would cowpox protect James Phipps from smallpox? On 1 July 1796 Jenner variolated the boy with smallpox. As Jenner had anticipated, and undoubtedly to his great relief, James did not develop the disease, either on this occasion or subsequently when Jenner repeated the procedure a number of times to prove that James Phipps was immune to smallpox.

It is accepted, however, that Edward Jenner was not the first person to use the material from cowpox in the hope of providing immunity to smallpox. A farmer named Benjamin Jesty from Yetminster, who had survived smallpox as a child, is given that accolade. Aware of the folklore surrounding dairymaids and cowpox, Jesty inoculated his family with cowpox material during a smallpox epidemic in 1774. As the disease raged through the surrounding countryside Benjamin feared that his pregnant wife Elizabeth, his baby daughter and two sons who were aged two and three would be stricken.[25]

When Jesty heard of an outbreak of cowpox on a nearby farm he immediately took his wife and sons there, leaving the baby behind as she was considered too young for what he was planning. Jesty then collected infected pus from a cow's udder and inserted it into a scratch he made with a stocking needle on Elizabeth's arm. His sons were next. All three developed cowpox and although Elizabeth became quite ill, probably from an infection, the two boys were soon well again. None of the Jestys caught smallpox during this epidemic or in later ones and Elizabeth recovered and lived for another 50 years. Several years after the cowpox inoculation, so the story goes, the family underwent variolation with smallpox and none of them suffered any ill effects from this either. Despite the success of his experiment Benjamin Jesty soon realised that he had risked more than his family. People were superstitious and they believed that Elizabeth and her sons would grow horns and turn into cows and Benjamin was reviled as some kind of sorcerer. It is little wonder that his inoculation method did not find favour amongst his neighbours. Years later the Jesty family moved to the Isle of Purbeck and in the parish church at Worth Matravers there is an inscription on one Mary Brown's memorial tablet stating that her mother, Abigail, had been inoculated by Benjamin Jesty.[26]

A similar incident occurred in Holland in 1791. A Dutch schoolmaster named Peter Plett, who was employed as a tutor for a family in Hasselberg in Holstein, had been told by milkmaids that cowpox protected them against smallpox. He inoculated his employer's two daughters and another child with material taken from cows that had cowpox. These children were amongst the few survivors of a smallpox epidemic that swept through

Holstein three years later.[27] Apparently Plett was deterred from performing any other inoculations because the hand of one of the children had become severely inflamed. As was the case with Elizabeth Jesty this was probably caused by an infection.

These early 'experiments' predated Jenner's inoculation of James Phipps and demonstrated that serum from a cow infected with cowpox could protect people from smallpox without them ever risking death through variolation with a virulent strain, but it was Edward Jenner who proved this scientifically and produced a vaccine which effectively combated smallpox. At the end of 1796, Jenner sent an article to the Royal Society describing the experiment with James Phipps and his earlier observations of thirteen people who had previously had cowpox and who after being variolated with smallpox had had no reaction.

And so began Jenner's struggle to have his work on the efficacy and safety of cowpox inoculation in preventing smallpox recognised and accepted. So much was at stake. Jenner was offering the world a miracle, a chance to defeat the great scourge that had afflicted humans since ancient times. Instead of accolades, he received his first rebuff. Sir Joseph Banks, president of the Society at that time, rejected Jenner's article for publication in the journal *Philosophical Transactions* despite the fact that two manuscript reviewers had strongly recommended it for publication.[28] An even greater insult was that the Council of the Royal Society, the same society of which Jenner was a Fellow, dismissed his research as being 'in variance with established knowledge' and not credible. He was warned not to 'promulgate such a wild idea if he valued his reputation'.

Jenner was bitterly disappointed and also frustrated because there were no new cases of cowpox in the vicinity of Berkeley until the spring of 1798, which meant his experiments had been put on hold. Armed with new material Jenner substantially revised his manuscript and, on the advice of friends, avoided further insults and financed its publication himself. The title of this groundbreaking 75-page book was almost as long as the book itself: *An Inquiry into the Causes and Effects of the Variolae Vaccinae, a Disease,*

discovered in some of the Western Counties of England, particularly Gloucestershire,
and known by the name of The Cow Pox.

Jenner used the term 'Variolae Vaccinae' for cowpox, and from this the
word vaccination is derived. Vaccinae comes from the Latin word *vacca*
meaning 'cow'. Cowpox was also called 'vaccinia'. It was in 1803 that 'vaccination' entered the English language when Richard Dunning, a surgeon
in Plymouth who had performed many cowpox inoculations, as they were
called, coined the term that is now used universally.

In his book *Inquiry*, Jenner described 23 successful vaccinations. He also
described a reaction now known as anaphylaxis, an allergic hypersensitiv-
ity of the body to a foreign protein or drug. He presented evidence that
cowpox material could be transferred from person to person to provide
protection against variolation with smallpox. He wrote, 'These experiments afforded me much satisfaction, they proved that the matter in
passing from one human subject to another, through five gradations, lost
none of its original properties.'[29] Far in advance of his time, Jenner suggested cowpox diseases were caused by some kind of infectious entity that
he called a 'virus', not a virus in the modern sense of a micro-organism,
but in its older sense meaning some kind of a poison.

After the publication of *Inquiry* in 1798, Jenner was fiercely attacked for
a second time. Even though his results were confirmed by other physicians
within the space of a year, the barrage persisted and Jenner's new technique did not catch on as quickly as he had anticipated and hoped. Firstly,
cowpox did not occur widely and doctors who wanted to test the new
process had to obtain cowpox matter from Jenner. Also there was a mixed
response from the medical profession. While some physicians were merely
sceptical, others who derived large incomes from variolation were suddenly threatened by Jenner's seemingly safer and more effective cowpox
treatment. Another cohort was motivated by bitter professional jealousy.
They responded with public ridicule.

A treatise written by Dr Benjamin Moseley in 1799 mocked Jenner's
work, referring to cowpox inoculation as 'cowmania' and 'cow's syphilis',

suggesting that like syphilis it could affect the brain. Dr William Rowley reported that after being inoculated with cowpox one child had developed an ox-faced deformity and another had developed mange, an animal skin disease.[30] Not only was the medical fraternity polarised but so too was the community. Some religious leaders denounced cowpox and people became fearful of the physical and religious consequences of being inoculated with material from what they considered God's lowlier creatures. Wild rumours spread that people had sprouted horns after being vaccinated. Political cartoonists made the most of the hysteria and published engravings of human bodies with cows' heads.

While fending off widespread scorn Jenner moved to London to gather volunteers for his cowpox vaccination program. After three months Jenner had made little progress but found some comfort in the fact that other physicians were succeeding where he failed. Henry Cline, Chief of Surgery at St Thomas' Hospital, was a personal friend and Jenner had provided him with cowpox material. In return Cline offered Jenner £10,000 if he would relocate his practice to London. This was a veritable fortune but Jenner declined the offer. At this stage of his life he was financially independent having inherited land and property. In a letter to another friend Jenner wrote that he did not need more money and that at no point would he attempt to enrich himself through his discoveries. Jenner's motives were truly altruistic.

At the London Smallpox and Inoculation Hospital William Woodville carried out extensive trials of Jenner's treatment, vaccinating approximately 600 people in the first six months of 1799. Many of his patients developed rashes that were not consistent with those exhibited by Jenner's patients and some contracted smallpox, which Jenner attributed to the use of contaminated lancets. Because the risk of infection was not properly understood the same lancets were used for both variolation and vaccination. It was also probable that mistakes were made during the development of the vaccine because smallpox rashes could be confused with cowpox rashes. This was later proven to be the case but initially led to claims that cowpox inoculation was no safer than smallpox variolation. It was an inexact science.

It was George Pearson from St George's Hospital who confirmed Jenner's findings. Pearson founded the Institute for the Inoculation of the Vaccinae and sent Jenner an invitation to the inauguration. When Pearson offered Jenner membership of the institute, Jenner was incensed believing not only that he should be in charge but that Pearson was trying to take credit for the discovery as well.[31] The politics of the time were particularly nasty, but as well as enemies, Jenner did have influential friends and they took action to have the institute boycotted.

Despite the personal and professional turmoil, a determined Jenner continued to experiment and publish results during this period. The title of one of his papers, *A Continuation of the Facts and Observations Relative to the Variolae Vaccinae*, was a message to his critics whose science was questionable. Jenner's fame spread rapidly. In 1800, the novelist Jane Austen wrote that she had attended a dinner party at which her host and hostess read one of Jenner's pamphlets on cowpox. Widespread interest reflected how important variolae vaccinae was in combating the ubiquitous and vicious smallpox disease and this was confirmed on 7 March 1800, when the Earl of Berkeley presented his local doctor, Edward Jenner, to the King of England. Jenner was granted permission to dedicate the second edition of *An Inquiry into the Causes and Effects of Variolae Vaccinae* 'To the King'.[32]

Only two years after the first publication of *Inquiry* the medical community had begun vaccinations on a large scale. As a result, deaths from smallpox plummeted. By the end of 1800 more than 5000 people in England had been successfully vaccinated using cowpox fluid and in Europe vaccination had reached over 100,000 people. In July 1800 the first vaccinations were carried out in the United States. Benjamin Waterhouse, a professor at Harvard Medical School, vaccinated his five-year-old son and six servants using vaccine from England. Soon after, President Thomas Jefferson organised the vaccination of his family and neighbours. In December 1801, Little Turtle, chief of the Miami tribe and several of his warriors were vaccinated in Washington DC, after Thomas Jefferson convinced them that 'the Great Spirit had made a gift to the white men in showing them how to preserve themselves from the smallpox'.[33]

For the saviour himself, however, life had become a series of ups and downs. In addition to the criticism and jealousy that he endured during his time in London while trying to establish his vaccine, Jenner suffered due to the separation from Catherine and his children, and because he was unable to continue his private practice. In a reversal of fortune he had amassed by 1802 an enormous debt of £12,000. Friends rallied and lobbied parliament on his behalf and after much debate Jenner was granted £10,000. His rivals were again vociferous, especially George Pearson who claimed that he was more deserving of a grant because he had inoculated many more people than Jenner, but his sniping went unheeded.[34]

In August 1803, Edward Jenner was granted the freedom of the City of London, (an historical and ceremonial honour bestowed on citizens considered worthy of veneration) and a month later the Royal Humane Society made him an honorary member. At the age of 54 the discoverer of vaccination had become a celebrity but over the next few years as Jenner's fame grew abroad, so did his tribulations at home. In London in 1803, having been given royal approval, the Royal Jennerian Institute was founded with Jenner as its president. The mission of the institute, the vaccination of the poor, accorded with Jenner's philosophy of medicine. In Berkeley, Jenner and Catherine had built a clinic adjacent to their cottage so that they could give free vaccinations. Eager for a chance at salvation, people queued in their hundreds and the clinic soon became known as the 'Temple of Vaccinia'.[35]

But there was a cost to Jenner's generosity. When Jenner's coffers began to run low again he made a fundamental error in asking a friend, Dr Walker, to take over the responsibility of inoculating the poor. Walker, who had a reputation for arrogance, compromised the success of the institute by obtaining the vaccine from patients' lesions. After Walker was dismissed he set up a rival institution, which eventually failed, but in the interim the

Royal Jennerian Institute was shut and Jenner came perilously close to being imprisoned for debt.

Old friends rallied again and another grant was requested from parliament. This time the process was stymied by petty professional jealousy between the Royal College of Physicians and the College of Surgeons. The former was asked by parliament to establish a vaccination commission to investigate the request, and the latter was not included and felt snubbed. So widespread was Jenner's reputation, however, that while the medical profession bickered, donations suddenly flooded in from Calcutta in India where Jenner was held in high esteem.[36] Jenner had been supplying cowpox material to the world, made possible by a technique he had developed. Cowpox matter was dried onto threads or glass making it easily transportable from one continent to another while retaining its efficacy in transit. Jenner was not only generous with his money. He gave his time and his advice freely to anyone who would benefit.

In the same way that smallpox had travelled around the globe the vaccine went in pursuit. During the period 1803 to 1806, King Charles IV of Spain had Jenner's vaccine transported to Spanish colonies in North and South America and Asia but the motive for this mass vaccination was not altruistic. The governor of the Council of the Indies had suggested that the economic benefits from vaccination would outweigh the costs because smallpox took such a huge toll and thus diminished tax revenues for Spain.[37] The method employed to transport the vaccine may not have met with Jenner's approval. On the ship sailing to the Spanish colonies were 22 orphan children who were sequentially inoculated arm-to-arm thus ensuring the viability of the vaccine.

Napoleon Bonaparte was also a believer and in 1805 all his troops who had not had smallpox were vaccinated with the 'Jennerian vaccine'. One year later he ordered that French civilians also be vaccinated. The vital importance of the vaccine was acknowledged in 1807 in the Grand Duchy of Hesse when the first smallpox vaccination law was passed. Bavaria and Denmark followed suit. Smallpox vaccine became the first mandatory vaccine in the United States in 1809 when Massachusetts required the entire state population to be vaccinated against the disease.[38] Only a decade after the introduction of the vaccine it was being widely used throughout Europe and the Americas and had been taken up in the Middle East, India, China and Australia.

With the success of the vaccine Edward Jenner had become so influential that the Emperor of Austria and the King of Spain freed English prisoners of war after Jenner personally mediated on their behalf. In 1813 when Napoleon was asked to release a captain in the English army who was a relative of Jenner's, Napoleon exclaimed, 'I cannot refuse Jenner anything! He has been my most faithful servant in the European campaigns.'[39]

Despite this stellar fame, Jenner's financial tribulations continued. In 1807 the British parliament finally granted him £20,000 and two years later in 1809, because the Royal Jennerian Institute had failed, they set up the National Vaccine Establishment with Jenner as director. But the carping and destructive opposition, the negative articles and professional jealousy that Jenner had endured since he first published *Inquiry* had not abated. There were members on the board of directors of the National Vaccine Establishment who had contrary views to Jenner, who was now 60 years old. The struggle had been long and hard. Enough was enough. Jenner resigned before the first official board meeting. The man who had come to refer to himself as the 'Vaccine Clerk to the World' retired from public life and until 1822 continued to practise as a country doctor.[40]

Edward Jenner's later years were marked by new difficulties. In 1813 when the University of Oxford awarded him an honorary medical degree, Jenner cantankerously refused to wear a cap and gown. This was interpreted as a symptom of his increasing age and his diminishing intellectual ability. The many battles he had fought had taken their toll. Even though he had triumphed over 'the most terrible of the ministers of death', Jenner's own life had not been immune from the tragedy of disease. His son Edward had died of tuberculosis when he was a young man, and perhaps when he needed her most Jenner also lost Catherine. Through much of their married life she had been plagued by poor health and in 1815 Catherine died from the same disease that had taken her son.

After Catherine's death Jenner was lonely and suffered increasing depression. He had little contact with his remaining son and daughter. He experienced a recurrence of a problem he had suffered in childhood, variously described as auditory hallucinations and neurological seizures. Whatever the nature of his mental disorder, Jenner was suffering and he became paranoid and withdrawn.[41] It was only when he began to pursue some of his old hobbies such as collecting fossils and gardening that his health improved somewhat, but his mind was no longer as incisive as it had once been. Medical articles that Edward Jenner wrote during this period were dismissed as second rate. However, in 1820, at the age of 71, Jenner, still fascinated by natural science, submitted an article to the Royal Society about the migration of birds. Deemed an exceptional piece of work, it was published in *Philosophical Transactions* after his death.[42]

In 1820 Jenner suffered a mild stroke but to the end, despite his tribulations, he was still a kind and gentle man. On the day before his death in the winter of 1823, Jenner walked to a neigbouring village to ensure that a number of poor families there were provided with fuel to keep them warm. On 25 January Jenner was found unconscious on the floor of his library. He had suffered another stroke which paralysed his right side and early the next morning Edward Jenner, the man who had liberated so many from the scourge of smallpox, died very much alone at the age of 73. He had received the freedom of many cities and honorary degrees and memberships from societies and universities worldwide; Napoleon had minted a medal in his honour; he had received a ring from the Empress of Russia and a belt of Wampum beads from the North American Indian chiefs. But, sadly, very few people came to farewell an old man at his funeral. Edward Jenner was buried near the altar in Berkeley church.

Edward Jenner did not receive a knighthood. The principal monument to commemorate his extraordinary contribution is a statue in Kensington Gardens in London inscribed simply with the name 'Jenner'. Other statues of this incomparable benefactor have since been erected in many countries, monuments that honour his legacy to humanity. A century after the introduction of the first vaccine, Louis Pasteur paid tribute to Jenner in an address to the International Medical Congress in London in 1891. In his speech Pasteur extended the term 'vaccination' to other agents that had been developed to protect against disease, 'as a homage to the merit of and to the immense services rendered by one of the greatest of Englishmen'.[43]

What Jenner achieved was indeed monumental. He was the first person to use science to produce a method of controlling an endemic infectious disease on a large scale. Although some argue he did not discover vaccination, Jenner made it viable and laid the foundations for many of medicine's greatest triumphs. His scientific genius enabled him through experimentation to demonstrate that a folk medicine tradition could be scientifically tested and verified. Jenner's methodology of injecting dead bacteria or their toxins, as well as dead or weakened viruses, into the human body to develop resistance to dreaded lethal diseases has since been used to fight diseases such as bubonic plague, rabies, anthrax, chickenpox, cholera, diphtheria, German measles, mumps, paratyphoid fever, pneumococcal pneumonia, poliomyelitis, tetanus, typhoid fever, typhus, whooping cough and yellow fever.[44]

Vital to the eventual eradication of smallpox was Jenner's perseverance despite the vehement opposition to his ideas. Jenner's pamphlet on cowpox vaccination, *The Origin of the Vaccinae Inoculation*, issued in 1801, ended with the prophetic words, 'the annihilation of the Small Pox, the most dreadful scourge of the human species, must be the final result of this practice'.[45] But it was to be almost 200 years after the vaccination of James Phipps that this prediction would be fulfilled.

As vaccination spread the dangerous practice of variolation fell out of favour and was forbidden by an Act of Parliament in Britain in 1840. In Europe, the cowpox vaccine was prepared in large quantities by growing the virus on calfskin and more and more countries introduced compulsory vaccination. Britain followed Europe in 1853. It did not take long for opposition to compulsory vaccination to arise. Anti-vaccinationists and civil libertarians organised protest marches and demanded freedom of choice. The vaccination debate that began in the 1800s continues today.

At the turn of the twentieth century, despite the proven effectiveness of Jenner's vaccine, smallpox remained a dangerous disease worldwide. Other methods of treatment and protection were tried. Especially popular, but somewhat arcane, was the use of red objects and light, a therapy that dated back to tenth-century Japan. The uptake of the vaccine was hampered initially because it was in short supply and hard to store, especially in hot climates. In 1926 the League of Nations' Smallpox and Vaccination Commission began to study the production, testing, standardisation, storage and delivery of the smallpox vaccine, while individual nations conducted their own research. During the 1920s French and Dutch researchers developed a dried vaccine for use in their colonies in the tropics.[46] It was hardier, but the quality was inconsistent.

In the United States, the more virulent form of smallpox, variola major, continued to be widespread throughout the nineteenth century before being controlled. An unexpected outbreak in New York City in 1947 led to the development of a new method of freeze-drying the vaccine in ampoules. The great advantage of this was that the vaccine could last for months without refrigeration, even in tropical climates. Consequently, after 1949 there were no endemic cases of smallpox in the United States and the increasing availability of this highly effective and more stable vaccine afforded new opportunities for the successful eradication of smallpox worldwide, which is what Jenner had conceived of and believed possible.

A coordinated campaign for global eradication was needed. In 1948 when smallpox was still a threat in at least 90 countries, the World Health Organization (WHO) took over the health functions of the League of Nations and in 1950 launched the first large-scale smallpox eradication effort with the goal of eliminating smallpox in the Americas. The Soviet

Union proposed a global campaign in 1958 but although some countries established smallpox eradication programs, there was no coordinated infrastructure and many of the programs faltered due to insufficient vaccine supplies and limited resources.

It was one step forward and two steps back. The WHO proposed the cessation of routine smallpox vaccination, which seemed contrary to the ideal of eradicating smallpox. There was an economic motive, the cost of the vaccine, but there were also complications associated with it. The calf-lymph vaccine was highly protective but could cause severe reactions, sometimes resulting in death. In the last natural smallpox outbreak in Britain, where outbreaks of smallpox continued up to the 1960s, the virus often carried by travellers from countries where it was still endemic, many more people died from vaccine reactions than from smallpox infection itself. Compulsory vaccination ended in Britain in 1971.[47] Following this a more attenuated, or weaker, vaccine was developed in order to minimise the risks and production of the calf-lymph vaccine was suspended in 1982.

It was in 1966 that the nineteenth World Health Assembly (WHA) finally adopted a resolution sponsored by several countries, including the United States and the Soviet Union, which set the specific goal of wiping out smallpox within ten years. After extensive debate, the WHA approved US$2.4 million for the global effort, but many countries thought it was an impossible and unrealistic task.[48]

Edward Jenner's goal, the extinction of the variola virus, came one step closer in 1967 when the World Health Organization embarked upon the Smallpox Eradication Program (SEP). In the preceding year, approximately 15 million people had contracted smallpox, 44 countries were still reporting the disease, in 33 of those smallpox remained endemic and the annual death toll was more than 2 million. Between 1967 and 1980 intensive mass vaccination campaigns were undertaken. The strategy was to achieve 80 per cent vaccine coverage in each country. The USSR contributed over 14 million doses of vaccine and the United States contributed 190 million doses.

As the campaign got underway, the invention of a vaccination gun that fired a jet of vaccine using compressed air was heralded because it eliminated needle replacement and sterilisation. But it was too difficult to maintain in dusty deserts. Then came the disposable 'bifurcated needle', which reduced the volume of vaccine required and simplified delivery. The needle's narrow, flattened fork end drew up the exact amount of vaccine and was then jabbed repeatedly into the skin to give a painless vaccination. Teams of SEP vaccinators from all over the world journeyed to remote communities with the ambitious goal of attempting to vaccinate every person at risk. It was unachievable and in many under-developed countries real progress was hampered by wars and political unrest.

It was a serendipitous discovery that led to a turning point in the campaign against smallpox. Insufficient vaccine supplies in Nigeria precipitated a strategy of aggressive case-finding. This involved locating people who had smallpox and then finding and vaccinating all their known and possible contacts to stop the spread. Coupled with this was surveillance containment, or ring vaccination, which meant that not every person had to be vaccinated.[49] The result was the disappearance of smallpox in eastern Nigeria even though less than 50 per cent of the population had been vaccinated.

Using the new tactics, medical teams travelled around looking for smallpox outbreaks and put up posters advertising rewards for people who reported cases. Once found, a smallpox sufferer was isolated at home with their family and they and all surrounding families were then vaccinated. The last case of smallpox in South America was reported in 1971. The last naturally acquired cases of endemic variola major were identified in Bangladesh and India in 1975 but the disease persisted in Ethiopia and surrounding regions of Africa.

The last case of smallpox, which was actually the less virulent strain, variola minor, occurred in Somalia in October 1977. Ali Maow Maalim, a Somali hospital worker, developed a smallpox rash. WHO officials guarded Ali's doorstep in his small village of Merka allowing no one near him until he had recovered and the last scab had fallen from his last pock. After this, no new cases of smallpox were reported in Somalia or elsewhere. Ali Maow Maalim was declared the last person on Earth to catch smallpox by natural transmission, that is, as a result of direct contact with another human being.[50] Eradication complete?

Not so. In 1978, two more cases of smallpox occurred in England as a result of incorrect handling of the smallpox virus in the medical school at the University of Birmingham.[51] When Janet Parker, a 40-year-old medical photographer, contracted smallpox and died in September 1978, experts were mystified. Because the disease had already been eradicated they surmised that she must have caught it from a laboratory sample. At that time smallpox was still used in many laboratories in the world, including a laboratory on the floor below the photographic unit where Janet worked.

An investigation showed how the virus could have moved up an unsealed ventilator shaft to a small room above the laboratory where Parker spent several hours on the day that a particular smallpox virus was cultivated. Molecular analysis of the virus that killed Janet Parker proved it was the same virus. Janet Parker's unnecessary death had a ripple effect. Her father died of a heart attack and her mother also contracted smallpox but fortunately recovered. The virologist in charge of the laboratory, Professor Henry Bedson, head of the Department of Medical Microbiology, felt so responsible that he tragically took his own life.

Smallpox had claimed its last victims but the incident revealed the danger that could erupt from smallpox virus stocks in laboratories. The argument for the destruction of all remaining stocks hotted up. In 1976 the World Health Organization had requested that all 76 countries holding smallpox virus either destroy or submit their stocks to one of two official WHO repositories in the United States at the Centers for Disease Control and Prevention in Atlanta, Georgia, or in the Soviet Union at the Moscow Institute. South Africa was the last to comply in December 1983.

THE MONSTER IS DEAD

The speckled monster was officially pronounced dead by the 33rd World Health Assembly in May 1980, when after two years of intensive surveillance in previously endemic countries no new cases had been found. Smallpox had been wiped from the face of the earth, thus fulfilling Edward Jenner's prediction. It is said that Jenner is responsible for saving more human lives than any other person. The global eradication of smallpox is acknowledged as one of the greatest accomplishments of the twentieth century, if not one of the greatest human accomplishments of all time.

But repositories of the virus still exist and it is not inconceivable that the work that took centuries to achieve could easily be undone, unleashing the unthinkable. These concerns plus the September 11 terrorist attacks in the United States in 2001 and the use of anthrax as a biological weapon later that year have led to a renewed interest in smallpox. There are fears that a weaponised smallpox virus may have been developed as well as recombinant strains of smallpox that have increased virulence and infectivity.

In May 1990 the secretary of the Department of Health and Human Services in the United States called on the Soviet Union to jointly determine the DNA sequences of selected strains of variola virus, followed by destruction of the virus stocks in Atlanta and Moscow.[52] The original plan was to destroy virus stocks on 31 December 1993. The history of smallpox should have ended then with the first deliberate elimination of a biological species from our planet, thus ensuring the extinction of the fatal disease. But the virus has gained a number of reprieves. The slow pace of research caused the planned date of destruction to be delayed until 30 June 1995 but it did not take place then either.

The World Health Organization's executive board again recommended to the 49th World Health Assembly in January 1996 that the last stocks of smallpox virus be destroyed. This was met with counter-proposals to retain 500,000 doses of a smallpox vaccine containing live vaccinia virus, which is closely related to variola virus, and to also keep the Lister Elstree strain of the virus as seed virus stock for future vaccine production. Scientific opposition to the destruction caused a further delay until June 1999.

The two main arguments against destruction of the virus were that it would eliminate the possibility of future studies and that destruction of the virus in the two known repositories (in 1994, Russia without consultation, moved its virus stocks from Moscow to Vector, a former research centre in Koltsovo) may not guarantee complete eradication.[53] The counter-arguments were that escape of the virus from the laboratories would pose a serious health risk because an increasing proportion of the global population lacks immunity to the disease (there is still no effective treatment once smallpox has been contracted), and that the sequence information and the availability of cloned DNA fragments of the full genome of several strains of the virus would allow most genetic questions to be resolved without the use of live virus stocks.

During 1998 and 1999 an intense debate over the destruction of variola virus stocks took place within the United States government. Arguments for retention won the day. The World Health Assembly passed a resolution to retain the stocks stored in the United States and Russia for three more years for the purpose of biodefence research. Again in May 2002, the WHA decided to extend the research program with live variola virus and not destroy the official stocks. The pattern has continued.

Amidst growing concern, in 2005 an international alliance of non-governmental organisations launched the 'Put Smallpox in the History Books Instead of the Genetic Engineering Lab' campaign and urged the WHO to carry out their original intention of destroying all virus stocks.[54] At the 59th World Health Assembly in May 2006 the smallpox issue emerged as the most controversial, creating friction between the representatives of various governments. Many developing countries advocated setting yet another firm date for destroying the virus stocks and stricter WHO controls over the remaining stocks and the research. Concerns were also expressed that the WHO Advisory Committee on Variola Virus Research lacked broad representation and suggested it should be independent of the scientists from the United States and Russian laboratories where stocks are held. Considering the previous delays it is not surprising that there was no agreement and no date was set for destruction. The next major review will be in 2010. And the smallpox virus lives on.

Thomas Jefferson, the third president of the United States, wrote to Edward Jenner in 1806 to thank him for 'erasing from the calendar of human afflictions one of its greatest', assuring Jenner that, 'Yours is the comfortable reflection that mankind can never forget that you have lived. Future nations will know by history only that the loathsome small-pox has existed and by you has been extirpated.'[55] It is true that one cannot forget what one has not learnt. Whole generations are now growing up unaware of Jenner and the disease whose name sounded doom. Perhaps this is his true legacy, that to not know about smallpox or Jenner means the disease has not returned.

Edward Jenner had great hopes for humanity and his scientific mind would no doubt grapple with the bitter irony that the eradication of small-pox, that thing which he desired most, has created a new vulnerability: the possibility that the virus could be used as a means of bio-warfare and ter-rorism. Today, few people have an understanding of how protracted and arduous the battle was to vanquish the speckled monster and fewer and fewer people have personal memories of the horror of the disease. Edward Jenner unselfishly gave to the world the first great medical breakthrough and the hope of perpetual salvation from the most terrible minister of death. Paradoxically, the end of the smallpox story is yet to be written.

POSTSCRIPT

In more recent times Edward Jenner has been accused of acting unethically in using James Phipps as a guinea pig in his experi-ments. These accusations arise, however, because of unfamiliarity with the medical standards of Jenner's day and interpreting his actions as putting the boy at risk, rather than protecting him. Jenner was a man of great generosity and he built a cottage for

James Phipps, his first vaccination patient. Even more telling is the fact that Jenner personally planted a rose garden for James. We can only surmise as to how James Phipps felt about the gifts that Jenner gave him but James was one of the very few mourners in attendance at the funeral of a man who was better known in his own time for his study of the cuckoo than for his contribution to saving humankind.

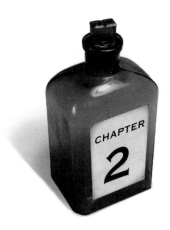

CHAPTER

2

ESTABLISHING THE
GERM THEORY OF DISEASE

LOUIS PASTEUR — THE FATHER
OF MODERN MEDICINE

I beseech you to take interest in these sacred
domains so expressively called laboratories. Ask
that there be more and that they be adorned for
these are the temples of the future, wealth and wellbeing. It is here that humanity will grow, strengthen
and improve. Here, humanity will learn to read
progress and individual harmony in the works of
nature, while humanity's own works are all too often
those of barbarism, fanaticism and destruction.[1]

Louis Pasteur

The wonders that the French chemist Louis Pasteur created in his laboratory, his temple, did much to advance the welfare of humankind in his own
time and made possible so many of the great medical advances that were to
follow. Scientific giants like Louis Pasteur and Edward Jenner laid the foundations of our knowledge of health and disease and made it possible for the
state-of-the-art temples of the future to produce even greater wonders.

Although Edward Jenner invented the first vaccine in 1796 and provided the means by which smallpox could be prevented and eventually eradicated, prior to the mid 1880s innumerable diseases could neither be prevented nor cured. So when news spread that a cure had been discovered for rabies, the horrific disease caused by the bite of a rabid animal, it followed that the scientist who discovered the cure, Louis Pasteur, became an instant cause célèbre. He was revered as a saviour and his name became familiar to people not just in his homeland, France, but all over the world.

However, Pasteur's contribution is by no means limited to the discovery of a cure for human rabies. It marked the culmination of a lifetime of work and a plethora of discoveries, and the legacy of Pasteur's superior intellect and scientific method continues to facilitate the progress of humanity. Louis Pasteur believed that his research was 'enchained to an inescapable, forward-moving logic', that one discovery, one concept, led inexorably to the next. This ethos drove him to an overwhelming breadth of research and accomplishments.

The Germ Theory of Disease is acknowledged by many as Pasteur's seminal work. His discovery that infectious diseases are caused by micro-organisms has been described as the most important in medical history. Diseases could not be defeated as long as the enemy, micro-organisms, remained unknown. With Pasteur's discovery the study of microbiology began. His discrediting of spontaneous generation, the 2000-year-old belief that life could arise spontaneously in organic material, is also seen as historically significant as it allowed science to progress. Both of these scientific breakthroughs would not have been possible without Pasteur's earlier groundbreaking work. Indeed, each of Pasteur's discoveries over a period of half a century, from the 1850s to the 1890s, represents a link in an uninterrupted chain, beginning with his early work on molecular asymmetry and leading to the pinnacle of his achievement, his rabies vaccine.

It would seem that many cures and advances since Pasteur's time have also been 'enchained', in turn leading to the discovery of the principles of acquired immunity and methods of being able to produce it artificially.

Pasteur ushered in a revolution in scientific methodology and research and is acknowledged as the founder of modern medicine and the father of microbiology and immunology.

Pasteur believed that the freedom of creative imagination must, by necessity, be subjected to rigorous experimentation. Not unlike the advice John Hunter had given to Edward Jenner, the maxim Pasteur preached to his students was, 'Do not put forward anything that you cannot prove by experimentation.'[2] Louis Pasteur was a humanist who put himself and science to work to improve the human condition. In so doing, he never hesitated to take issue with the prevailing ideas of his time when he believed them to be false. For this he often suffered at the hands of his critics and detractors. Even so, within his lifetime, Pasteurean theory and method were embraced well beyond French borders.

Genius of this type cannot help but incite envy and Pasteur's extraordinary discoveries were often met with scepticism, particularly when they seemed to contradict prevailing views. As Pasteur's fame grew so did professional and personal opposition, which caused anger and frustration for this zealous scientist. Pasteur alienated chemists, naturalists, physicians and surgeons alike. His professional life was marked by endless conflicts that on occasion precipitated breakdowns in his health.

Descriptions of Pasteur by myriad biographers and acquaintances vary. To many, Pasteur appeared cool, aloof and ungracious and was approachable only to people within his inner circle. These traits were suited to his work ethic and scientific rigour but often alienated his contemporaries. Unable to cope with any kind of criticism, the more he was challenged the more inflammatory he became. In return he challenged his opponents to disprove his claims, often causing offence when he scorned what he perceived as ignorance and lack of experimental skill. As Pasteur's career progressed and his output increased he had an ever-increasing amount to defend.

When Pasteur's research on fermentation challenged the established chemical theory of the day he won the ire of the arrogant and influential

German chemist, Baron Justus von Liebig. Pasteur came into conflict with the naturalist Félix Pouchet, director of the National History Museum in Rouen, over the theory of spontaneous generation, and was embroiled in a bitter quarrel with prominent physicians over the cause of contagion and disease. While experimenting on vaccination for animal and human diseases, Pasteur made enemies of other scientists, anti-vaccinators and anti-vivisectionists. The most scathing criticism came from Robert Koch, a German research physician. The rivalry between these two scientific icons was vitriolic, intense and lifelong.

Those who worked most closely with Pasteur, however, saw him as a humanitarian and a genius who, although fanatical about his causes, attacked falsehoods not individuals. The physician Emile Roux, who was one of Pasteur's closest associates, believed that Pasteur's work proved the brilliance of his mind, 'but one had to live in his house to fully recognise the goodness of his heart'.[3] Paul de Kruif, another contemporary of Pasteur, called him 'the scientific nonpareil, the microbe-hunting one and only'. Pasteur's grandson described him as intolerant of adversaries who refused to listen to the truth, but a man who in his private life was 'the gentlest, most affectionate and sensitive individual'.[4]

What cannot be contested is that Pasteur furthered the work of Edward Jenner, providing convincing evidence for both the theory and practice of vaccination, a link in the chain which would eventually lead to one of the greatest medical breakthroughs of all time: the development of antibiotics. Pasteur's discovery that most diseases are caused by germs, which seems so fundamental to us today, has made countless subsequent medical breakthroughs and cures possible. It is impossible to calculate how many lives have been saved as a result.

A QUAINT IDEA

It was not Louis Pasteur who first became aware of the world of microorganisms. That such destructive living microscopic creatures existed was acknowledged in ancient times. Around 46 BC, the Roman, Marcus Varro, advised that when building a house or a farm, it should be situated at the foot of a wooded hill where it would be exposed to 'health-giving winds'. Varro warned against building near swamps because creatures too small to be seen with the eye breed there.[5] In his writings he stated that these creatures float through the air and enter the body by the mouth and nose and cause serious disease.

What had been viewed for centuries as a quant idea became credible because of the scientific bent of a Dutch merchant, Antonie van Leeuwenhoek. Born in 1632, van Leeuwenhoek had no formal education but his passion for scientific observation and description took him in an unusual direction. Compound microscopes were first invented in the 1600s but because they had inherent difficulties with lighting and focal length, van Leeuwenhoek decided to construct his own. In his lifetime he made over 500 microscopes, only ten of which have survived. With a magnification of over 200, van Leeuwenhoek was able to enter a mysterious microscopic world.

Antonie van Leeuwenhoek found what he referred to as 'very little animalcules' in rain and pond water and in his own bodily fluids and excretions. He wrote descriptions of these micro-organisms and hired an illustrator to draw them. Between 1673 and 1723, van Leeuwenhoek wrote to the Royal Society in England detailing the wonders of his discoveries. The letters contained the first descriptions of an extraordinary cornucopia: bacteria, protozoa, spermatozoa, red blood cells, striations of muscle cells and the lifecycle of a flea. In the plaque scraped from his teeth van Leeuwenhoek observed 'an unbelievable great company of living animalcules, a-swimming more nimbly than any' he had seen previously.[6]

In 1677, after examining spermatozoa in the semen of a man suffering from venereal disease, van Leeuwenhoek examined his own semen and for the next 40 years continued investigating the spermatozoa from molluscs, fish, amphibians, birds and mammals. Van Leeuwenhoek concluded that fertilisation occurred when spermatozoa penetrated an egg and he considered this discovery to be one of the most important in his career.

Two centuries before Pasteur established the Germ Theory of Disease, Antonie van Leeuwenhoek's studies revealed a world where micro-organisms and human cells battled for dominance. His findings raised some doubt about the prevailing scientific notion that life could generate spontaneously. It was a common belief, for example, that weevils spontaneously generated in grain but van Leeuwenhoek's observation of corn weevils mating helped to disprove this. He also observed and described the life-cycles of other animals once thought to have been spontaneously generated out of materials such as mud and decaying matter.

Ironically, however, although Pasteur proved that germs cause disease, when he developed his vaccine for the fatal disease rabies, the rhabdovirus which causes it could not be seen because microscopes at the time were still not powerful enough.

Louis Pasteur was born in the French village of Dole on 27 December 1822. He was the only son of a poorly educated tanner, Jean Pasteur, a veteran of Napoleon's army. When Louis was still young the family moved to nearby Arbois where he attended primary and secondary schools. During his early education Louis was not an outstanding student but was artistic and at college painted professional portraits — his name can be found in compendia of nineteenth-century artists.[7]

Louis' father, however, had aspirations for his son other than art. Gradually, as Louis began to show an interest in chemistry and other scientific subjects, Monsieur Pasteur hoped that Louis would undertake an academic career at the college in Arbois. But Louis far exceeded his father's expectations. In 1840 he gained a Bachelor of Arts degree from the Royal College in Besançon, followed by a Bachelor of Science in 1842. The head of the college recognised Louis' prodigious ability and suggested that he apply to the Ecole Normale Supérieure in Paris, a prestigious university which had been founded specifically to train outstanding students for academic careers in science and letters. Louis gained entry in 1843, was awarded a Master of Science degree in 1845 and so began his incomparable scientific career.

Pasteur started as a chemist studying the shapes of organic crystals. In 1847, at the age of 26 when he began working for his doctorate, crystallography was emerging as a branch of chemistry. Pasteur worked on molecular asymmetry, bringing together the principles of crystallography, chemistry and optics. From his experiments Pasteur determined that asymmetric molecules were indicative of living or organic processes and therefore always a product of these. This discovery provided Pasteur with the 'inescapable forward-moving logic' that would soon lead him to his studies on alcoholic fermentation.[8] Louis was awarded his doctorate and in the following year, 1848, gained recognition when he presented a paper on his findings on asymmetry before the Paris Academy of Sciences.

After serving as Professor of Physics on the Faculty of Science at the Dijon Lycée for a brief period in 1848, Pasteur transferred to Strasbourg University and, as Professor of Chemistry, continued his studies on molecular asymmetry. But it was not all work and Louis fell in love with and married Marie Laurent, the daughter of the university rector. They married on 29 May 1849 and Louis and Marie remained devoted to each other throughout their lives. The couple had five children, but sadly only two survived childhood. Marie assisted Louis in his scientific pursuits in whatever way she could, although she did complain in a letter to her father-in-law that Louis spent too much time on his experiments. Throughout the times when Louis was beleaguered by controversy, however, Marie remained steadfast.

In 1854 Pasteur was appointed Dean and Professor of Chemistry at the new Faculty of Sciences in the industrial town of Lille, the economy of which depended on its distilleries and factories. It was at Lille that Pasteur showed in a practical way that he supported the view of the Minister of Public Instruction at the university that science should not exist only for its own sake. He encouraged members of the faculty to keep up with scientific theory, to be innovative and to apply their science to the real needs of the community. In accordance with these beliefs he trained his students to assist factory managers in solving the chemical problems they encountered in their production processes.

In the summer of 1856 one Monsieur Bigot, a distiller and the father of one of Pasteur's students, asked Pasteur for help. He and other manufacturers needed a chemist to examine why alcohol becomes contaminated with undesirable substances during fermentation. Their alcohol yields were erratic, wines unexpectedly became sour or turned to vinegar, lactic acid was sometimes produced instead of the desired vinegar and the quality and taste of beer was almost impossible to control. These problems had obvious economic consequences.

At the time that Pasteur agreed to help, the mysterious chemical processes of living animals were slowly being unravelled by scientists; Pasteur's work on crystals had contributed to this. A German organic chemist, Friedrich Woehler, had astonished the scientific world when he synthesised the organic compound urea, showing that organic compounds could be made in a test tube whereas previously it was thought that they could only be synthesised by living animals.

The process of fermentation was, however, believed to be a straightforward chemical breakdown of sugar that occurred due to the presence of inherent destabilising vibrations that could be transferred from a vat of finished wine to new grape pressings to restart the fermentation process. The yeast cells found in the fermenting vats of wine were recognised as being living organisms, but they were believed to be either a product of fermentation or catalytic agents that assisted during fermentation. A few lone voices had concluded that yeast was the cause and not the product of fermentation but they had been ridiculed by scientific experts who dismissed any biological theory that challenged chemical explanations of molecular reaction.[9] It was precisely because of these prevailing views that the brewers' problems had not been solved.

Pasteur's previous work prepared him to look beyond chemical explanations. Not long after beginning his investigations in the Bigot factory,

Pasteur found three clues that allowed him to solve the puzzle of alcoholic fermentation. Pasteur's methods, and his suspicion that only living cells produced asymmetrical compounds, led him to conclude and then prove that living cells, the yeast, were responsible for forming alcohol from sugar, and that contaminating micro-organisms turned the fermentations sour. Different micro-organisms, living creatures, caused normal and abnormal fermentations in the production of wine, beer and vinegar. Pasteur was able to demonstrate this by cultivating the various micro-organisms in an appropriate sterile medium. He discovered anaerobic life, a world of micro-organisms that can live without oxygen. This is the basis of microbiology and the discovery paved the way for his study of germs that cause septicaemia and gangrene and made it possible for techniques to be devised which could kill microbes and control contamination and infection.

But Pasteur's findings on fermentation challenged the established chemical theory of the day and brought him into direct conflict with Justus von Liebig. Liebig, nineteen years older than Pasteur, was an old-school expert in chemistry who refused to use a microscope. He dismissed Pasteur's biological view of fermentation and putrefaction as 'getting everything backwards'. When Pasteur criticized Liebig's methodology, a protracted battle began.[10] As Pasteur's reputation burgeoned so did the hostility that was directed at him and when he was proposed for a vacancy in the influential Academy of Sciences in Paris opposition came from many quarters.

According to Pasteur's nephew, one of Pasteur's many biographers, his uncle's objections to others were based on the science behind their work and were never personal in nature and for this reason, his nephew concluded, Louis was incapable of understanding envy and ill-will in others. In a letter that Pasteur wrote to his wife Marie, he stated without guile or conceit that everyone knew he was a valid candidate but that many of his opponents were afraid that chemists wished to subvert all other disciplines to chemistry. He believed this to be the reason that all the naturalists were against him, 'especially the ignorant ones' — but those in his own field were against him too.[11]

'SIMPLE EXPERIMENT' DELIVERS A MORTAL BLOW

In 1857, at the age of 35, Pasteur was appointed to his alma mater, the Ecole Normale Supérieure, as assistant director of both scientific studies and general administration. He moved to Paris with Marie and their three children but, despite his position, was given neither a laboratory nor funds. To continue his work on fermentation he set up a small laboratory in a rat-infested attic.[12] Pasteur used his own money to further his work while the frenzied excitement and controversy aroused by his research on fermentation swirled about him.

The ongoing debate in the scientific world surrounding the theory of spontaneous generation was also gaining momentum not only in the exalted French Academy of Sciences. The idea that beetles, eels, maggots, and now Pasteur's microbes could arise spontaneously from putrefying matter had been speculated upon since Greek and Roman times. Although the prevailing scientific elite supported spontaneous generation — if living tissue could turn into non-living matter then the converse should also be true — no definitive experiments had been undertaken. In January 1860 the academy offered a prize to anyone who could settle the matter.

Pasteur did not hesitate even though his colleagues and friends warned that challenging spontaneous generation could harm his reputation. Pasteur not only disputed the doctrine but took on its most prominent advocate, Félix-Archimede Pouchet. Pouchet had published a paper in 1858 and an authoritative book in 1859 on spontaneous generation and had conducted experiments that seemed to have produced micro-organisms from non-living matter. Pasteur suggested that Pouchet and other exponents of the spurious theory had achieved these results because their experimental methods were not exacting enough and germ matter from the air had contaminated their experiments.

From his work on fermentation Pasteur concluded that the yeasts and other micro-organisms that were found during fermentation and putrefaction came from the outside, via dust in the air. Pasteur designed and conducted a series of ingenious experiments that proved that if air carrying dust and dirt was excluded from a flask of nutritive broth, the broth remained pure and clear, but the same sterile solution when exposed to unpurified air or to a drop of water filled with micro-organisms was soon teeming with life.

In one experiment Pasteur showed that grape skins at the beginning of grape harvest were the source of the yeast. Grape juice extracted with sterile needles would not ferment. Covering the grape trellises to keep off contaminating dust resulted in grapes that would not produce wine. Pasteur then had to prove that contamination was carried in dust in the air. He devised the famous swan-neck flask. Air entered the flask through the opening but the curved neck trapped dust particles and micro-organisms ensuring the fluid within remained sterile. This showed that air alone could not trigger the growth of micro-organisms. When the flask was tipped the sterile liquid touched the contaminated walls and micro-organisms grew.

Never one to do things by halves, Pasteur worked with 60 flasks. He put twenty at the bottom of a mountain, twenty at approximately 2500 feet (762 metres) above sea level, and the remainder at the top of a glacier, at 6000 feet (1829 metres). These were the extraordinary lengths Pasteur went to in order to prove his hypothesis that it was possible to obtain air at any location in which micro-organisms would not generate spontaneously and thus dispute Pouchet's theory.[13] The higher the altitude the less dust in the air and the fewer flasks that showed growth.

Pasteur won the challenge and announced to the scientific world that the doctrine of spontaneous generation would never recover from the mortal blow of his 'simple experiment'. Some of Pasteur's preparations which are kept at the Pasteur Institute in France have remained sterile for over a century and are a testament to his scientific method. In 1862 Pasteur was awarded the Academy of Sciences prize and Pouchet withdrew, but not gra-ciously. He attacked Pasteur in a new book, accusing him of obstinacy and of not facing facts. Pasteur's retort was that he had science and 'true method' on his side, not 'fantasy and instinctive solutions'. In a lecture at the Sorbonne in 1864 Pasteur asserted that 'there is now no circumstance known in which it can be affirmed that microscopic beings came into the world without germs, without parents similar to themselves.'[14]

Although he had opponents, the esteem that others had for Pasteur was demonstrated in 1864 when Emperor Napoleon III requested that Pasteur investigate the diseases that were afflicting wine and causing economic losses for the wine industry.[15] In a vineyard in Arbois Pasteur demonstrated that wine diseases are caused by micro-organisms that can be killed by heating the wine to 55°C for several minutes. This process, now known as 'pasteurisation', also killed germs in beer and milk and was soon in use throughout the world.

In his eclectic findings, published in 1866, Pasteur discussed the causes and prevention of wine diseases, described pasteurisation and explained that some organisms like yeast can exist with or without oxygen. He also explained that putrefaction, the negative side of fermentation, is caused by an anaerobic microbe, which he called 'vibrio'.[16] Pasteur saw decay as a natural process that helps balance the environment by breaking down dead organic matter.

With each new phase of his work, Pasteur was compiling his dossier on micro-organisms. While continuing his study of fermentation and spontaneous generation, Pasteur was asked by the Department of Agriculture to head a commission to investigate a silkworm disease that was devastating the French silk industry. Even though initially Pasteur was unaware that silkworms suffered from disease, his research was to forge another link in his chain of discovery and save yet another industry. He began an intense five-year study in 1865.

Convinced that all putrefying processes were caused by micro-organisms, Pasteur concluded that putrefaction was destroying the silkworms. He identified at least two diseases and, elaborating on his study of fermentation, confirmed that each disease was caused by a specific foreign element, a microbe, and that the infection could be passed on.

The excessive workload and the unceasing criticism that Pasteur attracted began to take their toll and in 1868, at the age of only 46, Pasteur suffered a crippling stroke that almost ended his career. Astonishingly — and luckily, as many of his greatest discoveries were still to come — he recovered. While still partially paralysed, Pasteur completed his work on silkworms, often dictating his observations from an armchair. [17] As Pasteur regained his health so did the silk industry in France and other European countries.

It is both fascinating and astonishing that Pasteur would soon apply the findings from his landmark work on silkworms to human disease and infection and to the plight of the many women who died very soon after giving birth from puerperal fever or, as it was then commonly called, childbirth fever. This new scientific knowledge would soon bring huge benefits to humankind by establishing basic methods of sterilisation, or asepsis, to control contagion and infection, practices that would revolutionise surgery and obstetrics.

Pasteur was inching closer to formulating the Germ Theory of Disease and, the pinnacle of his achievements, finding a cure for rabies. It is almost impossible for us in the 21st century, in the age of cloning, mapping the genome and stem-cell research, to fathom the mindset of doctors who, through most of history, attributed infectious disease to foul air, harmful bodily fluids, comets and mystical forces. Pasteur was convinced that the microbes he studied were the agents of infection and he believed he had provided conclusive proof.

The discoveries that Pasteur made that saved many French industries led him to hypothesise on the possible connections between micro-organisms and disease in larger animals and humans. He proposed that micro-organisms such as bacteria, fungi and protozoan parasites did not occur spontaneously but reproduced within their own species in various ways, and that they were present in large numbers almost everywhere, in air, water and dust. Therefore germs caused fermentation, putrescence and disease, and ergo, different microbes cause different diseases. Although to

us this seems exceedingly simple and indisputable, in Pasteur's day —
because the idea that a living 'germ' could cause a chemical reaction would
be a retrograde step in scientific thought — to extrapolate that germs
cause disease was seen as a nonsense.[18]

Re-enter Baron Justus von Liebig, Pasteur's nemesis. He questioned
Pasteur's experiments and findings on Germ Theory in print in 1869. In
reply, Pasteur challenged the scientific world to decide between French
biology and Liebig's German chemistry. He suggested the Royal Academy
appoint a commission that would judge the validity of his experiments, but
there was no response from either Liebig or the academy. Undaunted,
Pasteur travelled to Munich and confronted Liebig face-to-face but the older
scientist dismissed Pasteur and bluntly refused to engage in any debate.

It was no holds barred for some of Pasteur's adversaries. The chemist
and historian Marcelin Berthelot published notes written by one of
Pasteur's closest friends and colleagues, Claude Bernard, to discredit
Pasteur's Germ Theory. Following Pasteur's methods, Bernard had used
the science available to him to question Pasteur's findings. Bernard could
not have imagined that after his death these same notes would be used to
publicly discredit his friend. Although distraught and reluctant to speak
against the colleague he had lost and whom he still held in high regard,
Pasteur, for the sake of his own reputation, refuted the accusations.

With each new sphere of research that Pasteur entered he polarised the
scientific community and the greatest enmity came from doctors who
were outraged and insulted by 'this chemist' whom they considered to be
their intellectual inferior. Pasteur was attacked by members of the
Academy of Medicine in Paris as a fanatic, afflicted with 'microbial madness'.[19] But he also had his supporters. Joseph Lister, the Professor of
Surgery at Glasgow University, was impressed by Pasteur's work.
Convinced of the link between micro-organisms and infection, Lister
began to systematically sterilise his instruments and bandages and sprayed
phenol solutions in his operating rooms. The result was a dramatic drop in
the number of infections following surgery.

By the mid 1870s many physicians acknowledged that some diseases were accompanied by specific micro-organisms, but the body of medical opinion was unwilling to concede that endemic diseases like cholera, diphtheria, scarlet fever, childbirth fever, syphilis and even smallpox could ever be caused by them. Although not a physician, Pasteur was aware of the huge mortality rate associated with childbirth fever. In order to further his studies he visited hospitals and morgues to obtain samples of blood and secretions from the uteruses of Parisian mothers who had died from the fever.[20] In the cultures he identified the micro-organisms that are now called streptococci.

As Pasteur wandered through hospital wards he became increasingly aware that infection was spread from sick to healthy patients by physicians and hospital workers. Pasteur, the chemist, began to hammer home this point to physicians. In a famous speech that he gave at the Academy of Medicine he stated:

> This water, this sponge, this lint with which you wash or cover a wound, may deposit germs which have the power of multiplying rapidly within the tissue … If I had the honour of being a surgeon … not only would I use none but perfectly clean instruments, but I would clean my hands with the greatest care … I would use only lint, bandages and sponges previously exposed to a temperature of 1300 to 1500 degrees.[21]

Not all those in the medical profession were quick to embrace Pasteur's findings or appreciated the blunt delivery of the message. Even after Pasteur had established that deadly microbes were the cause of infection, in the late 1870s an eminent physician, in a lecture to the Academy of Medicine, described childbirth fever as a metabolic disorder. Pasteur, unable to control himself, yelled from the back of the hall that it was doctors who carried microbes from sick women to healthy ones. The depth of the hostility towards Pasteur became evident when one elderly surgeon challenged him to a duel. But the medical profession soon came to accept the views of Pasteur and Lister and antiseptic medicine and surgery became the rule.

In April 1878 Pasteur presented a summary of his work to the French Academy of Sciences and made the point that the various branches of science could all gain from each other. Pasteur avowed that there was now 'absolute proof that there actually exist transmissible, contagious, infectious diseases of which the cause lies essentially and solely in the presence of microscopic organisms.'[22] He confirmed that he had found proof that for some diseases the idea of spontaneous generation must be abandoned, as should the idea that contagion and infection suddenly originate in the bodies of humans or animals. Pasteur described the hypothesis of spontaneous generation as gratuitous, as having no basis in observation and condemned it as 'fatal' to medical progress.

PASTEUR TACKLES ANTHRAX — AND KOCH

From the late 1870s Pasteur applied all that he had discovered in his study of microbiology to the battle against infectious diseases. Yet another phase of his research had begun. Anthrax, a disease of sheep and cattle, was destroying the livelihood of French farmers who were powerless to save their dying animals. The debate over Germ Theory was still raging when Pasteur entered the anthrax arena. The cause of anthrax, a bacillus (a type of rod-shaped spore-producing bacteria), had first been identified in 1849. Robert Koch, the German physician, had succeeded in growing the bacillus in pure culture in 1877.

Definitive proof was still lacking, however, that the cultured bacillus, and not something else that may have entered Koch's culture medium, was responsible for giving animals anthrax.[23] Pasteur provided the proof experimentally. He placed one drop of blood from a sheep dying of anthrax into 50 millilitres of sterile culture, grew up the bacterium, and then repeated this process 100 times. After the dilutions the last culture was as active as the first in producing anthrax. With this, Pasteur firmly established his Germ Theory of Disease.

Pasteur then applied what he had learnt from silkworm disease to help solve the mystery of how anthrax spread; why animals in one field remained healthy while animals in another succumbed. The answer: earthworms feeding on the carcasses of buried diseased sheep carried anthrax spores to the surface, contaminating the soil where healthy sheep graze and thus passing on the disease. Keeping animals away from contaminated fields would help control the spread of anthrax but was not the answer to preventing it.

'Chance favours the prepared mind' was an adage that Pasteur was fond of. A stroke of luck and Pasteur's prepared mind combined to bring about a major breakthrough — the discovery of the method for the attenuation of virulent micro-organisms. Attenuation is the basis of vaccination. Pasteur was researching chicken cholera at the same time as anthrax. Another serious problem for farmers, this disease could wipe out an entire flock in as little as three days. The experiments Pasteur carried out on chicken cholera led him to the development of specific vaccines against chicken cholera, anthrax and swine erysipelas. Once he had mastered the method of attenuation Pasteur would apply the concept to rabies.

In experiments in his laboratory at Arbois, Pasteur was growing chicken cholera bacillus in pure culture. Chickens injected with the culture invariably died within 48 hours. On one occasion, Pasteur took a chance and injected two chickens with a culture that was several weeks old. The chickens became ill and then recovered. During the summer Pasteur returned to Paris leaving the cholera cultures stored in the laboratory. When the staff returned, they conducted some experiments using these cholera cultures on two chickens and were surprised when the chickens did not become infected. New cultures of the bacillus were made and tested on new birds plus the two healthy birds that had survived. The results were astonishing. The previously injected birds were unaffected by the bacillus, while the new birds all died.[24]

When Pasteur saw these results he immediately realised that in a sense he was repeating the studies Edward Jenner had conducted 80 years earlier when he gave humans immunity to smallpox by vaccinating individuals with the milder disease, cowpox. Pasteur hypothesised that pathogens can be attenuated, or weakened, by exposure to environmental conditions such as high temperature, oxygen and chemicals. He then grew the cholera bacillus at 42–43°C, at which temperature the bacillus is non-infectious, and these attenuated bacterial cultures were used to successfully vaccinate chickens against cholera.

Pasteur had the key to preventing anthrax. By using various techniques involving oxidation and ageing, Pasteur developed attenuated anthrax bacillus and in laboratory trials anthrax vaccines successfully protected sheep. When Pasteur reported his findings it was déjà vu: both the scientific community and the general populous were divided. A well-known veterinarian challenged Pasteur to conduct a controlled public trial of his anthrax vaccine. Pasteur did what he always did, met the challenge head on. Risking his reputation, Pasteur organised a public demonstration on a farm at Melun, south of Paris.

Twenty-five sheep were controls and another 25 were vaccinated by Pasteur. All 50 were injected with a lethal dose of anthrax. Pasteur affirmed that only 100 per cent success would prove his theory, which meant that all of the control sheep must die and all the vaccinated sheep must live. When Pasteur's colleagues expressed their concern because the vaccines were still in the developmental stage, with bravado Pasteur declared that, 'What succeeded with fourteen sheep in our laboratory will succeed with 50 at Melun,'[25] but he knew he was taking an incredible risk. He had not had a 100 per cent success rate in the laboratory. Pasteur chided himself for acting impetuously but the trial went ahead.

This experiment attracted international attention. People came from everywhere. Farmers and scientists had a vested interest, some of the latter hoping to see Pasteur humiliated while the general public came to an event that seemed curiously like a circus. Once the experiment had begun newspapers in France and England published daily bulletins. Two days after the final vaccination on 5 May 1882, all 25 of the control sheep were dead while the 25 vaccinated sheep remained alive and healthy. This was

Pasteur's greatest experiment. He was a scientific superstar. Foes became fans and Pasteur's celebrity skyrocketed. At last the scientific elite and the hoi polloi believed in the existence of Pasteur's microbes.

Within ten years of the trial at Melun, throughout France 3.5 million sheep and half a million cattle had been vaccinated. The mortality rate dropped to less than 1 per cent, an enormous saving for the French economy. Pasteur's method of identifying the infectious agent, weakening it, and then using it to vaccinate a host was soon being applied to debilitating human diseases, by Pasteur and by others, thus ensuring the future salvation of millions. But if Louis Pasteur thought that finally all the sceptics and nay-sayers would be silent he expected too much. Pasteur was besieged by anti-vaccinators, who expressed similar views and objections to those who had opposed Jenner and his smallpox vaccinations.

Never able to avoid conflict for too long, Pasteur was soon embroiled again, this time with Robert Koch, who was working on contagious diseases. His publications in 1878 and 1879 had helped to confirm that bacteria were the cause and not the consequence of infection. An acrimonious dispute arose between Pasteur and Koch and his colleagues, who questioned Pasteur's scientific methodology and harshly criticised his work on the attenuation of viruses and his conclusions on anthrax vaccination.

In an article published in 1983, H.H. Molleret describes the relationship between Koch and Pasteur as 'hateful'.[26] The two great scientists first met in London in August 1881, during the International Congress of Medicine at which Pasteur presented his results on attenuation. The renowned Pasteur was 59, with a lifetime of work and discoveries behind him. Koch, who was only 38, already had impressive scientific credentials which Pasteur had previously acknowledged in April 1877 at the Science Academy in Paris when he referred to Koch's discovery of the anthrax spore as a remarkable achievement. In England both men attended demonstrations in Joseph Lister's laboratory at Cambridge University. When Koch presented the staining procedures that he had developed, a successful way of isolating micro-organisms, Pasteur again complimented Koch on a great scientific advance.

Molleret concludes that nothing in that first meeting justified the vicious attack that Koch launched in print a few months later. Koch discredited Pasteur's theory on the role of the earthworm in anthrax, calling it naïve and untenable, and claimed that scientific knowledge of anthrax had not been enlarged in any way by Louis Pasteur. Koch's colleague Friedrich Loeffler attacked Pasteur's attenuated vaccines, claiming that the cultures of the chicken cholera bacillus prepared by Pasteur were not pure because they were not done on gelatin, a method recently introduced by Koch. He also claimed that Pasteur's work on anthrax was based on poor science, and his experimental results were dependent on luck. Was there anything left to denounce?

Pasteur was deeply wounded by what he referred to as the 'strange ferociousness' of these attacks. Instead of responding in print as he usually did Pasteur hoped to debate Koch in person in Geneva at the International Congress of Hygiene in September 1882. At the congress Koch was enjoying the notoriety of having recently discovered the cause of tuberculosis, a momentous medical breakthrough. Pasteur, determined to make his point, gave a lengthy presentation on vaccination against anthrax. He pointed out that 'as brilliant as is demonstrated truth' he had met with 'contradictors' in France and in foreign countries and publicly named Robert Koch.

The audience was astonished when Koch interrupted Pasteur's speech. Koch dashed Pasteur's hopes for a public discussion and instead made a declaration that he had come to the Geneva conference hoping to learn some new facts but that once again he had learnt nothing new from Pasteur. Discussion would prove fruitless Koch said, because he did not speak French and Pasteur did not know enough German and therefore he would reply to Pasteur only in medical journals. Koch concluded with a stinging barb, saying that when 'Pasteur was celebrated as the second Jenner' for his questionable work on anthrax, the praise had been premature. 'Obviously in the desire to be enthusiastic it was forgotten that Jenner's beneficial discovery was not in sheep but in humans.'[27]

In December 1882 Pasteur wrote his reply, 'The Anthrax vaccination: Response to Dr Koch's Memoir'. Written with a tone as cutting as Koch's,

Pasteur told the German doctor that he was indebted to French science and accused Koch of misrepresenting him in previous papers. It had become bitter claim and counterclaim. In 1884, after Koch had made another breakthrough, the discovery of the cholera germ, he visited hospitals and laboratories in Paris and Toulon but deliberately avoided Pasteur's laboratory. Pasteur may have felt slighted but this did not prevent him some years later sending a telegram to Koch congratulating him on his discovery of the 'remedy against tuberculosis', which Koch announced at the Congress of Medicine in Berlin in August 1890.

Various suggestions as to the cause of the antagonism between Robert Koch and Louis Pasteur go beyond professional jealousy, brinkmanship and a personality clash. According to Molleret there was a climate of chauvinism and patriotism prevalent in the scientific community at the time. The rivalry over anthrax was an extension of an earlier patriotic quarrel that began well before Koch and Pasteur, with a debate over the discovery of the anthrax bacteria. The French attributed it to Rayer and Davaine in 1850 and the Germans credited Pollender who identified the bacteria in 1849 but did not publish his observations until 1855.

Another view is that the dispute between the two men and the scientific rivalry between the two countries was exacerbated by national loyalty and enmity between France and Germany after the Franco–Prussian War of 1870–71 which Germany won. Koch, who was anti-French, had volunteered for the Prussian Army in 1870 and had served in a military hospital near Orléans in France. Pasteur too was a passionate patriot who had wanted to join the National Guard. Pasteur's colleague, the Russian scientist Elie Metchnikov, wrote about how the war saddened and troubled Pasteur. Pasteur's own vitriolic words, written during the siege of Paris, reveal the depth of his animosity for the Germans, calling them 'vandals' who should 'perish from cold, misery and sickness' and vowing 'Hatred of Prussia, Vengeance, Vengeance!'. In January 1871 Pasteur returned the honorary Doctor of Medicine from the University of Bonn that he had been awarded in 1868 and a bitter exchange of letters with the Dean of the Faculty of Medicine followed. Pasteur was undoubtedly a man of deep passions.

In Geneva in 1882 Robert Koch had alluded to the language barrier between himself and Pasteur. Misconceptions could have arisen because neither scientist could read the work of the other in its original language. Documents from the time, held in the museum at the Pasteur Institute, suggest that the relationship between these two scientific giants was in fact affected by a lack of fluency in each other's language and that the altercation between them at the Congress of Geneva in 1882 may have resulted from a misinterpretation of one French word, *recueil*, which Koch interpreted as 'pride' rather than 'collection'. The word for pride is *orgueil*.[28] Koch may have felt insulted and it was at that moment that he had interrupted the meeting.

But nothing could keep Pasteur from his single-minded purpose and the forward momentum of his research. In the face of all opposition Pasteur was determined to apply the science that he had spent a lifetime mastering to curing human disease. Buoyed by his successes with anthrax and fowl cholera, over the next few years Pasteur employed the fundamentals of microbiology in a new battle. In 1882, aged 60 and partially crippled by the stroke that had weakened his left leg, Pasteur began to work on what Elie Metchnikov referred to as his 'swan-song' and what others have called his ultimate triumph.

MAD DOG DISEASE

Rabies, like smallpox, is a disease that has been known and feared since ancient times. A disease of the nervous system, rabies causes acute encephalitis (inflammation of the brain) in both animals and humans. The word rabies comes from the Latin *rabiere* meaning 'rage', which in turn is derived from the Sanskrit word *rabhas*, 'to be violent'. The Greeks call rabies *lyssa*, which means 'madness'.[29] All these words reflect the horrendous visible effects that rabies has on its victims. People suffering from rabies were often depicted as raving mad and frothing at the mouth.

Although rabies did not have the apocalyptic connotation of smallpox or bubonic plague, to people of Pasteur's time the horrifying disease evoked visions of victims raging, bound and howling, or being asphyxiated between two mattresses to subdue them, or having their bite wounds cauterised with a red-hot poker. Such treatments were as grotesque as the feared symptoms. A vaccine that cured the disease and eliminated such horrors would be considered nothing short of miraculous.

Rabies in humans is usually contracted after a bite from an infected animal because the virus can be present in the animal's saliva. By causing the infected animal to be exceptionally aggressive, the virus ensures its transmission to the next host. The disease is often associated with the stereotype of rabid, aggressive dogs. Other animals can carry rabies, including cats, ferrets, skunks, foxes, bears and bats. With bats, rabies can be transmitted via airborne liquid particles from their mucous. Following a bite by a rabid animal, if the virus is not inactivated by an immune response it enters the peripheral nervous system and can avoid recognition by the immune system by travelling gradually from nerve cell to nerve cell. When it reaches the central nervous system the virus is hard to detect and at this point is invulnerable to an immune response induced by vaccination. Viruses have developed cunning survival mechanisms and this one seems particularly cunning. Once the rabies virus reaches the brain, it rapidly causes encephalitis; symptoms appear — cerebral dysfunction, anxiety, insomnia, confusion, agitation and hallucinations — and death is certain.

As a boy living in Jura, Pasteur had witnessed the ghastly effects of the disease on several townspeople who had contracted rabies from a dog. The later stages of the disease are the most horrendous. People produce large quantities of saliva and tears, are unable to speak or swallow and develop hydrophobia, the fear of water, another name by which rabies is known. The final phase is delirium. The period between infection and the onset of symptoms is normally three to twelve weeks but it can be as long as two years. Despite the long incubation period, however, death usually occurs two to ten days after the first symptoms appear. Until Louis Pasteur developed his vaccine in 1885, the handful of people who are known to have survived the disease, except for one recorded case, were all left with severe brain damage.

Pasteur was aware that defeating rabies would be a defining scientific achievement and could lead to the conquest of other human diseases. Knowing that there were inherent difficulties in taking up this challenge Pasteur set to work with his colleague Emile Roux. The first hurdle was the lack of evidence that rabies was caused by a micro-organism, due to the fact that the virus was too small to be seen by microscope. This threatened Pasteur's Germ Theory, and was a point Koch would later use to attack Pasteur. However, convinced that an unseen microbe caused rabies, Pasteur followed his established procedures to find a way to weaken it. [30]

The work was slow and arduous. Pasteur and Roux initially attempted to transfer infection by injecting healthy dogs with saliva from rabid animals. The results were variable and unpredictable. Later, recognising that the active agent, even though it could not be seen, was in the spinal cord and brain, Pasteur and Roux applied extracts of rabid spinal cord directly to the brains of dogs. With this technique they could produce rabies in the test animals in a few days.

The aim, then, was to develop a vaccine that would provide protection before the virus moved from the bite site to the spinal cord and the brain. To do this Pasteur and Roux began by injecting dogs with spinal cord material taken from rabid rabbits. To attenuate the material it was air-dried over a twelve-day period. A strip of spinal cord was suspended from a hanger in the centre of what is now known as a Roux bottle. It had a hole at the top of the bottle and one on the lower side. Air entered from the bottom opening, passed over a drying agent and exited from the top. [31] The longer the cord was dried, the less potent was the tissue in producing rabies. Pasteur and Roux then injected the least potent preparation of minced spinal cord under the skin of their laboratory dogs. For the next twelve days the dogs were injected each day with an increasingly stronger extract, after which the animals were completely resistant to bites from rabid dogs.

In 1885 news got out that Pasteur and Roux had successfully made 40 dogs resistant to rabies by vaccination and the scientific fraternity was abuzz. Pasteur's name was again on everyone's lips. Although encouraged by the initial success, Pasteur was afraid to test the vaccine on humans because he was still unable to isolate the rabic microbe. Despite public pressure he insisted that years of additional research were necessary before human trials could begin. Two people did receive the vaccine, however; patients of physicians who were colleagues of Pasteur. Inexplicably, the first patient was discharged from hospital after receiving only one injection and his fate remains unknown. The second patient, a young girl, was in such an advanced stage of rabies that vaccination was too late and she died before the trial got properly under way.

Then events, as they so often do, took their own turn. On 6 July 1885, three people arrived unexpectedly at Pasteur's laboratory. Pasteur later related the events of that day in detail to the French Academy of Sciences. The three, he told the academy, were Theodore Vone, a grocer from Meissengot, who had been bitten on the arm on 4 July by his own rabid dog; Joseph Meister, a nine-year-old boy who had been bitten by Vone's dog on the same morning; and Joseph's distraught mother. Joseph was unable to walk properly because he had been knocked to the ground by the dog and bitten on the hand, legs and thighs and was covered with saliva and blood. The worst bites had been cauterised with carbolic acid by the town's doctor. Monsieur Vone had killed his dog but had not been at risk of catching rabies, Pasteur said, because his skin had not been pierced by the dog's fangs. Joseph's mother had pleaded with Pasteur to treat her son as he faced certain death.

The compassionate Pasteur agonised over the ethics of the situation and the risk to Joseph. He was reluctant to use the vaccine even though the prophylactic procedure had been successful in 'numberless experiments' over a three-year period and a series of 90 passages of the virus from rabbit to rabbit, at which point the incubation period of the disease was seven days. Using the same method he had made '50 dogs of all ages and breeds refractory to rabies' without a single failure. [32]

Two of Pasteur's medical colleagues examined Joseph, confirming that with fourteen wounds it was almost inevitable that Joseph would come down with rabies. Considering the success of Pasteur's recent experiments they suggested there was only one option. Pasteur said that he decided 'not without deep and severe unease, as one can well imagine, to try on Joseph Meister the procedure which had consistently worked in dogs'.[33] With nothing to lose, the boy agreed to be a test patient. Pasteur, putting his reputation on the line yet again (it had become a habit), began administering a series of fourteen painful injections of increasingly virulent material, the details of which Pasteur carefully documented in a written report that he later presented to the academy. Despite Pasteur's greatest fears, one month later Joseph Meister was healthy, symptom-free and had earned a unique place in history. He was the first person ever to be cured of rabies. Pasteur concluded that Joseph Meister had 'thus escaped, not only from rabies that his bites would have produced, but also from that which I had inoculated him with in order to check his immunity produced by the treatment, a rabies more virulent than that of ordinary canine rabies'.[34]

A few months later a young shepherd, Jean-Baptiste Jupille, who had also been bitten by a mad dog, made his way to Pasteur's door and another trial began. It was during the course of this treatment on 26 October 1885 that Pasteur reported to the French Academy of Sciences on the successful treatment of Joseph Meister and his progress with Jupille. He told of 'the courageous act and the great spirit of the young man which I have begun to treat last Tuesday'.[35] Pasteur related how the fifteen-year-old Jupille had thrown himself between a group of six much younger children and a rabid dog. When the dog seized him by the left hand, Jupille had wrested the dog to the ground, opened its jaws with his right hand to free his left, and then muzzled the dog with the cord of his whip. Without receiving too many more bites Jupille had managed to kill the dog by striking it with his shoes. Pasteur's vaccine ultimately saved Jupille as it had saved Joseph.

The speech that Pasteur delivered was startling in its implications for the treatment of the dreaded disease and did much to ensure Louis

Pasteur's exalted position in the annals of science and medicine. After the success of the vaccine was reported worldwide, victims of dog and wolf bites from as far afield as the United States flocked to Pasteur's laboratory hoping to be spared an agonising and certain death. The acclaim for Pasteur, saviour and hero both, knew no bounds. His name was soon to become legendary and his cure for rabies raised hope that cures for other infectious diseases such as typhoid, bubonic plague, cholera, diphtheria and syphilis were imminent.

No matter how great his achievements, Pasteur was never allowed to enjoy his moment of triumph. The old rivals still had not finished with him. When Pasteur published his results on rabies vaccination, there was immediate opposition from Robert Koch. As Pasteur had anticipated Koch accused Pasteur of failing to find the rabies microbe and therefore the 'methods followed by Pasteur must be called full of mistakes and cannot lead to successful results because they lack microscopic examinations, involve use of impure substances and use unsuitable experimental animals'.[36] Koch ridiculed French microbiology and voiced scathing doubts about the purity of the rabies vaccine. Not content with that, Koch also attacked the way in which Pasteur published his results, accusing Pasteur of withholding unfavourable findings even when they were important to the outcome of the experiment. This is a criticism that has also been levelled at Pasteur in more recent times.

Pasteur's response was characteristic, devising experiments that countered one objection after another. On 1 March 1886, Pasteur reported on the progress of his rabies treatments to the Academy of Sciences and called for the creation of a rabies vaccine centre. The now famous Pasteur Institute was established in Paris initially to treat the victims of rabies who were coming to Pasteur's laboratory in increasing numbers. However, in accordance with Pasteur's wishes, the institute was soon to become a research facility for infectious diseases and also a teaching centre. Funding to build the institute came from government grants, public subscriptions both local and international, (including 100,000 francs from the Russian

Czar expressing his gratitude for curing his subjects who had been infected with rabies) and the income from the rabies vaccine.[37] Although it was a private institute, it had government approval and was inaugurated in 1888 by the French president.

Louis Pasteur directed the institute that bore his name for the last eight years of his life despite suffering heart problems, no doubt exacerbated by the perpetual stresses of his life. As Pasteur's health deteriorated his rabies vaccine was restoring health to thousands of victims worldwide, ongoing proof of the significance of Pasteur's work. Pasteur's disciples, many of whom later created medical miracles of their own, began to set up a vast international network that still bears Pasteur's name. In 1891, the first Foreign Institut Pasteur was founded in Vietnam. It must have been of some consolation to Pasteur when his archrival, Robert Koch, finally acknowledged that the rabies vaccine was a success when he set up a rabies vaccination service using Pasteur's method at the Berlin Hygiene Institute.

In his latter years Pasteur was honoured throughout the world with prestigious decorations and awards. On 22 December 1892 prominent international scientists gathered to pay homage to the incomparable Pasteur at his 70th birthday jubilee. He received a standing ovation from hundreds of academics, doctors and members of scientific societies. Joseph Lister, a true believer who had applied Pasteur's Germ Theory of Disease to antiseptics in hospitals, praised Pasteur for having lifted the veil that had hidden infectious diseases for centuries. The two men embraced on stage to thunderous applause. Too overcome to speak, Pasteur allowed his son to deliver his humble address.

> *You delegates of foreign countries, who have come a long way to show your sympathy for France, have given me the greatest joy a man can feel who believes that Science and Peace will prevail over Ignorance and War, that the nations will learn to understand each other, not for destruction but for advancement, and that the future belongs to those who have done most for suffering mankind.[38]*

Robert Koch failed to attend the jubilee and personal reasons have been suggested for his non-attendance, rather than petty ones. (Ten years after Pasteur's death, however, Koch made a public visit to the Pasteur Institute in Paris where he received a more than enthusiastic welcome. According to Elie Metchnikov, Robert Koch, Pasteur's nemesis, returned to the institute later and privately visited Louis Pasteur's crypt.)

As director of his own institute, Pasteur turned his attention to developing a vaccine for typhoid, the disease that had killed two of his beloved daughters. But the master scientist would connect no more links in the chain. His failing health and the paralysis of his left side made working in the laboratory increasingly difficult. Pasteur's grandson's assertion that his health had been 'undermined by a life overcharged with ideas, emotions, work, and struggles' cannot be denied.[39] After suffering two more debilitating strokes, Louis Pasteur died on 28 September 1895, while holding the hand of his beloved wife.

Louis Pasteur was buried as a national hero by the French government. His funeral was attended by thousands of people, many of whom lined the Parisian boulevards to see his funeral cortege pass by. In England, the *London Illustrated News* published a full-page portrait of Pasteur on its front page. His remains, initially interred in Nôtre Dame Cathedral, were later transferred to a marble and mosaic crypt in the lower level of the Pasteur Institute.

Louis Pasteur was a man of contradictions — a modest man, a humanitarian who referred to himself as 'a mere chemist' and, conversely, an intractable, single-minded scientist devoted to his work and incapable of considering opposing opinions. Forced to defend his work at every turn, he withstood hardship, illness and character assassination and endured criticism decade after decade from those who considered him a 'crackpot', a 'charlatan', or just 'lucky'. However, Pasteur's brilliant mind, his tenacity and his belief that science should be used for the public good opened a door to a new understanding of infectious micro-organisms, immunisation and the body's amazing immune system. Because of the legacy of Louis Pasteur — immunisation, Germ Theory and attenuation — scientists today can target the genes that code for genetic diseases and are working to find molecular 'magic bullets' that can inhibit the toxins that germs produce.

Throughout his working life Pasteur demonstrated the importance of formulating hypotheses and of testing them through controlled experiments. A maxim he quoted often was: 'It is the worst aberration of the mind to believe things because one wishes them to be so.' Ironically Pasteur's detractors accused him of exactly this, of mere speculation that could not be tested. In a book, *The Private Science of Louis Pasteur* written in 1996, Gerald L. Geison makes similar claims to Pasteur's contemporaries: that there are discrepancies in Pasteur's science; in the vernacular — he fudged the results. Geison drew his conclusions from 102 of Pasteur's laboratory notebooks which had not been available before the 1990s and ignited a new and heated scholarly debate about the validity of Pasteur's scientific method. Other scholars in their turn now dispute Geison's findings, accusing him of the same selectivity that he accuses Pasteur of. [40] Claim and counterclaim seem part of a long tradition within the scientific world.

The more accepted view of Pasteur is that he embodied integrity and altruism. He used science to improve the lot of all he could, whether French provincial farmers whose livelihoods were threatened by anthrax or the desperate, afflicted with rabies, who as a last hope came to his laboratory seeking salvation. Because of Louis Pasteur, rabies is now a vaccine-preventable disease in both humans and animals. If people die from rabies today it is usually because they have not received adequate pre- or post-exposure treatment.

Although rabies has practically disappeared in most developed countries due to the vaccination of both humans and animals, it would sadden Pasteur to know that it continues to be a major public health problem in some parts of the world. Rabies is, in fact, the tenth most common fatal infectious disease worldwide. The World Health Organization now refers to rabies as a neglected disease. [41] On average, 55,000 human deaths from rabies are reported annually around the world, with more than 99 per cent of these occurring in Africa, Asia and South America. Most cases are caused by rabid dog bites. Of those fatalities approximately 50 per cent, or around 27,000, are children under fifteen years of age. Four million people annually in over 80 countries in which rabies is present require treatment following exposure.

Pasteur's original vaccine has been improved. In 1967 the human diploid cell rabies vaccine (HDCV) was introduced and by the end of 2006 it had been given to more than 1.5 million people worldwide. Vaccination remains the sole effective treatment against rabies. Currently pre-exposure immunisation is used to control rabies in domesticated and wild animal populations and given to humans in high-risk jobs such as veterinary surgeons, laboratory personnel, stable hands and foresters. Treatment after exposure is highly successful in preventing the disease if administered within fourteen days of infection. The vaccine overtakes the virus during the incubation period and neutralises it before it reaches the brain and becomes fatal.

In the United States the number of human rabies deaths is very low compared with the rest of the world. Over the last few decades more and more areas of Europe have been successfully freed from rabies but as international travel and animal importation has increased, so has the incidence of the disease. In the first quarter of 2006 in Europe, there were only two reported cases of rabies in humans and these were in the Russian Federation, but there were 173 reported cases of rabies in wildlife and 241 in domestic animals. [42]

In developing nations rabies continues to be a serious health issue because of large dog populations that have not been vaccinated. In China, rabies — which is called 'mad dog disease' — is the country's second-deadliest pathogen after tuberculosis. The number of cases has risen steadily in recent years because of a rise in pet ownership and a low 3 per cent vaccination rate. In 2006 after an outbreak of rabies in Shandong province, officials ordered the destruction of all dogs within a 5-kilometre radius of the outbreak. In a second cull in Yunnan province, 50,000 dogs were clubbed, electrocuted and buried alive sparking condemnation by the World Health Organization, which promotes humane methods of dog population management.[43]

In May 2007 an international conference, 'Towards the Elimination of Rabies in Eurasia', was held in Paris. It was attended by the World Organization for Animal Health, the World Health Organization, the European Commission and the three WHO-collaborating Centres for Rabies in Europe. It was agreed at the conference that the key to eliminating rabies remains preventing it, and eliminating it from animal populations. To raise awareness of the disease delegates supported the initiative to declare 8 September as World Rabies Day. The commitment was made to continue the battle against rabies with the only weapon available, the vaccine that was the product of Louis Pasteur's genius, a vaccine for both prevention and cure.

POSTSCRIPT

There is a tragic yet heroic end to Joseph Meister's story. As an adult Joseph was employed at the Pasteur Institute and served for many years as the gatekeeper. In 1940, during World War II, 45 years after his treatment for rabies made medical history, he was ordered by the Nazis, who were occupying Paris, to open Pasteur's crypt. Joseph Meister chose to commit suicide, shooting himself with his World War I service revolver, rather than allow the resting place of Louis Pasteur to be desecrated. The bond between the boy and the scientist had never been broken. Pasteur had given Joseph the gift of a long life and Joseph chose the time of its end to honour his saviour.

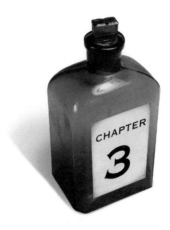

CHAPTER

3

OUTWITTING THE 'WHITE PLAGUE'
THE CHALLENGE TO CURE TUBERCULOSIS

> I was highly motivated to find antibiotics that could
> be used to treat gram-negative infections because
> I had seen soldiers die of such infections. I was
> also highly motivated to find an antibiotic that
> could be used to treat tuberculosis because when
> I was a boy in Passaic, New Jersey, in the 1920s,
> I had seen neighbors die of TB. We then called it
> 'consumption' because the disease literally con-
> sumed them. I knew people who coughed, and
> wasted away as they lost weight and died.[1]
>
> *Albert Schatz*

History testifies that cures for the major diseases that afflict humankind do
not come easily. Often, what is needed more than skill, ingenuity, knowledge
and intelligence are endless patience, commitment and years of repetitive
and painstaking work and sometimes sacrifice on the part of many individuals. This was certainly the case, and continues to be so, in the long battle to
combat tuberculosis (TB). In the last half of the twentieth century memories
of the dreaded lung disease that robbed millions of their lives began to fade

due to the discovery of a preventive vaccine and powerful antibiotics. A cautionary note, however: any declaration of victory is premature.

The continuing saga of finding a cure for TB is not without its own subtext of struggles, rivalries and tragedy and it began with the work of Louis Pasteur's archrival Robert Koch in 1882 in Berlin. The next episode was written by the French physician and bacteriologist, Albert Calmette, and his veterinarian colleague, Camille Guérin, who in the early 1900s laboured for twenty years to produce the first effective prophylactic vaccine. An ending was in sight when penicillin was developed during World War II but hopes that it would annihilate TB were soon dashed and the hunt was on for more powerful 'antibiotics'. The plot took a new turn in 1946 when the American biochemists Selman Waksman and Albert Schatz at Rutgers University developed streptomycin, the world's first broad-spectrum antibiotic. It seemed entirely feasible that tuberculosis, like smallpox, would be eliminated but it is a very determined survivor.

Mycobacterium tuberculosis, the cause of tuberculosis, is an ancient bacterium that once thrived in primeval mud and probably afflicted humans as far back as the Neolithic era. There is documentary evidence that a disease very like it was known to the ancient Egyptians.[2] But it was in eighteenth-century Europe, as urban populations grew during the Industrial Revolution, that a highly infectious form of tuberculosis, pulmonary tuberculosis, took hold because it spread easily through coughing, sneezing and spitting. By the beginning of the nineteenth century one-quarter of all deaths in England were caused by tuberculosis and as the century progressed TB became endemic amongst the urban poor. There was no cure. People afflicted with TB turned to old wives' remedies like cod-liver oil, pig's pepsin, iodine and copper which, not surprisingly, provided at best minimal relief from symptoms. As tuberculosis became more entrenched and took a greater toll, it caused grave public concern.

The disease did not become known as tuberculosis until 1839 when the German physician Johann Lukas Schönlein introduced the term.[3] It was derived from the word 'tubercle' which seems to have originated in

Sweden in the 1600s and entered the English language in 1689 when it was used by the English physician Richard Morton to describe the characteristic lesions that occur in the lungs of tuberculosis sufferers. In approximately 75 per cent of cases TB affects the lungs, the pulmonary form of the disease, where the bacterium slowly destroys lung tissue.

People can have tuberculosis for many years without knowing it. With pulmonary TB, when the infection becomes active the symptoms are a persistent dry cough, weakness, weight loss, fever and chest pains. Another form of the disease is disseminated, or miliary, TB — so called because in an X-ray the lungs resemble millet seeds. It is more common in people who have suppressed immune systems and in young children. Pulmonary TB can co-exist with extrapulmonary TB which can affect the central nervous system, the lymphatic system, the genito-urinary system, and bones and joints.

In industrialised Europe, the highly infectious pulmonary tuberculosis infected the poor in great numbers because of their impoverished living conditions. To stop the spread of the disease many were forced by public health authorities to enter sanatoriums, institutions that were more like prisons than hospitals and where there was little hope of recovery. The more affluent classes were not immune from the highly infectious disease but they could afford sanatoriums that offered excellent care and medical attention.

Despite the purported benefits of fresh air, exercise and the treatments provided in the sanatoriums, 50 per cent of patients still wasted away and were dead within five years of contracting the disease. It was the wasting that gave the disease one of its other names, 'the consumption', reflecting how sufferers appeared to be 'consumed' from within. Tuberculosis was also known as 'the White Plague' because sufferers appeared pale, a symptom that was associated with artistic sensitivity. It was seen as a disease that sought out the talented and creative as its victims — writers, politicians, musicians, artists and scientists. Cardinal Richelieu; Frederic Chopin; Robert Louis Stevenson; Amedeo Modigliani; Emily, Anne and

Charlotte Brontë; Sir Walter Scott; Lord Byron; Simon Bolivar; Paul Gauguin; Anton Chekov; Eugene O'Neill; Jean-Jacques Rousseau; Florence Nightingale; and Alexander Graham Bell are just a few of the gifted who suffered the misery of TB.

In a perverse and paradoxical way, tuberculosis became romanticised and took on its own persona in literature, art and music. The afflicted are tragic characters in novels, operas and films. The death of Little Nell in Charles Dickens' *The Old Curiosity Shop*, published in serial form during 1840 and 1841, caused genuine tears amongst readers of the tale on both sides of the Atlantic. The blood-soaked handkerchiefs and the tragic death of Margaret Gautier in Alexandre Dumas' novel *La Dame aux Camélias* are legendary, and the beautiful and consumptive courtesan, Margaret, became Violetta in Verdi's *La Traviata*, and Satine in the more recent film *Moulin Rouge*.

This fascination with the White Plague reflects its pervasive nature during the nineteenth century, but it was not until the 1880s when more was known about germs and infection that the very young German physician, Heinrich Hermann Robert Koch, laid the groundwork for the scientific battle against the disease. In March 1882, Robert Koch gave a lecture at the Physiological Society of Berlin to eminent doctors much more senior than himself. Showing a slide of animal tissue he pointed out the tubercle bacteria which were stained a beautiful blue.[4] These he announced were the cause of the 'White Plague', which at the time was responsible for one-seventh of all deaths in Europe.

It is ironic that Koch's announcement met with the same kind of scepticism and jealousy that he and his followers meted out to Louis Pasteur; and Koch, like Pasteur, also endured the professional jealousy of many of his contemporaries. What is also ironic is that Robert Koch did much to further the work of Louis Pasteur. The discovery of the tuberculosis bacillus *Mycobacterium tuberculosis* established Koch as one of the founders of the science of bacteriology and he devised many of the field's basic principles and techniques. Koch's scientific oeuvre earned him fame in his own lifetime and won him a place in the scientific pantheon. But one of his greatest triumphs would also lead Koch to his darkest hours and a humiliating fall from grace.

KOCH'S EARLY LIFE

Born on 11 December 1843 at Clausthal in the Upper Harz Mountains, Robert Koch was the third of thirteen children born to Hermann Koch, a mining official, and Mathilde Biewend, the daughter of an iron mine inspector. Robert's parents were astounded when they realised their son had taught himself to read from the newspapers at the age of five.[5] From this early age he displayed the methodical persistence which would be so characteristic of his professional life. Hermann Koch encouraged in Robert a fascination for the wonders of nature and also a desire for travel. He had a passion for collecting mosses and lichens and was fascinated by the anatomy of insects.

At the local high school Robert's interest in biology strengthened and in 1862 he began studying medicine at the University of Göttingen, which was considered to be a great achievement for a boy from his social background. During his studies, Koch was exposed to a revolutionary theory that the professor of anatomy, Jacob Henle, had published in 1840. Henle hypothesised that infectious diseases were caused by living, parasitic organisms. This concept, which was later proven by Louis Pasteur, underpinned much of Koch's research.

In 1866 Koch passed his final examinations with distinction and then passed the state medical examination in Hanover. After this he undertook studies in chemistry for six months at the Berlin Charité Hospital, the largest and oldest hospital in the city. Here Koch came under the influence of Rudolf Virchow, an influential pathologist, anthropologist and politician but from this time on Koch was never able to win the respect of the doyen of German science because of their variant views on the cause of disease.[6] Virchow proposed a cell theory of disease, believing that the presence of micro-organisms identified diseased tissue but he was convinced they were not the cause of disease.

At the age of 22 Koch, already exhibiting his peripatetic nature, took his first medical job as an intern at Hamburg General Hospital, where he saw first-hand the devastating effects of a cholera epidemic. People died in great numbers from this acute intestinal infection. In 1867 Koch became an assistant at an institution for intellectually disabled children in Langenhagen, a village near Hanover. At this time Robert Koch married Emmy Fraatz, the daughter of the Superintendant General of Clausthal, Koch's hometown. Emmy has been described as a domineering woman who during their married life together stifled her husband's desire to travel. But the marriage started well. After a brief sojourn in Niemegk, Emmy was happy when they settled at Rackwitz (now in Poland), where her husband established a flourishing practice.

When the Franco–Prussian War broke out in 1870, Koch volunteered for service but was rejected because of severe myopia. Perhaps it was his short-sightedness that made the microscopic world an appealing one for Robert Koch, one to which he would soon devote his life. On a second application to serve his country Koch was successful and was sent as a field hospital physician to France, where he worked first at a typhoid hospital at Neufchâteau and then a hospital for wounded soldiers near Orléans. Koch's war experience gave him an understanding of typhoid and later in his career he developed public health measures for the control of both this disease and cholera. The horrors that Koch witnessed no doubt entrenched his anti-French sentiments.

After the privations of war, Robert Koch returned to Emmy and Gertrud, the couple's only child, in the lakeside town of Wollstein, in a rural area near Berlin. While carrying out his duties as district medical officer from 1872 to 1880 Koch began his phenomenal research in a small laboratory he had built at the rear of his surgery, using a microscope that Emmy gave him for his 29th birthday. He converted a wardrobe into a darkroom and purchased microphotographic equipment that was crucial for the studies he was planning to carry out on micro-organisms.

Despite the much-documented antipathy that developed between Robert Koch and Louis Pasteur there were professional synergies:

independently of each other Koch and Pasteur investigated anthrax. Despite the demands of his practice and his isolation in the country away from libraries and colleagues, Koch took up his research on anthrax, a disease prevalent among farm animals, the consequences of which he had witnessed in the Wollstein district and which created significant problems for farmers in France and Germany. A number of studies had already been done on the disease. In 1850 the French veterinarian Pierre Rayer had reported discovering the anthrax bacillus in the blood of animals that were dying from the disease, and had succeeded in transmitting it. The German Franz Antoine Pollender had claimed the same discovery in a publication in 1855, reportedly based on observations he had made in 1849.

Things were already competitive when the French scientist Casimir-Joseph Davaine, who was inspired by Louis Pasteur's work, got involved. Like many early pioneers he did not have a proper laboratory and he kept his experimental animals in a friend's garden. Despite the privations, in 1863 Davaine proved that a healthy animal that did not have anthrax could contract the disease if it was injected with a minute amount of blood from an infected animal, blood which contained rod-like micro-organisms. Conversely, these organisms were not present in healthy animals and therefore it was highly probable that they caused anthrax.

It was at this point that Koch took up the challenge to prove scientifically that the rod-like bacillus did in fact cause anthrax. For three years, between 1873 and 1876, he spent all his spare time finding out what he could about the disease. Koch inoculated laboratory mice using slivers of wood to inject them with anthrax bacilli taken from the spleens of dead, diseased farm animals. These mice were all killed by the bacilli, whereas mice inoculated at the same time with blood from the spleens of healthy animals did not succumb. This confirmed Davaine's work, showing that the disease could be transmitted through the blood of animals suffering from anthrax.

Not satisfied with this, Koch wanted to know whether anthrax bacilli that had never been in contact with any kind of animal could cause the disease. To solve this problem he obtained pure cultures of the bacilli by growing them on the aqueous humour of ox eyes (the fluid between the cornea and the lens). By studying, drawing and photographing these cultures, Koch recorded the multiplication of the bacilli and noted that, when conditions were unfavourable to them, especially a lack of oxygen, they produced dormant spores that could remain viable for years. Even if they had had no contact with any kind of animal, under the right conditions the spores could develop into the bacilli and cause anthrax.[7] This finding explained why this surreptitious disease could recur in pastures that had not been used for grazing for a long time and why it is an inveterate survivor.

Louis Pasteur had introduced the concept that a disease organism might be cultured outside the body but the techniques for doing this, which were essential for his groundbreaking research and for many medical advances that were to follow, were perfected by Robert Koch. The genesis of Koch's pure-culture techniques was a discovery by Joseph Schroeter who worked with Ferdinand Cohn, the professor of botany at the University of Breslau. In 1872 Schroeter found that chromogenic, or colour-forming, bacteria would grow on what are called solid substrates such as potato, coagulated egg white, meat and bread, and that these colonies could form new colonies of the same type and colour.[8] Koch also invented the drop technique in which micro-organisms are cultured in a drop of nutrient solution on the underside of a glass slide, and so we have the stereotype of scientists dripping solutions onto slides and examining them under the lenses of their microscopes.

Koch's anthrax experiments gave the first real proof of a relation between a particular bacillus and a particular disease. When Koch demonstrated the results of this painstaking work to Professor Cohn at the university, Cohn called a meeting of his colleagues. They were impressed. Cohn, who was the editor of a botanical journal, published Koch's findings in 1876 and Robert Koch achieved instant fame.

As Pasteur had done Koch turned his attention to germs that specifically affected humans. He knew that infected blood contained septicaemia germs but he could not detect them under a microscope, which meant other scientists were unlikely to believe him. To prove that this specific germ causes blood poisoning Koch focused on improving his methods of fixing, staining and photographing bacteria and when it was stained with methyl violet dye he was able to see the septicaemia germ under a microscope.[9] As additional proof for the doubters Koch photographed the germs. This invaluable work on diseases caused by bacterial infections of wounds enabled Koch to provide a practical and scientific basis for the control of these infections. He published his results in 1878.

In the summer of 1879, Koch was appointed to the position of city physician at Breslau but found the salary inadequate, perhaps for Emmy more than himself, and after three months returned to Wollstein. As Koch's reputation and ambition grew, his patients took second place to his research and marital harmony was jeopardised as he spent more time closeted in his laboratory experimenting and reading research papers, and as an increasing number of menial tasks were delegated to his wife and daughter. More scientific apparatus was needed and the Koch household had to accommodate and feed the growing number of animals required for experimentation: innumerable mice, guinea pigs, rabbits, frogs, assorted birds and two monkeys.

By 1879 Robert Koch had perfected methods which made it easy to obtain and identify pathogenic bacteria in pure culture, free from other organisms. As a result Koch laid down the conditions that needed to be fulfilled in order to prove that particular bacteria cause particular diseases. Modifications that he made to these rules in 1882 resulted in what have become known as 'Koch's Postulates'.[10] The four postulates have since made it possible to accurately identify the causes of countless microbial diseases. They are: that the microbe or organism must be discoverable in every case of the disease; that once recovered from the body the microbe or organism must be grown in pure cultures for several generations; that the disease can be reproduced in experimental animals (i.e. a non-diseased susceptible 'host') through pure culture; and that the microbe or organism can be recovered from the inoculated animal or host that was experimentally infected, and then be recultured.

Robert Koch's circumstances changed in 1880 when he was appointed to the Imperial Health Bureau in Berlin. Initially given only a small room, Koch was soon provided with a laboratory where he worked with his assistants, Friedrich Loeffler and Georg Gaffky. In Berlin Koch refined the bacteriological methods he had used in his cramped home lab in Wollstein. He perfected the technique of growing pure cultures of germs using a mix of potatoes and gelatine on a specially designed flat dish that was invented by another of his colleagues, Julius Petri. We may not know of Julius but we are certainly familiar with his dish, which is still in common use today. Koch's techniques opened new horizons for future scientific discoveries.

For various reasons, some of which were purely economic, governments in many countries in the nineteenth century were becoming increasingly involved in the control of hygiene and public health and advances in science were providing the means to do this. Koch's reputation as a leading scientist was growing rapidly and in 1881, he and his team of researchers, under the health department's director Heinrich Struck, were assigned to develop reliable methods for isolating and cultivating pathogenic bacteria and to gather bacteriological data and establish scientific principles which could be applied to hygiene and public health. Koch's disciples worked tirelessly beside him and, according to Friedrich Loeffler, 'almost daily new miracles of bacteriology displayed themselves'; one of these was the discovery of the tuberculosis bacillus.

DEFEATING DISEASE — A GLOBAL PURSUIT

When Robert Koch was invited to address the seventh International Medical Congress in London in 1881, to demonstrate his technique for obtaining pure cultures on solid media, he was already working on tuberculosis, a great threat to public health. It was at this conference that Joseph Lister introduced Louis Pasteur to Robert Koch and the animosity between the French and German scientists began. Some critics say that when Pasteur congratulated Koch on his work in Lister's rooms, he did so with suppressed jealousy. Koch may also have been peeved because Pasteur had surpassed his anthrax work and developed a vaccine. This may have been the motivation for Koch's arrogance when he publicly announced that Pasteur had added nothing new to anthrax research, after which the two men never again spoke civilly to each other.

Abandoning anthrax, the new driving force behind Koch's research was to prove conclusively that tuberculosis was caused by an infective agent. This meant finding a way to identify and isolate the specific micro-organism. Koch began by taking tuberculous tissue from the body of a young man who in the space of three weeks had gone from being fit and well to having developed a cough and severe chest pains. Four days after being admitted to hospital he died, his emaciated body riddled with yellowish tubercles.

Koch worked with a passion, injecting ground tuberculous material into the eyes of rabbits and under the skins of guinea pigs. He also smeared the infected tissue on glass slides which he spent days observing, but the tubercle bacillus proved elusive. Koch then began to soak the tissue in various dyes and finally the bacteria took up sufficient colour to stand out from the diseased lung cells. The tiny blue-coloured rods that Koch observed were tubercle bacillus, one-third the size of the anthrax bacillus. When Koch dissected the animals he found identical yellowish tubercles and the same tiny blue-coloured rods. Convinced that he had identified the tubercle bacillus, Koch obtained infected tissue from the bodies of other hospital patients who had died of tuberculosis and meticulously and obsessively injected it into guinea pigs, rabbits, three dogs, thirteen cats, ten chickens, twelve pigeons, white mice, field mice, rats and two marmots.[11] In both diseased humans and animals Koch found the blue-stained rods.

Following his postulates, the next step for Koch was to grow the organism in pure culture. It was trial and error to find the right media. He inoculated a blood-serum agar, a gelatinous substance which he made from heat-sterilised animal blood combined with tissue from the lung of a diseased guinea pig.[12] His patient vigil continued long after others would have admitted defeat and begun again. After fifteen days Koch was rewarded when he observed minuscule colonies of bacteria on the surface of the agar. After working alone and secretively for six months, Koch had successfully isolated the bacteria on various media and was able to infect guinea pigs with tuberculosis.

On 24 March 1882, when Koch announced to the Physiological Society of Berlin that he had isolated and grown the tubercle bacillus that caused all forms of tuberculosis, the distinguished audience was silent. Rudolf Virchow left without saying a word, which must have come as no shock to Koch. When Koch had hoped to gain Virchow's support for his work on anthrax, Virchow had flipped through the report as Koch waited in suspense and dismissed the findings as highly improbable. However, Koch won the approbation of another rising star who was in the audience. Paul Ehrlich, a young German scientist, later recalled that evening as his greatest scientific moment. Ehrlich, who would become famous for finding a cure for syphilis in 1909 literally overnight, developed an improved method of staining tubercle bacilli, a method Koch soon adopted.

The day after Koch's announcement, the discovery of the tubercle bacillus was front-page news throughout the world and ushered in an era of 'microbe hunting' and a new generation of scientists who, like Ehrlich, were inspired by the work of both Koch and Pasteur.[13] They were the new guard, crusaders, determined to hunt down and destroy the disease-causing micro-organisms that most afflicted humanity.

Koch's work on tuberculosis was continuing when, in 1883, he was sent to Egypt as leader of the German Cholera Commission to investigate an outbreak of cholera in the Nile delta. The French scientific community was also involved, and because Pasteur was fully occupied in Paris with his rabies cure he sent a four-man mission in his place, which included his two assistants Emile Roux and Louis Thuillier. They reached Alexandria in mid

August. Koch's team, which included Gaffky and Bernhard Fischer, arrived nine days later equipped with microscopes and experimental animals. Old rivalries persisted and a race between the French and the Germans to find the cholera bacillus began.

Just as Koch targeted a comma-shaped bacillus as the specific cause, the cholera epidemic suddenly began to wane. The two French scientists who had had no success in isolating the bacilli from the cultures they worked on, became less focused on the quest while Koch and Gaffky laboured in the heat examining the last of the infected material that they could get hold of. Inadvertently they discovered the bacilli that cause amoebic dysentery.[14] Tragedy struck when Louis Thuillier was infected by the microbe he was hunting and died of cholera. Despite the rivalry between the French and German researchers, Koch acted as one of the pallbearers at Thuillier's funeral before rushing back to Berlin with specimens containing the prime cholera-causing suspect, the little comma-shaped, vibrating bacterium, or 'vibrio'.

To prove the vibrio was indeed the offending bug, Koch, Gaffky and Fischer went to India in 1884 to study cholera in regions where it was endemic. Two months after arriving in Calcutta they observed the same bacillus in 70 cholera victims. Despite being unable to produce the disease in experimental animals — one of his postulates — Koch asserted that the bacillus was the specific cause of cholera and could be easily grown on beef broth agar. More importantly Koch identified the method of transmission: via drinking water, food and clothing.

When Koch returned to Berlin in May 1884 banquets were held in his honour. Finding the cause of any disease that beleaguered people in all corners of the globe brought notoriety. The Kaiser awarded Koch the Order of the Crown with Star and the Reichstag granted him 100,000 marks. As could be expected, not all scientists were convinced that the vibrio caused cholera. One asked Koch to send him a vial of the bacilli, which he publicly swallowed, luckily — although Koch may not have concurred — without ill effect. Controversy continued to rage until August

1892, when Koch was asked by the city of Hamburg to help with a cholera outbreak. In a ten-week period 18,000 people had been infected and 8000 had died. Koch successfully implemented his measures for cholera containment — early detection and isolation of cases, the disinfection of patient excreta and the sanitisation of water supplies — measures that are still in use today.[15]

KOCH'S 'CURE' FOR TUBERCULOSIS

In 1885, the year after his triumphant return to Berlin, Koch was appointed Professor of Hygiene and Director of the newly established Institute of Hygiene at the University of Berlin but something was amiss. For the next five years Koch's scientific output paled in comparison to his earlier work. Koch's star was no longer ascending. Pasteur's international successes with the anthrax and rabies vaccines put Koch under great pressure from the German government and the press. He had become a symbol of German superiority.[16] Koch began working secretively again. He was seeking a cure for tuberculosis. What would provide salvation for the multitudes he hoped would also save him from anonymity.

Koch investigated the effect an injection of dead tubercule bacilli would have on a person who subsequently received a dose of living bacilli. He concluded that the local reaction produced might be the means by which the disease could be diagnosed and cured in the early stages. On 4 August 1890, at the tenth International Medical Congress in Berlin, Koch announced that, after testing many chemicals, he had isolated a substance that had the power to prevent the growth of the tubercle bacilli. Guinea pigs that had been injected with the substance he called tuberculin had become resistant to tuberculosis and he claimed that it could arrest the disease in humans.

Clinical trials began. In November 1890 Koch claimed success and again his name was on everyone's lips. Doctors and patients made pilgrimages to Berlin, filling hospitals, clinics and hotels, clamouring for his 'cure' for tuberculosis. Honours were again being flung his way by foreign rulers and prestigious societies. He was given the freedom of various cities including Berlin and received the Grand Cross of the Red Eagle from the Kaiser. In 1891 he became an Honorary Professor of the medical faculty of Berlin University and Director of the new Institute for Infectious Diseases located next to the Charité Hospital.[17]

It was soon realised, however, that tuberculin was not all that Koch had purported. His desire for success had influenced his science. In January 1891, Rudolf Virchow, ever the critic, revealed that 21 consumptive patients who had been treated with tuberculin had died riddled with miliary tuberculosis. Amidst the ensuing uproar Koch was forced to reveal the exact nature of tuberculin. To produce his 'miracle cure', Koch, for whatever reason, had used a method previously employed by Emile Roux to isolate diphtheria toxin. Koch had grown the tubercle bacilli on a glycerine broth for several weeks before killing the bacteria with heat, but the filtrate still retained active virulent organisms and many people died because not all the bacteria had.[18]

At the same time that Koch's professional life was disintegrating his personal life was in turmoil. His unhappy marriage to Emmy ended in divorce and scandal in 1893. At the age of 45 he had fallen in love with and married a beautiful seventeen-year-old art student, Hedwig Freiburg. Enemies were waiting in the wings and the divorce led to more criticism and censure for Koch. Vicious rumours circulated that he had sold his patent on tuberculin to a company in Marburg and allowed it to be tried on patients prematurely because he needed the money to support his second wife. Koch rode out the scandal and found happiness with his new wife.

By the 1890s it was widely accepted that TB was contagious and in response governments in many countries made it a notifiable disease and adopted health measures such as bans on spitting in public areas in the hope that this would help to control its spread. But a cure was still elusive. Although struggling to cope with his fall from grace, Koch was not entirely defeated by the humiliation of his failure and attempted to find a cure one more time. In 1896 he announced that he had developed a new tuberculin which proved to be a diagnostic tool, but not a cure. Koch noticed that within 48 hours of vaccination, tuberculous patients exhibited a reddish allergic reaction at the spot where tuberculin was injected into the skin. This reaction, called the Koch phenomenon, allows doctors today to determine through a skin test whether an individual has been infected with tubercle bacilli, even before symptoms develop.

With his reputation in a parlous state, in 1896 Koch accepted an invitation from the Cape Colony government in South Africa to investigate rinderpest, a disease which was ravaging cattle. Koch's thirst for foreign travel was revived and suddenly he saw new horizons for his microbial research and Hedwig was happy to go with him. As soon as they arrived in the Cape, Koch assembled a menagerie of experimental animals and began work. Although he did not identify the cause of rinderpest he succeeded in developing a method of vaccinating farm stock and limited the outbreak.

India was next. When Koch reached Bombay in May 1897, bubonic plague was epidemic in upper India. Various European governments had previously sent scientific missions in the hope of finding a cure. The bacillus *Yersinia pestis*, the cause of bubonic plague, had been discovered in Hong Kong in 1894 by both Alexandre Yersin, who led a French mission, and Shibasaburo Kitasato, who had worked in Koch's laboratory and was head of a Japanese team. While in Bombay, Koch concluded that rats were the source of the plague and that they spread the disease through cannibalism. Koch urged that measures be taken to control the rodents, unaware, as was everyone at the time, that it was the fleas on the rats that played the crucial role in the spread of bubonic plague.

Koch returned to Africa and in Tanganyika (part of modern-day Tanzania) discovered two protozoan diseases: surra, which affected horses, and Texas cattle fever. Malaria and blackwater fever were his next targets. Returning to Berlin in May 1898, after eighteen months away, Koch delivered an address to the German Colonial Society in which he described four types of malaria. Koch believed that malaria was a mosquito-borne disease but before he could prove his theory the British bacteriologist Ronald Ross published findings supporting the same conclusion. Koch next visited malarial districts in Italy where he confirmed Ronald Ross's discovery.

Koch's expedition then headed for the tropics. Although Robert Koch seemed indestructible, in German New Guinea, where malaria was prevalent, Hedwig became ill. Koch was desolate as he had no choice but to send Hedwig home and continue his work without her. He made huge inroads into controlling malaria by devising a control policy that aimed to destroy the parasite within its host. Although success was limited by a lack of drug supplies and trained physicians, the regimen was adopted throughout the German empire and Koch was again the centre of attention. The Kaiser Wilhelm Academy elected Koch to its senate because of the value of his discovery to the health of Germany's military forces.

The pace of travel and discovery was frenetic. After having spent only nine months in Germany over a period of four years Koch returned to Berlin in October 1900. By that time, Pasteur, Koch and their disciple microbe hunters, seeking salvation for humankind and perhaps a little glory for themselves, had in the space of just over two decades identified 21 germs that cause disease. 'As soon as the right method was found, discoveries came as easily as ripe apples from a tree,' Koch said.[19] And it was Robert Koch who had developed those methods.

Despite his myriad achievements Koch remained interested in tuberculosis and late in his career came to the conclusion that the bacilli that cause human and bovine tuberculosis are not identical. He suggested using the bovine bacillus as a human vaccine. Never far from controversy, his views met opposition at the International Medical Congress on Tuberculosis in London in 1901. He also proposed that infection of human beings by bovine tuberculosis is so rare that taking measures against it was not necessary. Koch's view, in time, proved to be correct and a strain of bovine tubercule bacillus was used some decades later to produce an effective vaccine.

As his sixtieth birthday approached, Robert Koch decided to retire from state service. His contribution to national health had been immeasurable and the Kaiser awarded Koch the Order of Wilhelm. But retirement was anathema to Robert Koch and after working as a consultant at the Institute for Infectious Diseases he headed off to remote locations, once again accompanied by Hedwig, who had made a full recovery. Early in 1905, on an expedition to Dar-es-Salaam, Koch investigated the lifecycle of the tsetse fly, the cause of the debilitating human disease African trypanosomiasis, or sleeping sickness.

Koch enjoyed a brief respite later that year when, in Stockholm, his work on tuberculosis was recognised internationally with the award of the Nobel Prize for Physiology or Medicine for his investigations and discoveries in relation to tuberculosis. There was no time for the ageing scientist to rest on his laurels, however. In 1906 Koch returned to Central Africa leading the German Sleeping Sickness Commission and travelled to the remote and dangerous Sesse Islands in Uganda and to north-western Lake Victoria where trypanosomiasis was rampant. Living and working in primitive conditions he confirmed that the drug atoxyl was somewhat effective in treating sleeping sickness.

Koch was a driven man to the end of his life. His passion for science was ingrained. The overwhelming contribution he had made to the advancement of humankind was acknowledged in his lifetime with innumerable prizes, medals, orders and honorary doctorates. Robert Koch was the first medical person to be awarded the German Order of the Red Eagle and was granted the rare honour of foreign membership to the Paris Academy of Sciences. In 1908 in Berlin he received the first Robert Koch Medal, instituted to commemorate the greatest living physicians. The inveterate traveller, while undertaking yet another overseas tour with Hedwig, was greeted as a hero wherever he went. In Japan he was welcomed by his former colleague Shibasaburo Kitasato and presented ceremoniously to the Emperor.

In 1907 after a celebration to commemorate the 25th anniversary of the discovery of the tubercle bacillus, a proposal to establish a Robert Koch

Foundation to combat tuberculosis had gained momentum. Funding came from the public, the medical profession, the German Kaiser, and the American philanthropist Andrew Carnegie in 1908 contributed funds for its establishment, reflecting the desire of the international community to combat the disease. Predictably, the last years of Robert Koch's life were devoted to tuberculosis control. Working daily at the Institute for Infectious Diseases, which had moved in 1897 to its present-day location in Nordufer in north-west Berlin, Koch supervised the production and clinical trials of new tuberculins.

On 9 April 1910, three nights after lecturing on the epidemiology of tuberculosis before the Berlin Academy of Sciences, Koch suffered a severe angina attack and on 27 May died peacefully at a sanatorium in Baden-Baden. In December his ashes were placed in a mausoleum at the institute, which the Kaiser renamed after him. Family, friends, and luminaries from the scientific and political community attended the ceremony, even erstwhile rivals. Elie Metchnikov represented the Pasteur Institute and presented a memorial plaque. It is possible today to visit Robert Koch's sepulchre on the ground floor of the institute. On the western wall there is a relief of Koch and on the eastern wall the important dates of his life are listed under the heading 'Robert Koch — Werke und Wirken' (works and achievements).[20] The list is indeed long. Although at times a victim of his own hubris, the good that Robert Koch bequeathed to future generations cannot be overlooked.

Paul Ehrlich dubbed Robert Koch one of the few princes of medical science, despite his arrogance, his failure to give credit where it was due and his reluctance to admit mistakes. Like Louis Pasteur, Robert Koch seemed suspicious and aloof with strangers but to friends and colleagues he appeared kind and considerate. Koch uttered words reminiscent of Pasteur's when he said in New York in 1908:

> I have worked as hard as I could and have fulfilled my duty and
> obligations. If the success really was greater than is usually the case,

the reason for it is that in my wanderings through the medical field
I came upon regions where gold was still lying by the wayside.[21]

Perhaps where tuberculin was concerned it was fool's gold, Koch's judgment having been temporarily clouded by personal ambition and his altruism pushed aside. In the first paper that he wrote on tuberculosis Koch expressed that his primary motivation for undertaking his research had been to benefit public health in the short and long term. He had built on the work of Louis Pasteur, finally extinguishing the belief that 'bad air' caused disease. Robert Koch isolated the germs that cause three feared diseases — the anthrax bacillus, *Mycobacterium tuberculosis* and *Vibrio cholerae* — and identified the method of transmission of bubonic plague and sleeping sickness. He demonstrated that a specific microbe causes a specific disease and developed research techniques that enabled other scientists throughout the world to find treatments and cures for many diseases. Koch's dedication was unflinching and, despite the failure and tragedy associated with tuberculin, he made future advances against tuberculosis possible.

CALMETTE TAKES UP THE CAUSE

Others were certainly ambitious to succeed where Koch had failed. Hope was raised that protection against tuberculosis could be found following the success of the German microbiologist Emil von Behring's work on diphtheria and the development of a vaccine for typhoid by Sir Almroth Wright in England in 1897. One of the researchers who decided to take on the tuberculosis challenge was the French physician and bacteriologist Léon Charles Albert Calmette.

Born in Nice in 1863, Albert Calmette, the son of a lawyer, wanted a career in the navy and became a cadet at the naval academy in Brest. After contracting typhoid fever he had to put his ambition on hold until 1881, when he was accepted for training as a naval physician at the School of Naval Physicians in Brest. Even as a student Calmette was keen to be involved in research projects and early in his career he developed an atom-iser for spraying antiseptic solutions.

Calmette's first post as a member of the Naval Medical Corps was to Hong Kong in 1883, where he met Patrick Manson, a Scottish parasitologist and founder of the London School of Tropical Medicine, whose malarial studies Calmette translated into French.[22] After Hong Kong, Calmette spent some years in West Africa investigating malaria and sleeping sickness (both of which Robert Koch would work on twenty years later) and then went to Newfoundland. In 1890 Calmette was transferred to the newly formed French Colonial Medical Service and he asked for leave to study at the Pasteur Institute in Paris. Here the young scientist worked under the supervision of Emile Roux but was also noticed by Pasteur, who recognised Calmette's potential and in 1891 nominated him for the job of organising the Saigon branch of the Pasteur Institute in what was then French Indochina. Calmette devoted himself to this task and soon after his arrival in the colony began pro-ducing smallpox and rabies vaccines. Like Pasteur and Koch, Calmette was able to keep many research balls in the air at one time. While in Vietnam he also undertook an extensive study of snake venoms and plant and bee poison and successfully developed a number of snake anti-venom serums.

Having an extensive knowledge of disease does not necessarily confer immunity and after two years in Saigon Calmette contracted a severe form of dysentery which forced him to return to France. His position at the Saigon institute was taken over by Alexandre Yersin whom Calmette had convinced to join the French Colonial Medical Service. Yersin, a Swiss biol-ogist, had previously been involved in the development of the rabies vaccine after joining Pasteur's research team in 1886, and in 1894 he would lead the French mission to Hong Kong and discover the cause of bubonic plague. There were many foes to conquer.

In Paris, when he was sufficiently recovered Calmette was given a part-time administrative post at the Ministry of the Colonies and spent part of his mornings and evenings in Roux's laboratory at the Pasteur Institute. In 1894, Louis Pasteur was asked by the city of Lille, where he had started his career in bacteriology, to establish a branch of the Pasteur Institute there.[23] Roux suggested Calmette for the director's position, a role that he fulfilled until 1919. Under Calmette's leadership the institute became prestigious.

While the Lille institute was being built, Calmette, a gifted organiser, started work in temporary laboratories which within a short time were producing sufficient smallpox and rabies vaccine to meet the needs of northern France. Also a talented inventor, Calmette developed a new commercial process for the conversion of starch into sugar and alcohol, the proceeds from which he would use to help finance a new project he was planning. After moving into the new building and ensuring that vaccine production was in full swing, Calmette turned his attention to the next major assault on tuberculosis.

Calmette's research followed Pasteur's practice of developing attenuated live vaccines. To do this he needed a veterinarian to maintain the stock of experimental animals. Professor Nocard, the veterinarian and microbiologist at the Pasteur Institute who had helped Pasteur and Roux in their classic anthrax experiments, recommended his assistant Camille Guérin, who joined Calmette in Lille in 1897.[24] Thus began a long association that would lead to the discovery and development of the successful tuberculosis vaccine, *bacille de Calmette et Guérin* (BCG). Camille Guérin, who had been born in Paris in 1872, spent most of his professional life at the Pasteur Institute in Lille, and later in Paris, where he continued to supervise the production of BCG after Calmette's death in 1933.

The research into tuberculosis was postponed for a year in 1899 when Calmette was sent to Portugal to help stem an epidemic of bubonic plague. A year was not a long time, however, because the research carried out by Calmette and Guérin was grindingly slow. By 1906 Guérin had demonstrated that resistance against tuberculosis is associated with the presence of living tubercle bacilli in the blood and two years later in 1908, after experimenting with different culture mediums, Calmette and Guérin had succeeded in obtaining an attenuated strain of the bovine tubercle bacillus.

The culture medium they used consisted of potato, glycerine and bile salts. The addition of ox bile to the mix, which may have been the result of trial and error, was to prove critical. The idea may also have come from a Norwegian physician Kristian Feyer Andvord, who was an expert on tuberculosis.[25] (In a lecture in 1991 on the 100th anniversary of the Veterinary Institute in Oslo in Norway, the chief physician, Gunnar Bjune, said that the idea of producing successively less virulent tubercle bacilli on a medium to which ox bile was added was suggested to Calmette in a discussion he had with Andvord in Paris.) Wherever the idea came from, Calmette and Guérin found ox bile was an effective agent for breaking up the clumps of bacilli and also changed the virulence and morphology, i.e. the form and structure of the organisms.

Prolonged culture of the bacilli in media containing bile did indeed produce a strain of organisms from which a safe and effective vaccine could be made. Calmette and Guérin had made great strides. Small doses of bovine bacilli injected into cattle produced accumulations of bacilli in parts of the abdomen but did not cause the disease. In December 1908 Calmette informed the French Academy of Sciences of this discovery. Over the next thirteen years, from 1908 to 1921, Calmette and Guérin conducted a series of historic experiments. Using a bovine strain of tubercle that had been isolated by Nocard in 1902, they sub-cultured the organisms a staggering 231 times, producing ever less virulent bacilli.

Totally committed to their goal, the two scientists took grave risks when they continued their work after Lille was occupied by the German army during World War I. Their research cattle were requisitioned by the Germans, putting an end to most of the animal experiments. Calmette secretly kept some pigeons but this was not the only regulation he flouted. The occupying authorities lost patience with Calmette and he was interned. His situation became even more tenuous when his wife was taken to Germany as a hostage and he was put under the threat of a death sentence. But Calmette was destined for greater things. A prominent German bacteriologist, Richard Pfeiffer, who was a general in the medical division of the German army, admired Calmette. Respect for a fellow scientist transcended national boundaries and Pfeiffer intervened on Calmette's behalf.

During the war, in 1917, Elie Metchnikov, who followed Pasteur as Director of the Pasteur Institute, died. Calmette was named Associate Director, in absentia, a great honour and a symbol of his standing in the scientific community. Despite the risks he took, Calmette survived and after the war ended in 1918 was free to go to Paris to devote himself completely to a cure for tuberculosis.

Working together again, Calmette and Guérin picked up the pieces of their research but it was some years before they could prove conclusively that the vaccine they had developed was safe for humans. The first prophylactic test of BCG on a human was carried out in 1921 when a physician persuaded Calmette to allow his vaccine to be used to protect a child who had been born to a mother who had tuberculosis. This unplanned test of the vaccine was completely successful and Calmette, in collaboration with medical colleagues, then carried out extended trials. The vaccine was initially used on newborn infants at the Charité Hospital in Paris.

In 1924 Calmette and Guérin published a historic paper in which they showed that vaccination trials on children undertaken in many parts of the world had clearly demonstrated the success and safety of the vaccine as a protective measure against tuberculosis. A new building was erected at the Pasteur Institute in 1928 specifically for the Service du BCG, signifying the importance of the cure. In the same year BCG was adopted by the Health Committee of the League of Nations. But in 1930, just at the time when BCG was gaining greater acceptance and thousands of children had been successfully treated, an unexpected tragedy occurred.

As with previous breakthroughs, there were critics who doubted the safety of the vaccine, fearing that the strain would not always remain avirulent. In what became known as the Lübeck disaster, 207 out of 259 children who had been vaccinated between the end of February and the beginning of April in 1930 contracted tuberculosis, and sadly, 72 of the infected children died.[26] This tragic event cast enormous doubt on the vaccine and created great personal anguish for its inventors. The whole world was profoundly shocked and Calmette was savagely attacked by many in the medical profession and in the press. Other doctors, however, particularly those in Germany who had successfully used the vaccine, rallied to his side.

The German health authorities held a rigorous and drawn out inquiry. Investigations revealed that the director of the public health laboratories at Lübeck had arranged for Calmette to send him a culture so that the BCG vaccine could be prepared in the city hospital laboratories but, because of careless practices during production, the vaccine they produced contained virulent bacilli. The German doctors who were found responsible were imprisoned and Calmette was absolved of any blame.

Production methods were overhauled and after another enquiry in 1932 the BCG was declared safe. Despite this clean bill of health, the vaccine was not widely used for some years which meant that tuberculosis remained a huge health problem globally in the first half of the twentieth century. After World War II there was an increased uptake, however, and from 1945 to 1950 relief organisations conducted an international tuberculosis campaign and vaccinated over 11 million children and adolescents in over twenty countries preventing a predicted increase in TB after the ravages of the war.[27] As a result of the introduction of BCG and the gradual introduction of a raft of health and hygiene measures in Europe, deaths from TB fell from 500 out of every 100,000 people in 1850 to 50 out of 100,000 by 1950.

Research into the vaccine continued and gradually its prophylactic value was accepted. Mass vaccination programs were eventually conducted in many countries including Japan, Russia, China, England, France and Canada. Although BCG was licensed in the United States in 1950, resistance to its use there has remained strong but in Great Britain the vaccine was widely accepted after a Medical Research Council investigation in 1959 guaranteed its safety. BCG is a safe vaccine because the virulence of the live bacilli it contains remains low and it is effective for both animals and humans because the tubercle bacilli of both bovine and human types are related closely enough to produce cross-immunity, as Robert Koch had suggested.

Camille Guérin outlived his colleague Albert Calmette by almost 30 years. Calmette died in 1933 a year after the tragedy at Lübeck. Although he was 70 years old, his death may have been hastened by the stress he suffered from the protracted enquiry and the responsibility he carried for the death of so many children when his hope had been to save them from a dreadful disease. Before his death in 1961, Camille Guérin, however, had the satisfaction of seeing the vaccine he had laboured over for two decades accepted as a safe prophylactic measure against tuberculosis. Today BCG is still a potent weapon against TB and is the most widely administered vaccine in the world. It reduces mortality from TB by about 90 per cent in vaccinated children.[28] How different things might have been if Albert Calmette had not survived World War I.

HOPES FOR A TB CURE GIVEN NEW LIFE

With the discovery during World War II of penicillin, the first antibiotic, the treatment of infections changed forever and hopes were raised that other drugs could be found to annihilate the micro-organisms that cause human disease. The quest to find a cure for TB was revived. Selman Waksman, a Russian-born American microbiologist, led the charge, initiating a calculated systematic search for antibiotics in the world of microbes. He spent his life studying the benign and dangerous micro-organisms that live in soil. Waksman coined the term *antibiotic,* which means 'against life', and was credited with giving the world streptomycin.[29] Although Waksman won the Nobel Prize for this achievement it was the work of his student Albert Schatz that made it possible. Acknowledgment of Schatz's contribution came somewhat belatedly.

Selman Waksman was born in 1888 in a Jewish village near Kiev, Russia. It was a difficult time for Jewish people in Russia. They were a persecuted minority which made Selman's goal to study at a university not easily attainable. Selman fought against the injustice of the pogroms initiated by the tsarist government. He organised a Jewish resistance group, a move that placed him in jeopardy. When Selman's mother died in 1910 there was nothing to hold him in Russia, and hoping for a less repressed life he emigrated to the United States where he had relatives and began his life there working on their farm.

Determined to acquire a university education, Waksman took advantage of the opportunities available to him in his new country and won a state scholarship to study agriculture at Rutgers University in 1911. He gained a Bachelor of Science degree in 1915 and a Master's degree the following year after which he undertook graduate studies at the University of California, being awarded a PhD in biochemistry in 1918.

In 1921 Waksman began work as a microbiologist for the New Jersey Agricultural Experiment Station and combined his academic pursuits with work in private industry. When he was just over 40 years old, in 1929, Waksman was appointed as a professor at Rutgers University. In the same way that Pasteur had gone against the accepted theories of his day, as with spontaneous generation, Waksman opposed the prevailing 'protozoan theory of soil fertility'.[30] This was based on the assumption that protozoa consumed bacteria, sometimes to such an extent as to destroy soil fertility. Waksman's evaluation of bacterial populations in the soil, their chemical properties and the complex balances between them seemed revolutionary at the time.

Before 1939, the year that World War II began, Waksman had not been interested in pharmacological research but his interest was piqued when one of his former students, René Dubois, discovered two soil-based antimicrobials (substances that kill microbes), tyrocidine and gramicidin. Although toxic to humans, these substances proved promising for treating some infections in animals. This discovery coincided with news that work was taking place in England on the development of penicillin, an anti-bacterial from a mould.

Waksman had long been interested in actinomycetes, a group of fungus-like bacteria, most species of which are harmless; so he made the decision to begin experimenting with soil-based fungi and bacteria.[31] He had already refined techniques that would enable him to isolate soil organisms, culture them and purify and crystallise soil-based substances. As was common practice, graduate students assisted Waksman with various aspects of his work, one of whom was Albert Schatz. It was Schatz who made a crucial discovery.

Born in 1920 in Connecticut, Albert Schatz was a graduate student at Rutgers University when he was drafted into the army in November 1942 during World War II. Working as a laboratory bacteriologist in an army hospital in Miami, Florida, he saw the miraculous success of the recently developed penicillin, which at that time was available in limited amounts to military personnel. Schatz's stint in the army was short-lived and after being discharged in June 1943 because of a congenital abnormality in his lower spine he immediately resumed his doctoral research. In an oral history recorded at Rutgers, Schatz gave an account of how he became involved in a project to find a cure for tuberculosis. Doctors at the Mayo Clinic, the world-renowned hospital and medical practice based in Minnesota, had suggested to Selman Waksman that he try to find an antibiotic that would be effective against TB.

> Dr Waksman was disinclined to take on that project because he was afraid of tuberculosis. This disease had by then killed about a billion people in the last two centuries. That was more deaths than were caused by all other infectious diseases combined. However, I persuaded Dr Waksman to let me do the TB project. He agreed, but, because I would be working with a virulent human strain of the tubercle bacillus, he transferred me from the laboratory adjacent to his office on the third floor of the Administration Building to the basement laboratory.

*He told me never to bring a culture of the tubercle bacillus to the
third floor. And he never visited the basement laboratory.*[32]

After researching alone in the basement for three and a half months,
Schatz found that the actinomycete *Streptomyces griseus* seemed effective
against the ancient survivor, *Mycobacterium tuberculosis*. Albert Schatz had
isolated the antibiotic that became known as streptomycin and he wrote
the first paper about it in which he described the discovery. However, in
January 1944 it was Selman Waksman, not Albert Schatz, who reported on
the antibacterial properties of *Streptomyces griseus* and as a result tests on
streptomycin were commenced in the Mayo Clinic. Favourable results with
streptomycin on tuberculous guinea pigs led to human trials. By October,
the first human patients were in treatment and streptomycin appeared to
be having unprecedented success in curing their TB.

In the wake of the tragedy of World War II, a cure for TB was hailed as a
timely miracle. Selman Waksman was catapulted into the limelight and revered
as the latest medical hero and disease fighter. He toured the world and his face
appeared on the cover of *Time* magazine. But amidst all of the publicity no
mention was made of Albert Schatz. Then in 1950 — a year that Waksman
describes in his 1954 autobiography, *My Life with the Microbes*, as the darkest of
his whole life — Schatz sued for royalties as a co-discoverer of streptomycin.[33]

This was not the first time, nor would it be the last, that the head of a
laboratory would receive the recognition for the work done by an assistant
under their aegis. In this case it was the diligent PhD student Schatz who
had brought *Streptomyces griseus* to his professor's attention. In more recent
times, Waksman has been accused of highlighting his own role to reporters
while not acknowledging Schatz's part in the discovery. However, Albert
Schatz and Selman Waksman jointly signed the patent for streptomycin.

Supposedly, it was rumours that Waksman was secretly providing information to a pharmaceutical company and receiving large royalties from the
patent of streptomycin in return that was the catalyst for Schatz taking legal
action. Waksman reluctantly agreed to settle and Schatz was declared

co-discoverer and awarded a small share of the royalties. With his much larger share Waksman established a Foundation for Microbiology and gave a small percentage to the other laboratory workers at Rutgers.

In 1952 when Waksman was awarded the Nobel Prize for Physiology or Medicine the Nobel Committee emphasised that his contribution to the advancement of medicine was paramount, even though he was neither a physiologist nor a physician, and that they as physicians regarded him as 'one of the greatest benefactors of mankind'.[34] It is said that at that time the committee had not heard of Albert Schatz.

Totally overshadowed after the discovery, Albert Schatz did receive his doctorate from Rutgers in 1945 and then spent his life working in various universities. During his academic life he published several books and more than 700 scientific papers. In 1994, Dr Schatz was awarded the Rutgers University Medal, the university's highest honour. It was for his work on streptomycin, a public acknowledgment of his discovery of a cure for TB. Albert Schatz passed away in 2005, 30 years after Selman Waksman had died suddenly from a cerebral haemorrhage on 16 August 1973.

Selman Waksman's tombstone at Wood Hole, Massachusetts, is inscribed with the words 'Out of the earth shall come thy salvation'.[35] The research carried out by Selman Waksman, Albert Schatz and their colleagues to produce streptomycin has indeed brought salvation to millions of people. It is still a mainstay of TB therapy and is effective against a number of bacteria, including some that are resistant to other antibiotics. Because resistant tubercle bacilli emerge during treatment, showing how determined they are to survive, antibiotics are usually used in combination with one or more drugs. Among these is isoniazid (INH), which kills the organisms and renders them non-infectious. The introduction of INH in the 1950s brought about the closure of separate TB hospitals.[36]

ANTIBIOTICS AND TUBERCULOSIS TODAY

The success of the antibiotic drugs penicillin and streptomycin has spawned a huge pharmaceutical industry that in turn has led to the 'commercialisation' of cures. Gone are the days of scientists experimenting in home laboratories and sharing their discoveries with the world at large. Sophisticated private laboratories have been set up almost in competition with those in universities and other non-profit institutions, and although new experimental drugs are being developed, mass-producing them is the domain of multinational drug companies. The first entirely synthetic antibiotic, an effective treatment for typhoid fever, was developed by the drug company Parke-Davis in 1949.

The fight against bacteria is ongoing. Many are becoming resistant to the drugs we use to attack them, including penicillin. The percentage of pneumococcal strains that are drug-resistant is on the rise and, in our chemotherapeutic era, thousands of hospital patients die every year because of drug-resistant bacterial infections. Five decades ago with the advent of streptomycin it was thought that by the year 2000 tuberculosis would have been eradicated and perhaps even be extinct. In 1965 Waksman published a book on the discovery of streptomycin, the title of which, *The Conquest of Tuberculosis*, reflects the belief at the time that TB would be defeated.[37] TB, however, is making an impressive comeback. New strains of the tuberculosis bacteria that are resistant to previously effective treatments surfaced in the 1980s and have become increasingly prevalent in poor and developing countries. The return of tuberculosis and the threat it poses is highlighted every year on 24 March, World Tuberculosis Day, which commemorates Robert Koch's discovery in 1882 of *Mycobacterium tuberculosis*.

A number of factors have contributed to the spread of TB in recent decades. In some countries, funds previously used to control the disease have been diverted to treat other public health problems, including HIV/AIDS. The emergence of this modern incurable disease which attacks the body's immune system has had a profound effect in two ways on the re-emergence of TB. People with a damaged immune system are 30 times more vulnerable to tuberculosis and, conversely, TB can accelerate HIV in a person who has both diseases.[38] Increased poverty, homelessness, travel and migration have also contributed to the spread of TB. Also, the efficacy of current TB therapies is limited because people with TB need a daily cocktail of drugs for up to six months which means keeping up with long-duration therapies is difficult.

The frightening statistics speak for themselves. In Britain in 1955 tuberculosis cases numbered around 50,000 but had dropped significantly to around 5500 by 1987 due to the availability of antibiotics. However, at the beginning of the new millennium there were over 7000 confirmed cases. Tuberculosis infects around 8 million people annually and kills 2 million of those infected. Virtually all TB deaths are in the developing world, where the victims are mainly young adults. Half of all new cases are in six Asian countries: Bangladesh, China, India, Indonesia, Pakistan and the Philippines; and a staggering 29 per cent of all TB cases occur in Africa where AIDS is also rampant.

In 1993 the World Health Organization, alarmed by the re-emergence of TB with multi drug-resistant strains, declared a 'global health emergency' and introduced a program called DOTs.[39] The acronym, standing for 'directly observed treatment, short-course', refers to the direct observation by trained personnel of TB sufferers taking their medications. Since 1995, some 183 countries have adopted DOTs and 22 million TB patients have been treated under the program.

In 2006 at an extraordinary conference convened in South Africa alarm bells rang when the WHO revealed that they were not winning the war against the new strains of TB. Of the 9 million cases of tuberculosis reported in 2005, 180,000 could be classified as 'extreme drug-resistant' and the WHO reclassified TB, along with HIV/AIDS and malaria, as a 'priority disease'.

The crusade to find better weapons to defeat TB has been taken up by the Stop TB Partnership which is comprised of more than 400 entities, including international organisations, individual countries, donors from the public and private sectors, governmental and non-governmental organisations and individuals. In January 2006, at the World Economic Forum in

Davos, Switzerland, the WHO Stop TB Partnership announced a new US$56 billion strategy, 'The Global Plan to Stop TB 2006–2015'. The aim is to stop the spread and reverse the incidence of TB, which now kills 1.7 million people each year, by 2015, by implementing effective TB care around the world and by assessing current research needs for the development of new drugs, vaccines and diagnostics. If fully implemented, the global plan will treat 50 million people for TB, halve TB prevalence and death rates and save 14 million lives.

As the saga continues, the best approach to preventing and combatting TB is still considered to be through continuing vaccination programs, but the search for new treatments has been taken up by various entities including public–private partnerships, government-funded researchers, industry and philanthropies. In partnership with Stellenbosch University in South Africa, the drug company GlaxoSmithKline is involved in a program to help identify 'biomarkers' in people who may respond to specific treatments.[40] Biomarkers can be used to predict whether or not patients will respond quickly to treatment or if TB is likely to recur. This kind of research certainly reflects the Koch tradition.

Despite the cumulative work of all those who have waged war on tuberculosis and the extraordinary scientific discoveries made by Robert Koch, Albert Calmette and Camille Guérin, and Selman Waksman and Albert Schatz, the curable White Plague remains invincible. It continues the struggle for its own survival while taking a toll of 5000 lives a day. It is estimated that every second someone in the world becomes infected with TB and one person dies every 15 seconds. There may yet be many challenges ahead before tuberculosis is finally vanquished.

POSTSCRIPT

There is no statute of limitations on the amount of time it can take to thank someone for saving your life. Fifty years after the discovery of streptomycin, on 21 March 1996, Senator Bob Dole, who was then a US presidential candidate, sent a letter to Albert Schatz written on United States Senate letterhead. 'During my recovery after World War II,' wrote Dole, 'streptomycin defeated an infection that threatened my life.'

In 1997, a year after Albert Schatz received the letter from Bob Dole he was contacted by a German-born woman, Inge Auerbacher, who 50 years after the event had read an article about Schatz being the co-discoverer of streptomycin and the controversy surrounding the events of that time. During World War II, Inge had been a prisoner at the Terezin concentration camp in Czechoslovakia where she contracted tuberculosis. After the war, as a refugee she emigrated to the United States where she was cured with the new, life-saving drug. Inge, like so many others wanted to express her gratitude to Albert Schatz. The two became friends and the product of that friendship is a book they co-authored, Finding Dr. Schatz, the story of a scientist who changed the world and a woman who lived because of him.

Until the end of his life Albert Schatz took quiet pleasure in the fact that he was still receiving letters from people all over the world who thanked him for saving their lives.

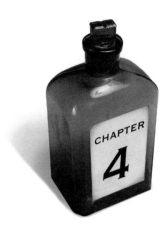

OF RATS AND FLEAS

SOLVING THE RIDDLE OF THE BLACK DEATH

> How many valiant men, how many fair ladies,
> breakfast with their kinfolk and the same night
> supped with their ancestors in the next world! The
> condition of the people was pitiable to behold.[1]
>
> *Giovanni Boccaccio*

Bubonic plague has an infamous place in history. No other disease can lay claim to its apocalyptic persona. A ferocious killer that can lay dormant for centuries, its horrific symptoms and pervasive, destructive consequences meant that the plague was feared far more than its nearest rival, smallpox. Bubonic plague was a scourge of epic proportions that arose sporadically and raced through mediaeval Europe and Asia, leaving countless millions dead in its wake. The great plague that devastated Europe in the fourteenth century was the most deadly of all and was aptly named the 'Great Mortality', the 'Great Pestilence' and the 'Black Death'.

In 1894, when plague broke out in Hong Kong, two research teams set off on a race to find a cause. The leaders of those teams, the eminent Japanese researcher Shibasaburo Kitasato and the unorthodox French bacteriologist Alexandre Yersin, were opposites in personality and in their scientific approach, and to this day controversy over the discovery of the micro-organism that causes plague persists. Without a cause there could be no cure and the development of a preventive vaccine for bubonic plague by the bacteriologist, Waldemar Haffkine, in a makeshift laboratory in India in 1896 is another dramatic story in the life of the plague.

To appreciate the enormity of the contribution made by these three scientists it is necessary to become familiar with the horror of the rapacious Black Death itself. Since ancient times plagues have decimated societies. An account in the Hebrew bible of a plague that struck the Philistines around the eleventh century BC describes symptoms which are consistent with bubonic plague, in particular large buboes, inflamed and painful swellings in the groin, armpits or neck. Also indicative, was that this plague followed an excessive number of rat deaths; throughout history there has been a link between rat plague and bubonic plague. The reason for this was not established until the early 1900s when it was proven that plague was carried by rodent fleas.

In 430 BC the Greek historian Thucydides wrote about a disease that struck Greece during the Peloponnesian War. In Athens alone, one-third of the population died, including Pericles, Athens' leader during its golden age.[2] With advances in science it is now possible for scientists to give a retrospective diagnosis. Cases have been made for the Greek plague being smallpox, typhus, measles and bubonic plague. A recent study of the DNA found in the dental pulp of plague victims from that time has led some scientists to conclude the disease was typhoid while others dispute this, suggesting that the DNA tests were flawed.

In the first century AD a plague broke out in Libya, Egypt and Syria and a Greek anatomist recorded the symptoms — acute fever, pain, agitation and delirium — in addition to the typical buboes behind the knees and around the elbows, again suggesting bubonic plague. There is no debate, however, about a plague that began in 540 AD in Pelusium in Egypt. It was bubonic plague and by 542 AD it had reached Constantinople, modern-day Istanbul. Ships from Egypt bringing massive amounts of grain to the bustling city also carried a cargo of contagion, rats and fleas, which soon infested the massive public granaries.

Called the Plague of Justinian, it is the first recorded pandemic in history. At its peak in Constantinople, 5000 people died daily and ultimately almost half of the city's inhabitants were wiped out. The pandemic was catastrophic, killing up to a quarter of the population of the eastern Mediterranean.[3] In 588 AD a second major wave of plague spread through the Mediterranean into what is now France. The death toll has been estimated at a staggering 25 million people.

It was eight centuries later that the Great Mortality swept through Asia and Europe, this time killing approximately one-third of the entire population and changing the course of history. It is almost impossible to conceive of death on this gargantuan scale. The Black Death began its killing spree in Constantinople in 1334 and spread inexorably through Europe and beyond for the next twenty years. It arrived in Alexandria, Cyprus and Sicily in the autumn of 1347 and by winter was rampaging through mainland Italy.

Giovanni Boccaccio's book, *The Decameron*, is a fictional work which opens with a description of the outbreak of plague in Florence in 1348.[4] Boccaccio describes how the first sign of having caught the plague was developing lumps in the groin or armpits. Following this, livid black spots appeared on the arms, thighs and other parts of the victim's body. He noted that people usually died within three days of the onset of symptoms.

An observation that the disease lay dormant for a while before infected people became symptomatic led the governors of Venice to pass a decree in 1348 that ships sailing into the harbour be isolated to allow time for the Black Death to reveal itself. A period of 30 days, *trentina* in Italian, was initially mandated but was later extended to 40 days, *quarantine*. This is the origin of the English word 'quarantine'.[5] By 1423 a dedicated quarantine station had been established on an island near Venice in an attempt to prevent the disease re-entering the city.

In 1348 the Black Death reached France and Germany, hit London in September and then spread rapidly through Scotland, Wales and Ireland. It is estimated that 1.5 million of England's 4 million people died. The plague was relentless, an invader like no other. Even the northern countries of Scandinavia were not immune. The plague found its way to Norway and then embarked on a journey through Eastern Europe. By 1351 bubonic plague had galloped across Europe and entered Russia.

THE NATURE OF THE PLAGUE

It is now known that there are three human forms of the disease commonly known as bubonic plague — bubonic, septicaemic and pneumonic plague.[6] Even though the first sign of having contracted plague is usually flu-like symptoms with all three forms, they do differ symptomatically and in the route of infection. This could account for the different descriptions of plague in historical accounts. The bubonic form is spread by fleas which deposit bacteria into a victim's lymphatic system when they bite. The bacilli then travel to the nearest lymph node, which becomes inflamed. After an incubation period of three to seven days the initial symptoms become evident: chills, fever, diarrhoea, headaches and painful swelling in infected lymph nodes where the bacteria replicate in high numbers in the buboes. Death can occur in less than a week after infection. Historically, 60 per cent of all people who were infected with plague had the bubonic type and the mortality rate ranged between 30 and 70 per cent.

Pneumonic plague, which is extremely contagious, is the most virulent but least common type of plague and in approximately 95 per cent of cases is fatal if untreated. It is not transmitted by fleas but is a secondary infection from the bubonic form spread from human to human. The bacilli are present in the water droplets from coughs or sneezes and they can also be present on clothing. The incubation period for pneumonic plague is usually between two and four days, but can be as little as a few hours. Symptoms include headache, weakness and coughing up blood from the respiratory tract. When the bacilli reach the lungs, victims develop severe pneumonia and death follows rapidly within one to six days.

Death is even faster with the septicaemic form of plague which is almost always fatal. Without treatment, victims usually die within 24 hours of the onset of symptoms. Victims of septicaemic plague do not develop buboes because the bacilli enter the bloodstream directly. Like bubonic plague, the septicaemic variety may be caused by flea bites or from direct contact with infective materials through cracks in the skin. There is haemorrhaging into the skin and other organs which creates black patches on the skin and in some cases red bite-like bumps as well. Today treatment with antibiotics can reduce the mortality rate of septicaemic plague dramatically to around 5 per cent.

In all three forms of the plague, internal bleeding causes large bruises to appear on the skin hence the appellation the Black Death. As there was no way to distinguish one form from another in the fourteenth century, many scientists and historians believe that the more contagious and virulent pneumonic and septicaemic varieties were present as well as the bubonic form during the pandemic, which not only increased the pace of infection but also facilitated the rampant spread of the disease into inland areas of many countries.

As is the nature of scientific enquiry and debate there are also claims that the plague that swept through England during the great pandemic was not plague at all and certainly not bubonic plague. A BBC news article published in 2002 discusses the proposition by anthropologists from Penn State University in the United States that the spread of the Black Death was far too rapid to have been bubonic plague and that the geographic reach of the disease supports this.[7] In England, for example, plague made its way along roadways and navigable rivers and its progress was not slowed by natural geographical barriers that would prevent the movement of rodents and thus the spread of bubonic plague.

Further to this the anthropologists, who subscribe to the theory that bubonic plague becomes rampant in the rat population before being carried to humans by rodent fleas, had found no historical records that referred to dead rats in sufficient numbers. Their conclusion was that the Great Mortality was not bubonic plague but could have been caused by any number of infectious organisms and was probably transmitted through person-to-person contact, not fleas. Because these findings were based on historical records, a bacteriologist at the London School of Hygiene and Tropical Medicine dismissed them as unscientific speculation. He suggested that unless bacterial DNA from that time could be found, tested and compared with various strains of plague bacteria that exist now, then the debate could not be resolved.

Debate is healthy and there is certainly an ongoing fascination with the Black Death amongst scientists, which says much about the status of this disease in history and the horror surrounding it. Susan Scott, a historical demographer, and Christopher J. Duncan, Emeritus Professor of Zoology in the School of Biological Sciences at the University of Liverpool in the United Kingdom, have also challenged the belief that the Black Death pandemic in the 1300s and the Great Plague of London in 1665 were bubonic plague.[8] Their book, *Biology of Plagues*, published in 2001, combines epidemiology, molecular biology and computer modelling with historical records to show that rats were not the source of infection. Scott researched the parish records of the English town of Penrith in Cumbria and discovered that the disease that reached this remote spot during the Middle Ages was spread by person-to-person contact and was unlikely to be any form of plague but it may have been the dreaded Ebola virus.

So, was the fearsome bubonic plague responsible for inestimable deaths in the Middle Ages? The consensus is that because of the rapidity and extent of its spread and the range of symptoms that have been recorded, the Black Death was in fact a combination of all three forms of the plague.

THE GREAT MORTALITY RESHAPES MEDIAEVAL EUROPE

In mediaeval times people believed that the Black Death was a punishment from God. As we now know, the cause was far more terrestrial than celestial. In towns and cities people lived cheek by jowl in squalid, unhygienic conditions and knew nothing about infection and contagious diseases, although there was a common belief that rats caused the disease in some way. Streets littered with refuse and sewage provided a perfect breeding ground for rodents and they carried plague fleas into shops, houses and churches. Fleas bit into their victims, literally injecting them with bubonic plague. The problem of contagion was further exacerbated by the unhygienic disposal of bodies and those who handled the plague-infested dead were particularly at risk.

Medical knowledge was minimal and superstition was rife. As a result people would try anything to save themselves from falling victim to plague. One extreme measure was flagellation.[9] To show devotion to God, people whipped themselves viciously in the hope that their sins would be forgiven, sparing them a gruesome death. Mediaeval literature is littered with macabre illustrations of flagellants with their whips.

As the Great Mortality diminished populations throughout Europe, the established order of mediaeval society was utterly disrupted. Crops rotted, fields went unploughed and farm animals died because there was no one to tend them. The inhabitants of towns and cities faced food shortages because the surrounding villages could not provide them with enough food. Grain farming became less popular because the noble class who owned the land had turned to sheep farming, which was less labour intensive. Inflation was rife and exorbitant food prices created additional hardship for the poor.

Those who survived the Black Death believed that they had been chosen by God and began to question the status quo. The feudal system under which they lived was restrictive and had been introduced to tie peasants to the land. Peasants could not leave their village without their lord's permission. As labour shortages became critical due to the plague, laws were relaxed and peasants began to move to areas where work was available, some even demanding higher wages. There came a realisation amongst the nobility that the system they relied on to maintain power was breaking down. In England the *Statute of Labourers* was introduced in 1351 to limit wages that could be paid and received and to reinstate the law restricting the movement of peasants. The resultant anger and discontent led to the Peasants Revolt of 1381.

Although it may seem paradoxical, it is believed that the Great Mortality was immortalised in the original version of the English nursery rhyme 'Ring-a-ring o' roses'.[10] The 'roses' refer to the red spots that appear on a victim's skin over the buboes; 'A-tishoo! A-tishoo!' mimics the flu symptoms and 'We all fall down!' reflects the swift death that accompanies the pneumonic form of plague. The song may also allude to the fact that the plague made everything fall down — the political, economic and social structures of many countries.

The Black Death continued to strike parts of Europe throughout the fourteenth, fifteenth and sixteenth centuries with varying degrees of intensity and fatality. In May 1665 the famous, or infamous, Great Plague of London began. Only 43 people died during May of that year but the death toll for June was 6137. This figure almost trebled in July when 17,036 succumbed. The mortality rate doubled again in August, with a staggering 31,159 deaths. Then in 1666 a fire, the Great Fire of London, raced through the city purging it of its infestation of plague-carrying rats and fleas and the slums that harboured them. With widespread destruction came temporary salvation.

In 1679 plague devastated central Europe and erupted again in England but this was the last major outbreak ever experienced there. During the eighteenth century outbreaks of bubonic plague in the rest of Europe also diminished, probably partly due to improvements in public hygiene and sanitation. Gradual genetic adaptation which provided humans with resistance to the disease may also have contributed to stopping the spread of plague.

The Black Death had not finished with other parts of the world, however. A third bubonic plague pandemic began in China in 1855 and by 1877 had become a serious problem in India, China and Russia, ultimately killing more than 12 million people in India and China alone.[11] There were two likely sources for this pandemic. The bubonic form of plague was carried around the world via ocean-going trade which transported infected people and cargoes infested with rats and fleas. A more virulent strain that was rampant in Manchuria and Mongolia was probably pneumonic, highly contagious from person to person.

The pandemic persisted in China and India until the mid 1890s and it was because of this continuing threat that Alexandre Yersin and Shibasaburo Kitasato set off with their research teams to go microbe hunting in Hong Kong in the hope of finding the cause of the plague. What was to follow is as intriguing as fiction.

THE HUNT FOR THE CAUSE

Alexandre Emile Jean Yersin was born in 1863 in the Swiss town of Aubonne, not far from Lake Geneva. His father, who had been a professor of natural history, died a few days before his birth. As a child, Alexandre showed an aptitude for scientific studies and had a keen interest in nature (a recurrent theme), often spending time collecting and studying insects. Yersin received his secondary education in Lausanne and began his early medical education at the university there but later attended the University of Marburg and completed his training at the Paris Faculty of Medicine.

Right from the start of his medical career Yersin eschewed routine clinical work and decided to specialise in pathology. He became an assistant to Professor André Cornil, the pathologist at the Hôtel-Dieu Hospital in Paris, and it was while he was here that he suffered an accident that determined his future medical career and brought him in contact with Emile Roux. Yersin cut himself while performing an autopsy on a patient who had died of rabies.[12] An injection of Pasteur's new rabies vaccine was administered by Emile Roux at the Pasteur Institute and this one event saved Yersin from an agonising death, and changed his life.

Yersin saw the vaccine as miraculous and he was in awe of Pasteur and the scientists who worked with him. It became Yersin's ambition to join both them and the quest that was taking place in the major European laboratories to find ways of combating the major diseases that humankind had always accepted as being a part of living and dying. Before joining Pasteur, Yersin spent some months during 1877 in Berlin continuing his bacteriological studies under the tuition of the other demi-god of science, Robert Koch. While there Yersin was able to learn and practise the new research methods and technical aspects of tissue staining that Koch had introduced and it was Yersin who introduced many of these to Pasteur's laboratory.[13]

In 1888 Emile Roux hired Alexandre Yersin as his assistant and, having been influenced by Robert Koch, Yersin began his first research project working on tuberculosis and the action of antiseptic and heat treatment on tubercle bacilli. Roux at this time began to focus on diphtheria and invited Yersin to collaborate with him. Some early research had been done on diphtheria and the bacillus had been discovered in 1883. The two scientists spent an arduous three years examining the toxic properties of the diphtheria bacillus and developing a procedure that enabled them to produce diphtheria toxin. During the time that they worked so intensively together Yersin and Roux became good friends. The results of their groundbreaking work were published in three classic papers, one in 1888, the next in 1890 and the last in 1891.

Although Yersin's standing in the scientific community was increasing rapidly, once the diphtheria project had been completed he was struck by a desire for travel and adventure, another trait many of the early medical pioneers had in common. He had found it difficult working within the constraints of a laboratory and did not approve of the imperious way in which Louis Pasteur directed the institute. Yersin was described as boyish and admitted to a desire to follow in the footsteps of Dr Livingstone, the British explorer.[14]

After resigning in 1889, Yersin signed on as a ship's doctor on a steamer bound for Saigon and Manila. Yersin made several voyages to Saigon, and like Albert Calmette, who had set up the Saigon branch of the Pasteur Institute, became fascinated by Indochina. He happily took charge of the institute when Calmette had to return to France in 1891. This position gave Yersin an opportunity to help fight disease in the country he had come to love and it also meant he could pursue both his scientific interests and his passion for exploration. He did travel to Europe in the winter of 1892 to visit both family and colleagues but found it so depressing and cold that he knew he could never return permanently to a conventional life. Emile Roux had planned a warm welcome for his young friend hoping to lure him back, but he soon became resigned to the fact that Yersin's heart was now in the Far East.

Yersin undertook three expeditions to the remote central region of Indochina, the first in 1892. The inveterate explorer often set out with inadequate supplies but despite the many hazards he encountered, which included a violent skirmish between armed Vietnamese and the French colonial authorities, he collected valuable information on the topography, flora and fauna of the region. He discovered the source of the Dong Nai River and the high plateau of Langbiang, where he established the village of Da Lat. The village would eventually become a city and, perhaps regrettably for Yersin, a vacation destination for Europeans. One thing that Yersin never failed to do on his journeys was to treat the sick wherever he found them and he believed it was his moral duty never to ask the poor for payment.

While Yersin was immersed in his work in and around Saigon, in May 1894, during the third pandemic, plague spread from the mainland of China to the colony of Hong Kong and the death toll began to rise. As an employee of the colonial health service, the Corps de Santé des Colonies, Yersin was sent to Hong Kong to conduct research on the plague. He was not the first bacteriologist to arrive, however. The Japanese government's mission landed in Hong Kong a few days earlier. Led by the eminent and experienced Shibasaburo Kitasato, the mission was well staffed and well organised and immediately gained the upper hand when they began work on 14 June, the day before Yersin arrived.

Shibasaburo Kitasato, who was born in 1853 in Kumamoto on the island of Kyushu in Japan, had been educated at Kumamoto Medical School and completed his medical studies at the Imperial University of Tokyo in 1883. Following this, as a young researcher he did groundbreaking work when he moved to Berlin to work in Robert Koch's laboratory from 1885 until 1891, research that contributed enormously to the understanding of disease and how the body fights infection. In 1890 Kitasato discovered a method of growing the tetanus bacillus in a pure culture and, with the bacteriologist Emil von Behring, developed tetanus and diphtheria antitoxins, substances that neutralise poisons produced by micro-organisms.

After returning to Japan in 1891 the respected Kitasato founded an institute for the study of infectious diseases and he was working there when asked by his government to take up the challenge against the plague in Hong Kong as it represented a direct threat to Japan. The authorities in Hong Kong had ignored the early signs of the plague and by the time Kitasato and Yersin began work the disease was spreading rapidly, ravaging the colony. Because of his world-renowned research skills, and because it was in their interest to do so considering the enormity of the crisis, the British government allowed Kitasato unrestricted access to patients and to supplies. He was given personal support by Dr James Lowson, the Superintendent of the Government Civil Hospital, who immediately provided Kitasato's team with a functioning laboratory.[15]

Yersin's situation in Hong Kong was the antithesis of Kitasato's. There was no laboratory for Yersin. He and his 'team', a misnomer really, as there was only Yersin and two assistants, set up what equipment they had in a straw hut. Yersin had even less to work with when one of the assistants disappeared with the meagre funds Yersin had been allotted. Two great minds were trying to solve the same puzzle but any hope of collaboration on Yersin's part was dashed when he paid a courtesy visit to Kitasato.[16] The meeting failed not just because of language difficulties but because reputations were at stake.

The odds were stacked very heavily in Kitasato's favour. Yersin found himself ostracised by the authorities and deliberately obstructed in his research. Because material from autopsies on plague victims was reserved for the Japanese mission, Yersin had great difficulty acquiring the specimens he needed to make progress with this research. With all the advantages Kitasato had, it is not surprising that within a few days of his arrival in Hong Kong he had isolated what he believed to be the bacterium that causes bubonic plague. He then confirmed his finding after applying Koch's postulates to tests on experimental animals. Without delay and using the new communication medium, the telegraph, Kitasato cabled the Japanese Interior Minister and announced his discovery of the bacillus, *Pasteurella pestis,* to the local English press.

What is astonishing is that despite his difficulties Yersin seems to have made the same discovery at the same time. However, before Yersin was able to get his findings into print in French journals, Kitasato had sent a paper on 7 July to London and his article appeared in *The Lancet* on 13 August 1894 complete with photographs.[17] It was barely two months after the discovery.

And so the controversy about who discovered the bubonic plague bacillus began. People in different parts of the world credited one or the other scientist with the discovery, depending on the source of their information. Since then the validity of Kitasato's original findings has been the subject of debate and the topic of much scientific literature. In 2002 Edward Marriott published *Plague: A story of science, rivalry, and the scourge that won't go away,* in which he tried to piece together the events surrounding the discovery of the plague bacterium and the rivalry between Kitasato and Yersin. (The title also alludes to the fact that the plague, despite the best efforts of science is determined to stay with us.)

Rightly or wrongly, Kitasato was originally acknowledged as the discoverer of *Pasteurella pestis*, named after Louis Pasteur, and Yersin's work was seen as a confirmation of this.[18] It is impossible not to feel some sympathy for Yersin who, with grossly inadequate resources, solved one of the world's greatest disease mysteries but because of circumstances was sidelined. It is interesting to note, however, that the pendulum has swung and Yersin and Kitasato are now credited with discovering the bacteria at the same time. The public affirmation of this is that since 1970 the bacillus has been known as *Yersinia pestis*, 'Yersinia' after Yersin, and 'pestis' after the Great Pestilence.

Shibasaburo Kitasato returned to the institute he had founded in Tokyo as a hero, and continued his work on disease. Four years after isolating the bubonic plague bacillus, he and his student Kigoshi Shiga discovered the organism that causes dysentery, an infection of the lower intestinal tract. Seven years after starting his own laboratory in 1892 the Japanese government took control but Kitasato agreed to stay on as director at the time. However when the laboratory was consolidated into the University of Tokyo in 1914, Kitasato resigned. A scientist of Kitasato's calibre needed autonomy and so he founded the Kitasato Institute, which he headed for the rest of his life.[19] Revered in his homeland, Kitasato was named the first president of the Japanese Medical Association in 1923 and was made a baron by the Emperor in 1924. After a long and distinguished career Shibasaburo Kitasato died in his homeland in 1931.

As for Alexandre Yersin, after the monumental disappointment of not being acknowledged as a discoverer of the plague bacillus, he returned to his adopted country of Vietnam. In 1895 Yersin established a new laboratory in Nha Trang, a small fishing village set on an idyllic bay. Putting his frustrations aside he continued his research into diseases. To finance the laboratory, which had been given in 1903 the imprimatur Pasteur Institute of Nha Trang, Yersin began cultivating grain crops and coffee, which led him to a new field of research: agronomy.

In 1904 Yersin was recalled to Paris to continue his research at the Pasteur Institute, where Emile Roux had become director. With Albert Calmette and Amédée Borrel, he made the important observation that certain animals can be immunised against the plague through the injection of dead plague bacteria.[20] On his return to his modest laboratories in Nha

Trang, Yersin perfected an anti-plague serum that appeared to be success-ful in reducing the death rate significantly in both animals and humans. He then began to set up a network of laboratories and vaccination centres throughout Vietnam to facilitate the production and administration of the new vaccine.

Yersin was always deeply concerned with the needs of the sick and the poor. He lacked the ego of many of his contemporaries and as a true humanitarian fought against the exploitation of the lower classes. With the assistance of Paul Doumer, the governor-general of Indochina, a medical school that Yersin directed for many years was founded in Hanoi. Because of his work and his commitment to his fellow humans, many of the epi-demics that spread through Indochina were controlled. In the early 1920s Yersin was responsible for planting the first quinquina plantations in Vietnam.[21] Quinine was the only effective treatment against malaria at the time and Yersin distributed it throughout the country. He never tired of new endeavours, also introducing the Brazilian rubber tree to Vietnam and at one time working for the Indochina Meteorological Service producing maps and tidal charts of the country's coastal waters.

In recognition of Yersin's medical achievements, the French government appointed him an honorary director of the Institut Pasteur in 1933. As a member of the Scientific Council, once a year he made the journey to Paris by air to fulfill his official duties, his last visit being in 1940 when he was in poor health. Alexandre Yersin died in 1943 at Suô'i Giao, south-west of Da Lat, at the age of 80 and his request in his will that he be buried at his beloved Nha Trang was carried out. And so ended the life of another great microbe hunter.

TOWARDS A PLAGUE VACCINE

With the discovery of *Yersinia pestis* the first step in eradicating the Black Death had been achieved but the disease would continue to take its toll until a successful weapon against it was available. The first vaccine for bubonic plague predated Yersin's and was developed by Waldemar Haffkine two years after *Yersinia pestis* was identified. It was one of two vaccines developed by Haffkine which greatly advanced the lot of humankind. His first vaccine proved to be successful against cholera, caused by the bacterium *Vibrio cholerae* that Robert Koch had isolated in Egypt in 1883.

Waldemar Mordecai Wolff Haffkine, known in Russia as Vladimir Khavkin, was the son of a Jewish schoolmaster. He was born on 15 March 1860 in the Black Sea port of Odessa, which was then an intellectual and prosperous commercial centre of Russia. Haffkine went to school in Berdiansk and after graduating from high school in 1879 he enrolled in the Department of Natural Sciences in Odessa Malorossiysky University and studied physics, mathematics and zoology.

As for many Jewish people, life was difficult for Haffkine in anti-Semitic Russia during the Jewish pogroms. While at university Haffkine fortunately came under the influence of the prominent scientist Elie Metchnikov. Also during his university years Haffkine joined the Odessa Jewish self-defence league and when he was arrested and tried by the Russian authorities, the high-profile Metchnikov intervened on his behalf and he was released. However, the experience brought home to Haffkine how unsafe it was for Jewish intellectuals in Russia. However, Haffkine managed to complete his studies and in 1883 was awarded his degree in Natural Sciences.

After graduating in 1884, Haffkine joined the staff of the Zoological Museum in Odessa where he spent the next five years. His early research on infusoria, minute aquatic creatures including protozoa and unicellular algae, led to the publication of several papers in Russian and French scientific journals and pointed him in the direction of future research.[22] Despite such early scientific accomplishments Haffkine was denied a teaching position at a university, having refused to denounce his own religion and be baptised as a Christian. Haffkine's response was that he had been a Jew before he became a bacteriologist and that there was a greater honour in remaining a Jew than in denying who he was to get ahead in his chosen field.[23]

Realising how precarious his situation was, Haffkine made the decision to leave his homeland. There was no future for him in Russia and certainly no way to advance his career. In 1888 the authorities gave him permission to emigrate to Switzerland and during his first year there Haffkine worked as an assistant at the medical school at the University of Geneva. It was the right move. At the age of 28, Haffkine became Assistant Professor of Physiology under Professor Schiff, and after eighteen months in this position, Louis Pasteur invited him to join the prestigious Pasteur Institute in Paris.

The day after his arrival, in 1889, Pasteur came to welcome Haffkine and found him nailing something to the doorpost of his laboratory. When Pasteur quipped that Haffkine had wasted no time in renovating his lab, the young scientist explained that he was putting up a *mezuzah,* a quotation from the Torah that is customarily nailed to the doorpost of a Jew's living quarters or workplace. Pasteur seemed quizzical about why Haffkine was doing this in a laboratory, 'a place of science'. Haffkine is reported to have replied that it was important to do so, 'particularly in a place where we search for truth and need God's guidance in the quest'.[24] This certainly accorded with Pasteur's philosophy.

Elie Metchnikov, Haffkine's mentor, had preceded him to the institute and was already working on the cellular defence mechanism of the human body against microbial diseases. Haffkine went to work on producing a cholera vaccine. During the nineteenth century five cholera pandemics ravaged Asia and Europe, taking a heavy toll of human life. Some scientists were still sceptical that the micro-organism *Vibrio cholerae* was the sole cause of the disease, but Haffkine produced his vaccine from an attenuated form of this bacterium by exposing it to blasts of hot air.

After successful animal trials Haffkine, prepared to make the ultimate sacrifice for science, performed the first human test on himself, injecting himself with cholera bacteria and then with his serum. Two days later he reported to Pasteur that the serum he had produced was not toxic to humans, and a few weeks after this, still suffering no effects, he reported his findings to the Biological Society.[25] Although his discovery caused excitement in the press, there was resistance in the medical establishment in France, Germany and Russia. Even more perturbing for Haffkine was the lukewarm response of his senior colleagues, including Metchnikov and Pasteur.

Perhaps prompted by disappointment at this point in his career and also by altruism, in 1893 Haffkine moved to India where hundreds of thousands of people were dying from ongoing epidemics. The Indian government was intensely interested in Haffkine's new prophylactic vaccination for cholera and asked him to conduct trials. Little did Haffkine know that it would not be long before he would be directing his scientific zeal towards developing a vaccine for the seemingly invincible bubonic plague.

Haffkine made Calcutta his headquarters. At first in many communities, Haffkine, his vaccine and his motives were met with deep suspicion and he survived an assassination attempt by Islamic extremists. Haffkine's commitment was greater than his fear, however, and during his first year in India he managed to vaccinate approximately 25,000 volunteers, most of whom did not contract cholera. It almost goes without saying that local medical bodies were critical of Haffkine's cholera vaccine, but the phenomenal results could not be ignored for long. Within a short space of time Haffkine's vaccine was saving lives all over the world. While successfully fighting one disease, Haffkine contracted another one, malaria, which left him no choice but to return to France to recover.

In a report on his Indian expedition to the Royal College of Physicians in London in August 1895, Haffkine dedicated his successes to Pasteur, who had recently died. Pasteur may not have supported Haffkine in the way he had expected but he had given Haffkine opportunities that were denied him in Russia. Haffkine was acknowledging that his association with Pasteur and other eminent scientists had shaped the direction of his research.

Although still suffering from the effects of malaria and against his doctor's advice, Haffkine returned to India in March 1896 and threw himself once more into his crusade. He performed 30,000 cholera vaccinations over a period of seven months. And then as a reminder of how formidable a foe disease is, in October of that year a bubonic plague pandemic flared and struck Bombay. People throughout the entire country began to panic as thousands fell victim to the disease and died and thousands more fled the city. At this critical moment, the government turned to Haffkine for help once again. He immediately left Calcutta for Bombay to launch an assault against the age-old Black Plague.

On arriving in Bombay on 7 October 1896, Haffkine started work immediately to develop two vaccines, one that would prevent the disease and one that could cure it, as he felt this two-pronged approach would be the best way to control the plague. In a makeshift laboratory in a corridor of Grant Medical College Haffkine began the arduous work.[26] After four months a curative vaccine was ready for testing but it was not reliable so Haffkine turned his focus to producing a prophylactic vaccine using dead bacteria. The first obstacle Haffkine successfully overcame was to find a way to grow the plague bacilli, which he did in small glass containers. Once this was achieved the preparation of plague vaccine became feasible.

After another three months of persistent and fatiguing work, one of Haffkine's assistants became ill and two others resigned. Haffkine ploughed on regardless and a vaccine was ready for human trials by January 1897. On 10 January Haffkine, as he had done with the cholera vaccine, vaccinated himself publicly to demonstrate the vaccine was harmless. The following month tests were carried out on volunteers at the Byculla jail. All the prisoners who were vaccinated survived the epidemic, while seven inmates from the control group who did not receive the vaccine died.[27] The government immediately embarked on vaccination campaigns and by the turn of the century, the number of people vaccinated in India alone reached 4 million.

Recognition followed quickly for Haffkine and his vaccine. The Aga Khan provided a building for a dedicated plague research laboratory. Haffkine was appointed as Director of the Plague Laboratory and prominent citizens of Bombay supported his research. Apart from producing and providing the vaccine for the whole of India the laboratory prepared many thousands of doses of vaccine for various tropical countries and Haffkine's method of producing the vaccine remained basically unchanged for decades.

At times Haffkine must have wondered how much he had to achieve to win acceptance. After all his successes he still faced opposition from officials in several countries, including Russia. Even so, hedging their bets, two of Haffkine's Russian colleagues visited him in 1898 in Bombay during a cholera outbreak in Russia. The significance of Haffkine's cholera vaccine was immediately obvious. Called *limfa Havkina* (Havkin's lymph) in Russia, the vaccine subsequently saved thousands of lives across the empire.

So many of the early medical pioneers had careers that were roller-coaster rides and Haffkine was no exception. He suffered greatly during an incident that became known unofficially as the Little Dreyfus Affair because of similarities with events that occurred in France in 1894 concerning a Jewish army officer, Alfred Dreyfus. (Tried for treason and sentenced to life imprisonment, it was many years before it was proven that Dreyfus was innocent and had been convicted on false evidence. The Dreyfus Affair split French public opinion and there were accusations that Dreyfus had been persecuted because he was a Jew.) Haffkine's Little Dreyfus Affair began in a Punjabi village in 1902, when nineteen villagers who were vaccinated from the same bottle of bubonic plague vaccine died from tetanus.

A commission of inquiry indicted Haffkine. He was relieved of his position as Director of the Plague Laboratory and travelled to England where the Lister Institute reinvestigated the claim against him.[28] The original findings were overruled and the blame placed at the door of the doctor who administered the injections. It was discovered that an assistant had failed to sterilise a bottle cap that was contaminated with tetanus spores.

In July 1907, a letter published in *The Times* in London called the case against Haffkine 'distinctly disproven'. It was signed by Ronald Ross, the Nobel Prize winner for his malaria research who spearheaded the campaign to exonerate Haffkine, and other medical luminaries and Nobel laureates, among whom were William Smith who was the President of the Council of the Royal Institute of Public Health, and Simon Flexner, the Director of Laboratories at the New York Rockefeller Institute. This was an affirmation of the esteem in which Haffkine was held in the scientific world.

After being absolved of any wrongdoing Haffkine returned to India to find that he had been replaced at the Plague Laboratory in Bombay. Once again overcoming disappointment and wanting to stay in India, Haffkine moved to Calcutta, where he worked until his retirement and his return to France in 1914. He settled in Boulogne-sur-Seine, occasionally writing articles for medical journals. In 1925, Haffkine must have felt both vindicated and valued when the Plague Laboratory in Bombay was renamed the Haffkine Institute in his honour. The Haffkine Biopharmaceutical Corporation Ltd and the Haffkine Institute for Training, Research and Testing in Mumbai continue to be important centres for public health.[29] Haffkine later wrote that 'the work at Bombay absorbed the best years of my life'.[30]

Haffkine returned to Russia only once. In 1927 he visited Odessa briefly but found it difficult to adapt to the tremendous changes wrought by the Russian Revolution. In 1928 Haffkine moved to Lausanne and spent the last two years of his life there. He remained a practising Jew and in 1929, shortly before his death, still painfully aware of the persecution he had suffered, used some of the fortune he had amassed to establish the Haffkine Foundation in Lausanne to foster Jewish education in Eastern Europe.

The gifted scientist Waldemar Haffkine, who according to those who knew him had a strong personality but also possessed unusual charm, died on 26 October 1930. Apart from stemming the tide of epidemics with his vaccines for cholera and bubonic plague Haffkine had made many other significant contributions to science. He had conducted research on monocellular organisms, infectious diseases associated with infusoria, the adaptability of microbes to their environment and Asiatic cholera. In India, the government was indebted to Haffkine for his contribution to public health and he was the recipient of a number of honours. On the 104th anniversary of his birth, the Indian Posts and Telegraphs Department brought out a special commemorative stamp in memory of 'this great bacteriologist, whose work was of immense value to India'. In issuing the stamp the department also made the point that, 'Perhaps the greatest tribute our countrymen have paid to him is by naming after him the Bacteriological Laboratory at Bombay, which he established.'[31]

In the 1960s the people of Israel commemorated the centenary of Haffkine's birth with the establishment of the Haffkine Park. He was also honoured on an Israeli stamp issued in 1994. Featured on the stamp is the title of one of Haffkine's manuscripts: 'What to do against the plague in India'.[32] Waldemar Haffkine had worked out what to do and what he did was immeasurable. Much of Haffkine's work as a bacteriologist was carried out in India in difficult conditions and with inadequate funds and equipment, a familiar theme amongst the stories of the medical pioneers. He was committed to helping in the endless fight against disease and to achieve this was not averse to personal risk-taking. Whatever his methods, Waldemar Haffkine was referrred to by Joseph Lister as 'a saviour of humanity'.

UNDERSTANDING TRANSMISSION OF THE PLAGUE

Shibasaburo Kitasato and Alexandre Yersin had discovered the cause of the abominable Black Death and Waldemar Haffkine had developed a miraculous vaccine but the way in which plague was transmitted was still not understood. In many countries disinfection campaigns were undertaken, homes were washed with lime, suspected carriers were herded into camps and hospitals and travel restrictions were introduced. In some places carbolic acid was run through sewers, a practice which actually spread the disease even more rapidly because it flushed out rats that lived there, the very rats that carried plague flees.

In 1894 during the Chinese epidemic, Dr Mary Miles, a physician working in Canton, had reported on the widespread death of rats during plague epidemics. But people assumed the rats caught the disease from humans. Robert Koch had also pointed to rats as the cause. In 1897, a Japanese physician, Masanori Ogata, wrote: 'One should pay attention to insects like fleas for, as the rat becomes cold after death, they leave their host and may transmit the plague virus directly to man.'[33] Someone was needed to put all the clues together. In the United States, Paul Louis Simmond collated various observations and experimented with the bacillus, rats and fleas, observing that rat fleas bit people and that a sick animal could not transmit the disease if it didn't have fleas. Simmond's conclusions, published in 1898, were ridiculed (as was so often the case), but in 1905 a British commission published similar findings. The commission issued another report in 1908 that confirmed Simmond's conclusions without crediting him. At last the blame was directed where it belonged. Fleas transmitted bubonic plague, not rats or humans.

The last plague pandemic ended in China and India in the late 1800s but sporadic outbreaks continued to occur throughout the twentieth century. In 1899 the plague was carried to America by stowaways on a ship sailing from Hong Kong to San Francisco. The following year there were outbreaks of plague in Portugal and Australia and another scare in San Francisco when during an autopsy a city health officer found organisms that looked like plague bacilli in the body of a deceased Chinese man. In the next few years over 100 people died from plague in San Francisco. An effort was made to quarantine and clean up parts of the city, but in 1906, when San Francisco was devastated by an earthquake, people were left homeless and so were the rats.

During the rebuilding program thousands of people lived in refugee camps that were highly conducive to rat and flea infestations. In 1907 new cases of plague were reported. Armed with the new knowledge about the method of transmission, officials launched a different kind of campaign: they offered a bounty on rats. A similar rat-catching campaign had been used successfully to fight plague in New Orleans and it proved successful again in San Francisco.[34] The widespread outbreak was brought to a halt in 1909.

There were outbreaks of plague in other parts of the world as well. China was particularly hard hit. In 1910, the year after plague had been controlled in San Francisco, 60,000 people died in Manchuria of the pneumonic strain. Ten years later in 1920 it struck Manchuria again, killing just as many. Much more recently, in the summer of 1994, 5000 cases of pneumonic plague occurred in Surat in India, killing approximately 100 people.[35] According to World Health Organization figures there are 2500 new cases of the bubonic plague annually and 180 annual deaths, of which 75 per cent occur in Africa.

Today plague is successfully treated with antibiotics although about 1 in 10 cases can still be fatal because rapid diagnosis is essential. Despite the great inroads since *Yersinia pestis* was outed by Kitasato and Yersin, plague remains endemic in many countries in Africa, in the former Soviet Union, the Americas and Asia. It also exists in animal populations across vast areas of southern and central Russia; Mongolia; parts of China and southern Asia; southern and east Africa including Madagascar; North America; Mexico; the Andes and the mountains of Brazil. There are no plague-infected animal populations, however, in Europe or Australia.

In 1996 the World Health Organization, after having recorded 24,000 plague cases over a fifteen-year period, reclassified the plague as a 're-emerging disease'. Like tuberculosis, it is making a comeback. The WHO continues to report on and monitor outbreaks of plague in various parts of the world. This was the case in Zambia in 2001, and Malawi and India in 2002. In the Indian village of Hat Koti in Himachal Pradesh sixteen cases of pneumonic plague were confirmed.[36] Under the guidance of the National Institute of Communicable Diseases (NICD) the local health administration took various measures, including vaccination and fumigation, to control the spread of the disease.

The Algerian Ministry of Health reported an outbreak of plague in June 2003 in Tafraoui, on the outskirts of Oran. Of the ten cases there were eight cases of bubonic plague and two of septicaemic plague, one of which was fatal. Patients were treated with antibiotics and once again preventative measures stopped the spread.[37] Overall in 2003, nine countries reported 2118 cases of plague and 182 deaths. This is a far cry from the Great Mortality of the fourteenth century.

In February 2005, WHO received reports of 61 deaths of pneumonic plague in the Democratic Republic of Congo and dispatched a multi-disciplinary team to deal with the outbreak. The WHO was still dealing with outbreaks of plague there in late 2006; control has proved difficult because of the country's ongoing internal conflict.[38] Various news sources reported on 19 April 2006 that in Los Angeles a woman had been admitted to a hospital with a fever, swollen lymph nodes and several other symptoms, the first case of bubonic plague in Los Angeles County since 1984. The woman was successfully treated with antibiotics. In 2006 there were two deaths attributed to plague in New Mexico, the first fatalities in that state in twelve years.[39] With plague still present in animal populations in various countries, humans remain at risk.

Today the control of bubonic plague does not rely on the vaccine developed by Waldemar Haffkine in 1896. With various modifications a plague vaccine was available until the mid 1990s, but because of short-term effectiveness and many side-effects, production ceased. Plague vaccination is no longer recommended for immediate protection in outbreak situations except as a prophylactic measure for high-risk groups such as laboratory personnel who are constantly exposed to the risk of contamination. Surveillance strategies and a range of control measures — taking precautions against flea bites, avoiding direct contact with infective tissues and people infected with pneumonic plague — are tools used by the WHO and other health agencies for preventing outbreaks of plague.

In 2005 the World Health Organization introduced the Epidemic and Pandemic Alert Response, the aim of which is to prepare for global health emergencies by ensuring there are adequate laboratory capabilities and warning and alert systems in place, by implementing national and international training programs and by developing standardised methods for responding to epidemics. The category of epidemic diseases includes plague but also emerging diseases such as SARS, avian influenza and viral haemorrhagic fevers which have been the cause of panic in recent years.[40]

Despite the breakthroughs achieved by scientists like Waldemar Haffkine, the struggle for existence between humans and disease is far from over. The WHO continues to build on the discoveries of the medical pioneers to ensure that the world never again experiences the horror of a pandemic such as the Great Mortality. Sadly, the medical miracles performed by scientific geniuses a century ago have been undermined. As with smallpox, bubonic plague has a reputation for being used as a biological weapon and in the current climate of the early 21st century the threat has not lessened.

Historical accounts from Mediaeval Europe detail the use of infected animal carcasses and human bodies to contaminate enemy water supplies during times of war. Particularly gruesome are accounts of plague victims being tossed by catapult into cities under siege. During the Japanese occupation of Manchuria from the early 1930s until the end of World War II, the Japanese army developed weaponised plague. Civilians and prisoners of war were deliberately infected with plague bacterium and some were dissected in macabre experiments while still living and conscious. Science is not always used for the greater good. It has been suggested that after World War II both the United States and the Soviet Union developed methods for weaponising pneumonic plague including strains resistant to antibiotics. More recently, developments in genetic engineering have led to new experimentation and there is fear that strains of plague bacilli resistant to all drugs, including penicillin, may have been developed.

The disappearance of three mice infected with *Yersinia pestis* in September 2005 from a Public Health Research Institute laboratory located at the University of Medicine and Dentistry of New Jersey was cause for alarm. The laboratory conducts anti-bioterrorism research for the United States government. Authorities launched a search for the animals and an investigation into how they might have escaped.[41]

Suggestions ranged from the feasible to the very worrying: the mice may have been stolen; the mice may have cannibalised each other; the mice were 'unaccounted for' due to a paperwork error. The institute's director said that the disappearance was more likely the result of 'an honest mistake', a response which probably requires some qualification. Some experts expressed surprise at the idea that the mice could escape because of the tight security at the lab, which is categorised as biosafety level 3 out of a possible 4.[42] Although the issue was played down — the public were assured that the mice posed very little risk even if they had escaped — the FBI joined in the investigation, as did the Centers for Disease Control and Prevention.

The mice have not been located. There are suggestions that research into plague and plague vaccines has tripled in the United States following the fears of bioterrorism sparked by September 11. Whatever the trend, it is impossible to know how many laboratories throughout the world currently hold infected animals — potential escapees.

In October 2001, the science journal *Nature* announced that the complete genetic structure of the plague bacilli had been unravelled by scientists at the Sanger Centre in Cambridge in the United Kingdom.[43] Brendan Wren, a scientist who helped to sequence the DNA of the plague bacterium, said that the 'missing mice' incident was extraordinary, but he pointed out that there are many animals in the wild that carry the bacterium. The real worry he noted is that there may be animals carrying a plague bacterium that has been engineered in a clandestine laboratory to be resistant to any form of treatment.

It is not all doom-saying, however. According to the leader of the team that sequenced the 4.65 million DNA letters, the successful unravelling of the complete genetic structure of *Yersinia pestis* will be 'the basis of all future work' on plague.[44] It is critical for the design of more effective antibiotics and vaccines to treat the disease. The knowledge is also insurance against potential new plague threats whether created by natural selection or weapons of bioterrorism, a concept that would have been anathema to Alexandre Yersin, Shibasaburo Kitasato and Waldemar Haffkine. To these scientists, plague was a scourge of nature. Their concern was to save humanity, not destroy it.

POSTSCRIPT

Alexandre Yersin lived a simple life in Nha Trang and was respected by people in the region for his humility and for all that he did to improve their lives. The locals affectionately called his home Lau Ong Nam, 'Home of Fifth Uncle' (the First Uncle is Ho Chi Minh, the man who led Vietnam to independence from France) and it has become a national shrine. His legacy is remembered in many different ways in Vietnam today. Throughout the country there are many towns where streets are still named after this selfless scientist. In 1935 the municipal authorities in Da Lat established a school, the Lycée Yersin, to honour Yersin's medical achievements. The French international school in Hanoi, Lycée Français Alexandre Yersin, is named in his honour. And in Nha Trang, every year on the first day of March, over 50 years after Yersin's death, many of the local people still come to his grave, bringing joss sticks and fruit as offerings to show their gratitude to this dedicated scientist.

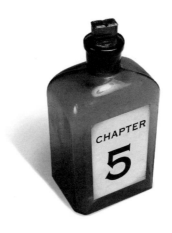

BANISHING THE 'STRANGLING ANGEL'

DIPHTHERIA, TETANUS AND
BEHRING'S BLOOD SERUM THERAPY

Both Pam and Poppy became very ill with sore
throats and could hardly swallow ... In spite of my
mother's and Betty's round the clock nursing, poor
Pam died a week later followed by Poppy the day
after ... my mother was in a state of deep shock
and had been confined to bed by the doctor but
worse still it was feared that Mary the baby had
also caught the dreaded diphtheria ... We must
have a curse on us.[1]

Benjamin Edward Walker

The disease diphtheria swept through Europe during the seventeenth
century and struck the American colonies in the eighteenth century, killing
1 in 10 of its victims. Tragically most of them were children, their deaths
usually the result of suffocation. Diphtheria, an upper respiratory tract
infection, was called the 'strangling angel' because it came unexpectedly
and took so many young lives. Tetanus, an acute infectious disease that was

also rampant at that time, had another name as well. It was dubbed 'lock-jaw' because of the uncontrollable and painful muscle spasms it induced in its victims. With both these diseases it was the manner of death that was most frightening.

The discoveries of 'cures' for tetanus and diphtheria are inextricably linked, not only because of the scientists involved in discovering treatments to combat these diseases but also because of the science that made the cures possible in the late 1800s. The lead roles in this story are taken by the German physician Emil von Behring, whose brain-child was Serum Therapy — treating tetanus and diphtheria using antitoxic blood serum — and the Japanese bacteriologist Shibasaburo Kitasato, who began working on tetanus five years before he discovered the cause of bubonic plague.

From the time Shibasaburo Kitasato arrived in Berlin in 1885 to join Robert Koch's team at the Berlin Institute of Hygiene it was immediately obvious that he was a superior scientist. Kitasato focused on typhoid, cholera and anthrax for the first three years after his arrival and began his research on tetanus early in 1889. In April of that year, at the eighteenth Congress of the German Surgical Association, Kitasato was able to announce that he had isolated the tetanus bacillus, *Clostridium tetani*, after only three months of work. It was possible for Kitasato to do this in such a short space of time because of his fastidious approach to his work. Before he began in earnest Kitasato had thought through the experiment as a whole, designed the experimental procedure and protocols and predicted the results.[2] Perhaps he applied this method later to finding the plague bacillus, which he isolated even more quickly.

Prior to Kitasato's breakthrough, in 1884 the Spanish researchers Antonio Carle and Giorgio Rattone had injected animals with pus from a man who had died of tetanus, and proved that the disease could be transmitted. Also that year, the Berlin physician Arthur Nicolaier produced tetanus in animals by injecting them with samples of soil, indicating that an organism was the cause. Under a microscope the tetanus bacterium looks like a slender rod and it is the toxin produced by this micro-organism that causes tetanus. The bacteria are generally found in manured soil, are sensitive to heat and cannot live in the presence of oxygen. However, *Clostridium tetani* can survive these conditions by developing spores that are very resistant to heat and to many antiseptics and chemicals. In fact, they can survive autoclaving (heating) at 121°C for up to 15 minutes.[3] This goes some way to explaining why tetanus has survived for aeons.

The most common way of contracting tetanus is when the spores enter the body through a skin wound, even a simple cut or prick with a thorn. *Clostridium tetani* produces two exotoxins, tetanolysin and tetanospasmin. (Exotoxins are soluble toxic substances secreted by some species of bacteria that are released into the host.) The function of tetanolysin is not really known, but tetanospasmin is a neurotoxin which causes the tetanus symptoms. An interesting statistic is that, on the basis of weight, it is one of the most potent toxins known. The minimum human lethal dose is estimated to be 2.5 nanograms per kilogram of body weight (one-billionth of a gram), an amount that is almost impossible to conceive.[4]

Tetanus can be contracted almost anywhere in the world because of the ubiquity of the spores but they are more common in hot, damp climates where the soil is rich in organic matter. This is particularly the case with manure-treated soils because the spores can be carried in the intestines and faeces of both large and small animals. Also in agricultural areas it is easy for humans to carry the organism internally and on the surface of the skin. Today, as a by-product of the society in which we live, the spores are increasingly being found in contaminated heroin. Spores can lie dormant in the soil and remain infectious for more than 40 years.

There are four different clinical forms of tetanus that humans can contract: cephalic, local, generalised and neonatal tetanus. Both the cephalic and the local form are quite rare. The generalised form of tetanus is the most common and accounts for 80 per cent of cases. The fourth type, neonatal tetanus, is a common cause of infant mortality in developing countries. Neonatal tetanus can occur when a baby's umbilical cord is severed with an unsterilised instrument contaminated with *tetani* spores and when the cut is sealed with contaminated substances.[5]

The incubation period for tetanus varies depending on how far the wound is from the central nervous system. It can be as little as three days or as long as fifteen weeks but the average is eight days. The longer the incubation period the less likely a person is to die as a result of the infection. A deep wound allows the bacteria to flourish and causes a quick, aggressive infection that is much more life-threatening. It is when the bacteria multiply in the wound that they produce tetanospasmin, the neurotoxin that attacks the nerves. Symptoms include an increase in body temperature by 2–4°C, excessive sweating, elevated blood pressure, muscle rigidity and severe muscle spasms. The spasms begin in the neck and jaw muscles, hence the name 'lockjaw'. As the spasming spreads to other muscles, victims find it difficult to swallow and suffer breathing difficulties, and when the spasms reach the abdomen victims go into painful and powerful convulsions that can tear muscles and fracture bones.[6] It is horrifying to witness these spasms and as they progress abnormal heart rhythms can develop, causing death in many cases. For those who survive, muscle contractions and spasms last for three to four weeks but complete recovery can often take months.

Today, despite a vaccine being available, for which we are indebted to Emil von Behring and Shibasaburo Kitasato, both generalised tetanus and the neonatal form remain a significant public health problem in developing countries where the mortality rate for people contracting tetanus can be as high as 60 per cent, although on average the rate is closer to 30 per cent. Of the approximately 1 million cases of tetanus that are reported annually worldwide, an estimated 300,000 to 500,000 people die as a result, the main reason being that they have not been vaccinated.

A HIGHLY CONTAGIOUS DISEASE

When deciding which formidable diseases to challenge with the new and growing scientific knowledge that had been acquired in the late 1800s in Louis Pasteur's and Robert Koch's laboratories, tetanus certainly presented as a likely candidate. Tetanus had survived unchallenged since ancient times. The Greek physician Hippocrates had written about tetanus in the fifth century BC and there are clinical descriptions of the disease in other documents from that time. In a post Germ Theory of Disease world tetanus was at last in the firing line.

Shibasaburo Kitasato's achievements were already significant when Emil Adolf von Behring, who began his career as a doctor in the army, was assigned to the Berlin Institute by the military authorities in 1888 as an assistant to Robert Koch. Born on 15 March 1854 in Hansdorf, West Prussia, which is now in Poland, Emil was one of thirteen children in the Behring family and the first child of nine born to August Behring, the village school teacher, and his second wife, Augustine Zech. Even as a child it was obvious that Emil was intellectually gifted, so much so that the village minister took an interest in Emil's education and arranged for him to attend the high school in the village of Hohenstein.[7] Influenced by his patron, Emil then began to study theology.

With his quick mind, Emil found his interests broadening and his focus moved from religion to medicine. Fortunately he was able to begin medical studies at the University of Berlin due to the assistance of a family friend who was a military doctor. When it soon became obvious that the salary of Emil's school teacher father was inadequate to keep Emil at university, Emil entered the Academy for Military Doctors at the Royal Medical-Surgical Friedrich-Wilhelm Institute in Berlin in 1874 to complete his studies, even though it meant serving for several years in the military after qualifying as a doctor. Behring was awarded his medical degree in 1878 and was entitled to practise medicine after passing the mandatory state examination in 1880.

It was during the early years of Behring's career as a military doctor that he first became interested in infection and how substances in the blood fight disease. While working at the chemical department of the Experimental Station in Posen in Poland he gained valuable practical experience as a doctor and in his spare time delved into the study of septic diseases. During the years 1881 to 1883 the young doctor carried out important investigations on the action of the chemical iodoform (a crystalline solid of the organic halogen compounds, first prepared in 1822 and used as an antiseptic in medications). He determined that it did not kill microbes as a vaccine does, but had the capacity to neutralise the poisons given off by them and was thus antitoxic. This early research was crucial to his later studies of tetanus and diphtheria toxins. Behring began publishing his findings in 1882.

With the advances in medical science the German government began to realise the benefits that could be gained for military health if epidemics could be prevented and combated. Because of Behring's expertise and his interest in disease he was promoted to the rank of captain and assigned to the medical corps at the Pharmacological Institute at the University of Bonn where he was tutored in experimental methods by the respected pharmacologist Karl Binz. Together they worked on iodoform, which was considered as a highly effective topical treatment for skin ulcers.

In 1888 Behring received orders to transfer to the Berlin Institute of Hygiene, considered at the time to be at the cutting edge of research. Thrilled with this appointment Behring began his close association not only with Robert Koch but also with Shibasaburo Kitasato and Paul Ehrlich, who had joined the institute in 1890. Many of the young and eager 'microbe hunters' later followed Robert Koch when he moved to the Institute for Infectious Diseases in 1891. Behring's research was inextricably tied to the epoch-making work of these scientists and others — Louis Pasteur, Friedrich Loeffler, Emile Roux, Alexandre Yersin and Elie Metchnikov. Collectively they laid the foundations for the study of bacterial diseases and the science of immunology.

When Emil von Behring began his work at the Institute of Hygiene other scientists were already conducting research into diphtheria. It had become a serious concern in many countries and the fact that it was a child killer added an emotional urgency to the desire to find ways to fight the disease. Today, most of us in the developed world would never have experienced the disease or even know someone who has had it. But diphtheria was, in the not too distant past, one of the most dreaded diseases and there were frequent large-scale outbreaks in many parts of the world. The diphtheria epidemic that hit the New England colonies in North America between 1735 and 1740 was said to have killed, in some of the towns, as many as 80 per cent of the children under ten years of age.[8] Often whole families died of the disease in the space of a few weeks. No one was safe from the 'strangling angel', whether rich or poor.

By the nineteenth century, as many as 1 in 10 people were afflicted by diphtheria, many of whom died horribly from suffocation, paralysis and heart failure. Ten years before diphtheria research began in earnest in Paris and Berlin, the disease struck the British royal family. Queen Victoria's daughter, Princess Alice, who was married to the German Prince Louis of Hesse, contracted diphtheria from her children while she was caring for them during their illness. One daughter, Princess Marie, died in November 1878 and Princess Alice herself died a month later.[9]

The French physician Pierre Bretonneau had given the disease its name in 1826. It is derived from the Greek word for 'leather', which alludes to the leathery, sheath-like membrane that grows on the tonsils, throat and in the nose of the afflicted, often blocking the airway and causing them to choke to death. In 1883 Edwin Klebs, a professor of pathology at Zürich University between 1872 and 1892, had discovered and described the diphtheria bacillus, *Corynebacterium diphtheriae*. The following year, 1884, Friedrich Loeffler, who applied Koch's postulates in his research, had successfully cultivated the bacillus and proved that it caused diphtheria by injecting it into animals.[10] This was an important milestone in finding a way to prevent the highly contagious disease which was spread so easily through direct physical contact or breathing the secretions of those already infected with *Corynebacterium diphtheriae*, which also became known as the Klebs-Loeffler bacillus.

Diphtheria has an incubation period of two to five days. The early symptoms are a sore throat, low-grade fever and the growth of a membrane that adheres to the tonsils, pharynx and, in some cases, the nose. Pharyngeal diphtheria, which takes its name from the pharynx, is the most common form. Laryngeal diphtheria, which involves the voice-box, or larynx, is the form most likely to produce serious complications. In children who become infected symptoms can include nausea, vomiting, chills and a high fever, although some do not show symptoms until the infection has progressed significantly. In 10 per cent of cases victims experience neck swelling, sometimes referred to as 'bull neck', which indicates a high level of exotoxin in the bloodstream and is associated with a higher risk of death due to obstruction of the airways.[11]

In addition to these symptoms, a person who has contracted diphtheria may become pale and listless and develop a fast heart rate. As with tetanus the symptoms are caused by the toxin that the bacterium releases. Some people also develop low blood pressure. Longer-term effects of the diphtheria toxin include cardiomyopathy, a heart muscle disease that impairs the heart's ability to pump blood, and damage to the sensory nerves in the peripheral nervous system, the network that transmits information from the brain and spinal cord to every other part of the body.

One of the first early effective treatments for diphtheria was developed in the 1880s by an American physician, Joseph O'Dwyer. He inserted specially designed tubes into the throats of victims to prevent them from suffocating from the membrane sheath that obstructed the airways. But this development did nothing to prevent or cure the disease. However, the collaborative research conducted by Emile Roux and Alexandre Yersin at the Pasteur Institute was a significant stepping stone. Building on Friedrich Loeffler's discovery, Roux, who had assisted Pasteur in his research on the anthrax and rabies viruses, made the first analysis of the chemical properties of the bacillus's toxin.

Over a three-year period Roux and Yersin had shown that filtrates of diphtheria cultures which contained no bacilli contained a substance which they called a 'toxin'. They found that when it was injected into different animals — guinea pigs, rabbits, dogs, cats and horses — all developed diphtheria symptoms. The symptoms were caused by the toxin released by the bacteria, which remained in the filtrate even after the bacteria had been removed.[12] This finding was critical to Emil von Behring's development of an antiserum to the toxin, which he called an 'antitoxin'.

Roux and Yersin published their findings between 1888 and 1891. In their first publication they confirmed Loeffler's methods of cultivating the bacteria. They presented their conclusion that the diphtheria bacillus was capable of producing a poison, or diphtheria toxin, and had proved this by passing cultures of the diphtheria bacillus in a broth through porcelain Chamberland filters. The bacteria were trapped but the sterile filtrate caused the disease when it was injected into experimental animals. In their second paper, published in 1890, Roux and Yersin described in detail their procedure for producing the toxin and reported the results of their in-depth and complex investigations into its pathogenic effect on various experimental animals.[13] A technique for the laboratory diagnosis of diphtheria was outlined in their third paper, which came out in 1891.

Today a diphtheria diagnosis is confirmed by taking a swab of material from the infected area and placing it on a microscope slide where it is stained using a procedure called Gram's stain. The diphtheria bacillus is called gram-positive because it holds the dye after the slide is rinsed with alcohol. Under the microscope, diphtheria bacilli look like beaded rod-shaped cells, grouped in patterns that resemble Chinese characters. Another laboratory test involves growing the diphtheria bacillus on what is called Loeffler's medium, after Friedrich Loeffler.[14] He had developed a new medium in which to isolate and cultivate the diphtheria bacillus as Koch's gelatin method did not work with the diphtheria pathogen. So many of the great scientists have given their names to procedures and protocols and often the connection between the name and what was achieved has been lost over the years.

A MONUMENTAL BREAKTHROUGH FOR IMMUNISATION

In 1889 Emil von Behring realised that Yersin and Loeffler had given him a starting point from which he could work to develop an immunising serum for diphtheria. It was also at this point that the collaboration between Behring and Kitasato began. Informed by the observations Behring had made some years earlier on the action of iodoform, the two scientists, experimenting mainly with diphtheria and tetanus bacilli, set out to find whether they could disinfect the living organisms with various disinfectants.[15] What they did find was that when animals were injected with graduated doses of attenuated forms of toxins, their blood produced antitoxins which would neutralise the invading bacilli. This meant that animals injected with the bacilli that cause tetanus and diphtheria produced substances in their blood that neutralised the toxins produced by the bacteria.

Behring and Kitasato repeated their experiments with rats, guinea pigs and rabbits, injecting them with attenuated forms of diphtheria and tetanus bacilli. The next phase was to inject blood serums produced by these animals into non-immunised animals that had previously been infected with the fully virulent bacteria. The antitoxins miraculously cured the ill animals. The third breakthrough was that healthy animals became immune to the diseases when they were injected with the blood serum and they remained resistant for long periods of time. Antitoxin serum extracted from their blood could then be used to treat other animals.[16] This finding was to prove monumental in explaining the workings of the immune system and in the development of future vaccines.

In 1890, Kitasato and Behring jointly published their classic paper, 'The Mechanism of Immunity in Animals to Diphtheria and Tetanus', reporting on their discovery that for the first time the passive immunisation method was used to fight infectious diseases because the presence of tetanus and diphtheria toxins in blood causes the blood to produce antitoxins that neutralise the poisonous substances.[17] Emil von Behring called this new procedure 'Blood Serum Therapy'. What made it vastly different to vaccination was that in Blood Serum Therapy it was possible to provide an animal with passive immunity by injecting it with the blood serum of another animal infected with the disease, not with a vaccine made from the infective organism. The news of a 'real cure' created a sensation. Behring and Kitasato continued to repeat their experiments so that there could be no doubt about their findings. Other scientists did likewise which resulted in a flurry of publications confirming the original results.

Hard on the heels of his joint publication with Kitasato in 1890, Behring — now as a sole author — published an authoritative paper dealing with immunity against diphtheria and outlining five ways in which this could be achieved. He had conceived of the idea that curing both tetanus and diphtheria in humans might now be possible by producing an antitoxin against them. To achieve this, Behring collaborated with his university friend Erich Wernicke on the first therapeutic serum for diphtheria, and with Shibasaburo Kitasato he developed an effective therapeutic serum against tetanus.[18] The tetanus antitoxin was made by first injecting the tetanus bacteria into an experimental animal, such as a rabbit or guinea pig. The blood was then removed from the infected animal. Next, that blood was injected into a second animal, such as a horse. Finally, the blood was removed from the second animal, and from this blood the vaccine to be used on humans was made.

In 1891 the tetanus serum was introduced but not entirely in the way Behring had hoped. The Institute of Hygiene had the support of the Agricultural Ministry to develop tetanus serum but the ministry's main concern was with protecting valuable agricultural animals.[19] Behring's primary motive had been to help humans and it was not based on economics. Elation gave way to disillusionment when it became obvious that he had no support for large-scale clinical testing of the serum on humans. A program for protecting animals went ahead and the considerable amounts of blood serum required were obtained through immunising horses.

A wonderful opportunity to help humankind had been squandered and some twenty years later when World War I broke out in 1914, because there had been insufficient 'proof of the pudding', the military were reluctant to use the life-saving tetanus serum. During the first months of the war the Germans suffered massive losses and thousands of those lives, lost to tetanus, could have been saved. There were some hit-and-miss attempts to use the tetanus antitoxin serum in a number of military hospitals which failed dismally. There was very little of the precious blood serum available and what little there was, was often mishandled because many practitioners had not been adequately trained in its use.

At the end of the first year of the war Behring could no longer stand by and accept the unnecessary deaths. He waged his own campaign to have the authorities support the use of the serum. By this time he was in a position to exercise some influence and by April 1915 the earlier setbacks of distribution and control were overcome as he was personally involved in the production of the serum at his own laboratory.[20] In army hospitals the serum was used for both treatment and prophylaxis and the numbers of soldiers succumbing to tetanus fell dramatically. Emil von Behring was hailed as the 'Saviour of the German Soldiers' and his contribution was recognised with the award of the Prussian Iron Cross medal. This was the proof that tetanus could become a preventable and a curable disease.

The development of the diphtheria serum took a different course. Emil von Behring developed his therapeutic serum for diphtheria in 1891. The antitoxin did not kill the bacteria but neutralised the toxic poisons that the bacteria released into the body. More than 50,000 children in Germany were dying every year from diphtheria and 1891 was a particularly bad year as the vicious disease with the mellifluous name was taking a huge toll on the young.[21] There was no time to waste and the serum was used for the first time to treat a seriously ill child. She made a full recovery. In 1892 the Hoechst chemical and pharmaceutical company at Frankfurt am Main became interested in the therapeutic potential of the diphtheria antitoxin (and no doubt in the financial potential as well) and began working with Behring to develop the serum to make it viable.

By 1893 Behring had successfully treated a group of human diphtheria patients with antitoxin but there were constant setbacks because the toxin did not yield consistent results. Enter Paul Ehrlich. He who had improved Koch's method of staining the tubercle bacilli in 1882 was chiefly responsible for standardising the diphtheria antitoxin, thus making its widespread therapeutic use possible. Ehrlich had determined that the toxin–antitoxin reaction, which is a chemical reaction, was accelerated by heat and retarded by cold and that the content of antitoxin in antitoxic serums varied greatly for a range of reasons. Therefore it was necessary to establish a standard by which the antitoxin content could be measured exactly. The method that Ehrlich devised for determining the effectiveness of serums, not just diphtheria serum, was soon adopted all over the world.

Because of Ehrlich the potential for the diphtheria serum to save lives on a mass scale was now feasible and Behring entered into a formal partnership with Ehrlich, one which would come to an acrimonious end. They had a contract drawn up which laid down the terms of their future collaboration. Together they organised a laboratory under the railroad circle, the Stadtbahnbogen, in Berlin, so that diphtheria serum could be produced in sufficiently large amounts.[22] Even though the diphtheria serum and the antiserum could be standardised using guinea pigs, in order to extract enough antitoxin it was necessary to use large animals, as had been the case with the tetanus serum, and they began with sheep.[23]

After a series of experiments, Ehrlich and Behring determined that high-quality antitoxin could be obtained from horses as well as from sheep and this opened the way for large-scale production. In 1894 the Hoechst pharmaceutical company began the production and marketing of the diphtheria therapeutic serum and a successful commercial partnership was established between Behring and the company. But this was to have a detrimental effect on the partnership between Behring and Ehrlich.

While working on the development of the diphtheria serum Behring was given the opportunity to leave the army and start an academic career. One of the leading officials from the Prussian Ministry of Education and Cultural Affairs, Friedrich Althoff, who wanted to improve the control of epidemics in Prussia by supporting bacteriological research, secured a position for Behring at the University of Halle-Wittenberg in 1894. After a short time in the position of Professor of Hygiene, he was again recruited by Althoff to take over the vacant chair of Hygiene at Philipps University of Marburg in April 1895. [24]

Behring's appointment as a full professor followed shortly after but the moment was marred when professional snobbery raised its head. There was vehement opposition to Behring from members of the faculty who, although acknowledging his outstanding discoveries, believed that the position of university lecturer in hygiene would be better filled by someone from within the field (no doubt one from amidst their ranks) not by Behring, who came from a medical background. Althoff rejected all the counterproposals, however, and Behring took over as Director of the Institute of Hygiene at Marburg University. His position included giving lectures on hygiene and on the history of medicine. In 1896, the institute moved to a new location which gave Behring the opportunity to divide it into two departments: a Research Department for Experimental Therapy and a Teaching Department for Hygiene and Bacteriology. He remained director of the institute for the next twenty years until his retirement in May 1916.

During his early career Behring had been totally committed to his work and for whatever reason had not married, although lack of funds has been suggested. The year 1896 brought another change to Behring's life when at the age of 40 he married Else Spinola who was half his age. Else was the daughter of Werner Spinola, the administrative director of Charité, the university medical hospital in Berlin.

During their life together Else and Behring had seven children. [25] Friends described Behring as a contented family man, although somewhat patriarchal, which was entirely in keeping with society in the early twentieth century and with his stature in the scientific world. Behring's passionate devotion to his work meant that Else and the children had to share him. Behring had a vast number of contacts and belonged to an eclectic and distinguished discussion group called 'the Marburg Circle'. Among its members were the zoologist Eugen Korschelt, the botanist Arthur Meyer, the physiologist Friedrich Schenk and the pathologist Carl August Beneke, to name a few.

The incestuous nature of the scientific elite becomes evident when looking at who the early medical pioneers had as their friends and sometimes their enemies. The list of godfathers Behring chose for three of his sons reads like a who's who from the Berlin Institute of Hygiene and the Pasteur Institute. Behring chose his friend and co-worker Erich Wernicke and the bacteriologist Friedrich Loeffler to be godfathers to his first son, Fritz. The godfather of his third son, Hans, was the Prussian Under-Secretary of Education and Cultural Affairs, Friedrich Althoff, who supported Behring's career. The godfathers of his fifth son, Emil, were Elie Metchnikov, founder of the theory of phagocytosis, with whom Behring had a continuous scientific exchange of ideas, and Emile Roux who, like Behring, conducted groundbreaking research on diphtheria.[26]

Paul Ehrlich was not on the list. Despite their early scientific collaboration and friendship, tension developed between the two and they fell out. After Ehrlich was made director of a government-supported institute near Berlin the relationship never recovered. When the institute was transferred to Frankfurt am Main in 1899 it was called the Royal Institute for Experimental Therapy and Ehrlich was given a free rein in his research there. This irked Behring, who wanted his colleague to continue specialising in immunology and serum therapy but Ehrlich was moving in a different direction. Inherent personality differences had also strained the relationship. Ehrlich was utterly indifferent to monetary rewards and he saw Behring as having aligned himself with wealthy industrialists. He resented Behring's ambition and was content to immerse himself in research for its own sake and that of the greater good. Friedrich Althoff attempted to mediate but the friendship between the two scientists was never really restored. It is interesting to note that what was believed to be the only photograph showing Behring and Ehrlich together, which appeared on the cover of a Berlin newspaper to celebrate their 60th birthdays in 1914 — Ehrlich was born on 14 March 1854 and Behring was born on the 15th — was actually two separate photographs spliced together.[27]

Because of what they had achieved together, however, diphtheria was no longer invincible and despite some early difficulties with production, widespread use of the diphtheria antitoxin followed. Some specific problems with the serum also had to be overcome. It had to be administered soon after infection but this was not always possible because getting an accurate diagnosis was not a straightforward matter. As with anything new in the medical field the antitoxin soon had its critics, who spoke out in a very audible and public way. Resistance did not last long, however. Several studies published in the 1890s attested to the serum's miraculous success and even with the delays in administering the antitoxin, the number of deaths from dipththeria was soon almost halved.

In fact, the fall in the diphtheria death rate around the turn of the twentieth century was one of the sharpest ever recorded for any treatment. In Germany alone, an estimated 45,000 lives per year were saved. It is for this unprecedented contribution to humankind, and to children in particular, that Emil von Behring was celebrated throughout the world when he was awarded the very first Nobel Prize in Physiology or Medicine in 1901 for his work on Serum Therapy. It was the decision of the Nobel committee that Behring, through his discovery of Serum Therapy and its particular application against diphtheria, 'had opened a new road in the domain of medical science and thereby placed in the hands of the physician a victorious weapon against illness and deaths'.[28]

BEHRING RESEARCHES TB, CONTINUES DIPHTHERIA WORK
Established in his position at Marburg University, settled in his domestic life and celebrated for his contribution to humanity, Behring turned his

mind to one of his other research interests, the fight against tuberculosis. Robert Koch had failed disastrously with his tuberculosis therapy, tuberculin, in 1893, so Behring began to search for an effective therapeutic agent against this disease. However, very soon, he had to admit that combating tuberculosis using Serum Therapy was not feasible. He changed course and began to concentrate on a preventive vaccine. For reasons that were not positive Behring was able to spend more time on tuberculosis research from 1901 onwards: he began to suffer from poor health and was no longer able to sustain his rigorous academic work.

Assuming that the different forms of tuberculosis found in humans and in cattle were actually closely related, Behring experimented, immunising calves with a weakened strain of the human tuberculosis bacillus but the results were disappointing.[29] Although his bovine vaccine was widely used for a time in Germany, Russia, Sweden and the United States, it was found that the cattle later excreted micro-organisms that were still virulent and could cause further infection. Nevertheless, Behring's basic idea of using a bacillus from one species to benefit another influenced the development of later vaccines. Each piece of new information added to the armoury of disease-fighting weapons.

While working on tuberculosis, Behring did not entirely abandon his work on diphtheria. In 1898, while collaborating with Erich Wernicke, Behring had found that immunity to diphtheria could be produced in animals by injecting them with diphtheria toxin neutralised by diphtheria antitoxin. In 1901, Behring, for the first time, used a vaccination of diphtheria bacteria with reduced virulence. Whereas the first therapeutic serum he had developed could prevent diphtheria for only a short period of time, Behring hoped that with this active immunisation the body would be stimulated to produce its own antitoxins.[30] It is well-established knowledge today that active vaccination stimulates antitoxins, which we now call antibodies.

Research on diphtheria had also been carried out in other laboratories during the 1890s. In 1891, a pathologist in New York City, Anna Wessels Williams, isolated a stronger and more effective strain of diphtheria antitoxin.[31] In 1894, Emile Roux developed a diphtheria antitoxin serum using horses. He used this serum to successfully treat more than 300 diseased children in the Hôpital des Enfantes-Malades in Paris and was hailed as a hero throughout Europe.

The development of an active vaccine took some years as Behring was unable to work consistently. The demon that drove him to work also plunged him into the depths of depression and he sought treatment in a sanatorium between 1907 and 1910. Behring was also coping with a condition that increasingly impaired his mobility, the result of fracturing one of his thighs. He was far from finished, however. By 1913, the year before war broke out in Europe, Behring had managed to resume his work and had successfully completed the new phase of his diphtheria research. He then publicly announced his diphtheria protective agent, toxin–antitoxin (T.A.).[32]

T.A. contained a mixture of diphtheria toxin and therapeutic serum antitoxin. The toxin was meant to cause a light general response from the body, without causing the disease itself. In addition, it was a longer lasting vaccine designed to provide long-term protection. A range of trials proved it to be non-harmful and effective. In the same year that T.A. was announced, the Hungarian scientist and paediatrician Bela Schick produced another medical marvel: a simple and reliable test to determine whether a person is susceptible to diphtheria.[33] The Schick test involves injecting a small amount of toxin under the skin. If a red, swollen rash appears around the injection, the person is susceptible and should be immunised.

Subsequent modifications which refined Behring's toxin–antitoxin mixture resulted in the modern methods of immunisation that have largely banished the blight of diphtheria. Behring himself saw this as the crowning achievement of his life's work. In the same way that Jenner believed that smallpox could be eradicated, Behring believed in the possibility of ridding the world of diphtheria.

Emil von Behring was a man of great intellect and he was a tireless worker both in research and in academia, for which he enjoyed many financial rewards. Unlike many of his peers he also had business acumen and his commercial arrangements with private pharmaceutical firms added to his prosperity. Behring owned an impressive estate at Marburg which was large enough to accommodate the livestock he needed for use in his own experiments. He and Else opened their house as a gathering place for society and the couple also owned a vacation home on the island of Capri in the Mediterranean, where they had honeymooned.

In 1914 Behring took stock and changed tack. To regain autonomy over his scientific work he founded the Behringwerke in Marburg, an institute where the manufacture of serums and vaccines could be under his control and he could also determine the nature of research that was undertaken.[34] His independent wealth made this possible. Today the Behringwerke is a large corporation with worldwide operations in pharmaceutical manufacture. Research is still conducted there, mainly in the field of immunology.

When the war began in 1914, Behring was able, because of the Behringwerke, to make the decision to cease his efforts to combat tuberculosis and dedicate himself entirely to the development of the tetanus serum as this was the greater need. The overwhelming success of the serum during the war went some way towards consoling him for the wanton waste of life that he was witnessing. The obscenity of war saddened him. His life's work had been dedicated to wiping out diseases, the enemy of the human species, but he had no vaccine that could be used to prevent humans turning on each other.

Emil von Behring, the 'Saviour of the German Soldiers', like many soldiers, did not live to see the end of the war. Behring was already in a precarious state of health when he contracted pneumonia in 1917. His frail body was unable to withstand the added strain and he died on 31 March in Marburg and was entombed in a mausoleum at the Marburg Elsenhöhe. Else von Behring lived on without her husband until 1936 when Germany was witnessing the rise of Adolf Hitler and the National Socialist Party. Else died from a heart attack at the age of 59.

Apart from receiving a Nobel Prize in 1901, Emil von Behring was honoured in many ways during his lifetime for his extraordinary medical achievements. He was elevated to the status of the nobility and in 1903 he was elected to the Privy Council with the title of Excellency. He was granted honorary memberships of societies in Italy, Turkey, France, Hungary and Russia; he became an officer of the French Legion of Honour and an honorary freeman of Marburg.[35] However, despite all outward appearances of wealth and personal and professional success Behring had endured his share of difficulties, disappointments and ill-health.

DIPHTHERIA INTO THE TWENTIETH CENTURY AND BEYOND

In the early 1900s death rates from diphtheria remained high in countries where immunisation was not widespread. In the United States in the 1920s there were an estimated 100,000 to 200,000 cases of diphtheria per year, resulting in 13,000 to 15,000 deaths. Children still represented the large majority of cases and fatalities.[36] Behring's work was taken up by new pioneers. A new vaccine for diphtheria, a formalin-inactivated toxin (formalin rendered the toxins harmless) was developed in the United States by Alexander Glenny and Barbara Hopkins in 1923. Standardisation was required, as with Behring's toxoid, and was carried out using guinea pigs. In the same year, Gaston Ramon, working at the Pasteur Institute in France, chemically detoxified diphtheria toxin by using formaldehyde — and provided the world with one of its safest and most reliable vaccines.[37]

The uptake of diphtheria vaccination was patchy from the mid 1920s onwards. Behring had hoped for more. Progress was slow in Britain but successes in various local health districts eventually led to acceptance. Widespread vaccination began to occur across the country in the 1940s when the death rate from diphtheria was still at about 10 per 100,000 of population. Over the following ten years the incidence of diphtheria dropped to virtually zero. There was a similar pattern in the United States:

by 1989 there were only 24 cases of diphtheria reported and only two were fatal. Astonishingly, only one case of diphtheria was reported in the United States in 1999.

Diphtheria has now been largely eradicated in developed nations due to the combined DPT (diphtheria–pertussis–tetanus) vaccination programs. DTP is a combination vaccine that was developed in the 1940s containing weak toxins that serve to stimulate the growth of antibodies to diphtheria and tetanus combined with inactivated pertussis (whooping cough) bacterial cells.[38] However, in areas where the immunisation rate has fallen, such as Eastern Europe and the newly independent states of the former Soviet Union, tens of thousands of people have suffered from diphtheria in recent years. In 1990, an outbreak began in Russia and over a period of four years spread to every state of the former Soviet Union. By the time the epidemic was contained, over 150,000 cases and 5000 deaths had been reported.[39] A vast public health immunisation campaign was implemented and had largely confined the epidemic by 1999.

In 1991, the Food and Drug Administration in the United States licensed the DTaP (diphtheria–tetanus–acellular pertussis) vaccine. While DTP vaccine was made using whole cells of the pertussis germ, DTaP is made using only small, purified pieces of the germs. Fewer side-effects have been reported with the DTaP vaccine than with DTP, which is no longer recommended for use in the United States. DTP is currently still widely used in other countries and is equally effective.

Today 1 out of every 10 people who get diphtheria still dies from the disease. Universal immunisation is the most effective means of preventing and eradicating it. With DTP it is recommended that three injections be administered two months apart, beginning at about two months after birth. Booster shots are given at fifteen months and four to six years. The most important treatment for diphtheria remains a prompt injection of diphtheria antitoxin which neutralises any circulating exotoxin. It is still made from horse serum because a human antitoxin is still not available for the treatment of diphtheria. Antibiotics such as penicillin, ampicillin or erythromycin are given to wipe out the bacteria, to prevent the spread of the disease and to protect the patient from developing pneumonia but they are not a substitute for treatment with antitoxin.[40]

As with other diseases, the World Health Organization monitors the incidence of diphtheria internationally. In 2003 there was an outbreak in Afghanistan in a resettlement camp for internally displaced persons in Kandahar. Around 75 per cent of the cases were children aged five to fourteen. In response the WHO undertook a mass vaccination of around 40,000 people.[41]

The acceptance of immunisation has also led to a significant decline in tetanus in many countries. The first tetanus vaccine to be made from tetanus toxoid, an inactivated toxin, was produced in 1924 and was successfully used to prevent tetanus during World War II.[42] The same procedure used to develop the diphtheria vaccine was used to protect against tetanus: first, passive immunisation using horse anti-tetanus serum — Behring's Serum Therapy — followed by active immunisation with the tetanus toxoid. In this form it became part of the DTP vaccine. A tetanus booster is recommended every ten years, with an additional tetanus injection administered if a person suffers a severe wound.

Globally, tetanus mortality dropped from between 20 to 50 deaths per million per annum between 1945 and 1950, to less than 0.16 per million in 1996.[43] War is certainly an ally of disease. Tetanus remains a problem in countries with very low rates of immunisation, as well as those that are at war or experiencing civil unrest where there are often high rates of injury.

A very disturbing statistic is that in developing countries approximately 200,000 young babies and 30,000 mothers die each year from tetanus, which represents the second-highest cause of death by vaccine-preventable diseases. The true extent of the tetanus death toll is not really known. Eight countries account for about 73 per cent of neonatal tetanus deaths: Bangladesh, China, the Democratic Republic of the Congo, Ethiopia, India, Nigeria, Pakistan and Somalia. Many women live in rural areas in these countries and have little access to healthcare. Newborns and mothers die at home and neither the birth nor the death is reported. For this reason, tetanus is now often called the 'silent killer'.

In 1989 the World Health Assembly called for the elimination of neonatal tetanus worldwide. By necessity, the objective was redefined in 1993 to achieving less than one case of neonatal tetanus per 1000 live births in all at-risk countries by the year 2000. In 2000, 104 of the 161 developing countries that were targeted had achieved this. The result was accomplished by improving the immunisation rates of pregnant women — rates in the target population jumped from 4 per cent to 66 per cent in 1997 — and by improving sanitary conditions during childbirth.[44] In 2006 a new campaign to provide up to 6 million tetanus vaccinations to protect vulnerable mothers and their new babies was launched by UNICEF because studies have shown that 100 per cent of children born to mothers who are vaccinated during pregnancy possess protective antibodies to tetanus.

It was the discovery of Blood Serum Therapy by Emil von Behring and Shibasaburo Kitasato which led to the development of vaccines and cures for diphtheria and tetanus and also laid the foundations for the understanding of the body's immune system. Their research into bacterial diseases at the end of the nineteenth century and the beginning of the twentieth also paved the way for the later development of penicillin and other antibiotics.

Although they had parted company, in the Croonian Lecture delivered at the Royal Society of London on 22 March 1900, Professor Dr Paul Ehrlich, Director of the Royal Institute for Experimental Therapy, acknowledged that with 'Behring's remarkable discovery, that in the blood serum of animals immunised against diphtheria and tetanus, there were contained bodies which were able to specifically protect other animals against the toxines [sic] of these diseases', he had introduced an entirely new factor into the study of immunity and provided a promising prospect of immunising humankind against the majority of infectious diseases.[45]

POSTSCRIPT

On 4 December 1940, in the second year of World War II, the Philipps University at Marburg celebrated the 50th anniversary of the original publication of Emil von Behring's discovery of Serum Therapy. Present at the ceremony were leaders of Adolf Hitler's National Socialist Party, the elite from numerous German universities, many distinguished scientists and Behring's friends, some of whom had travelled from other countries for the occasion.

One of Behring's sons participated in the ceremony but he was not greeted by any of the official speakers. The reason for this was that the Nazis had regarded Else von Behring as a 'half-Jew', because her mother came from a Jewish family. Fearing for her children, with the help of a number of friends Else had managed to have her six sons accepted by Hitler as 'Aryans'. After her death in 1936, the Nazi party claimed Emil von Behring as an exemplification of national socialist 'Germanic' science. It was all part of Nazi propaganda.

During the celebration at Marburg a new Behring Memorial was unveiled and at a two-day scientific meeting that followed, scientists discussed developments in immunology and the battle against infectious diseases. It is hard to imagine such enlightened discussion about medical discoveries to advance human health when we consider the progress of World War II and the medical experimentation that was conducted during the Nazi period.

At the meeting, only the Danish researcher Thorvald Madsen, who had previously been chairman of the Health Organization of the League of Nations, dared to mention Emil von Behring's personal and professional relationships with researchers from what had become enemy countries, including those at the Pasteur Institute in Paris. Courageously, Madsen also recalled how the brilliant Paul Ehrlich, despised by the Nazis because of his Jewish origin, had contributed significantly to Behring's success.

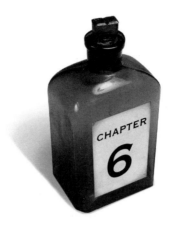

CHAPTER

6

Magic Bullets

PAUL EHRLICH, SERENDIPITY, SYPHILIS AND THE BEGINNING OF CHEMOTHERAPY

It is unthinkable for a Frenchman to arrive at
middle age without having syphilis and the Cross
of the Legion of Honour.[1]

André Gide

In the first decades of the twentieth century the medical profession's understanding of health and disease was expanding. Louis Pasteur's Germ Theory of Disease had provided specific enemies for researchers to target and vaccines had been developed for some of humankind's most vicious foes: smallpox, rabies, bubonic plague and cholera. With the emergence of immunisation and subsequent developments such as Emil von Behring's Blood Serum Therapy, it had become established that antibodies could be produced in response to specific microbes — antibodies that were toxic only to those microbes, but harmless to the patient.

This was the theoretical basis for the development of 'designer' drugs, drugs that target a specific pathogen. In the early 1900s the German bacteriologist and medical scientist Paul Ehrlich, who had worked with Emil von Behring, predicted the future of pharmaceutical research. After the introduction of Blood Serum Therapy he envisioned that chemists might soon be able to produce substances which he called 'magic bullets' that would have the capacity to target specific disease-causing agents. And it was Paul Ehrlich himself who set the designer drug revolution in motion when, in 1909, while he was looking for a cure for the microbial disease sleeping sickness, serendipitously discovered a cure for syphilis.

The origins of syphilis have been a subject of much contentious debate. Some scientists suggest that syphilis — and the micro-organism that causes it, *Treponema pallidum* — existed in isolation in the New World and was brought back to Europe after Christopher Columbus discovered the Americas in 1492. The evidence for this is that an epidemic in Europe coincided with Columbus' return in 1493. Some historians propose that the disease was carried by sailors who contracted it from indigenous people in the West Indies. Since war was common in Europe during this period, the constant movement of troops was a perfect conduit for spreading an epidemic. Historians who disagree with this theory point to ancient accounts in a range of sources from the Bible to Chinese documents which describe symptoms that seem consistent with late-stage syphilis. Because documentary evidence does not exist of illnesses compatible with syphilis amongst the indigenous peoples of the New World before European imperial expansion, other historians conclude that it was Europeans who brought the disease to the New World. A third view is that syphilis emerged in the Old World and the New World independently.[2] Wherever it came from, syphilis spread like wildfire throughout Europe during the 1600s.

Confusion about its origin is reflected in the many names syphilis had prior to the one by which it is now known. The Italians called it the French disease, the name which had the widest currency. The French, refusing to lay claim to it, called syphilis the disease of Naples. The English used several names that implicated both the French and the Spanish among others. In the Middle East it was referred to as the European pustules. It was an international game of blame and name calling. The disease actually received its modern name from the Italian physician and poet Fracastoro. In 1530 he wrote about a shepherd suffering from 'the great pox' in his poem *Syphilis, sive morbus gallicus*.[3] The word 'syphilis', the name of the shepherd, was adopted by some physicians for the disease but it was not widely used until the nineteenth century.

The descriptions of symptoms associated with syphilis written in the late fifteenth and early sixteenth centuries indicate that it was initially more rapacious than it is today. It was debilitating, spread rapidly and killed quickly. Known as the great pox, in contrast to smallpox, the pustules which developed on the body of the afflicted could be the size of large acorns and were described as dark green in colour and foul smelling.[4] Other symptoms included rashes, mouth ulcers, severe fevers and bone pains and in many cases death was the result.

At the beginning of the twentieth century there were very few chemical treatments for the plethora of infectious diseases that humans endured and there was no cure for syphilis. For more than three centuries mercury, which was also used for ringworm, was the only treatment available for syphilis.[5] It was first used in the late fifteenth century and could be administered orally or rubbed onto the skin. The mercury induced heavy salivation, which was thought to remove the 'bad humours' that caused the illness. Hot vapour baths supposedly had the same effect and syphilitics were often plunged into scalding baths.[6] Treatment was more akin to torture. Often almost lethal doses of mercury were given, causing symptoms that were similar to those of the disease itself. Trained physicians were still using mercury in the mid nineteenth century for syphilitic patients.

There was money to be made from the afflicted in a time when superstition prevailed and there was little understanding of disease. The unscrupulous touted fantastic remedies. In 1858 William Earl claimed that treatment with mercury could be supplanted by his new method which he called an 'Anti Detersive Essence', a complete cure which, he said, needed no recourse to deleterious drugs or chemicals.[7]

The method of transmission, through sexual intercourse, made syphilis a taboo topic. The desperate fell victim to claims that went unchallenged partly because of strict attitudes in Victorian times towards sexuality and the human body. In an age when chair and table legs were covered with fabric skirts to preserve modesty and decorum, open discussions of venereal disease were unlikely to happen.

Until the 1800s, gonorrhoea and syphilis were assumed to be different types of the same disease. In 1837 the French scientist Philippe Ricord, as a result of carrying out experiments on syphilitic *chancres*, or lesions, discovered that they were in fact two specific diseases. Ricord also discovered that syphilis goes through three distinct stages of infection: primary syphilis, secondary syphilis and tertiary syphilis. At the time Ricord was studying the disease it was common for syphilitics to experience a period of latency, in which no symptoms are visible.[8]

Two discoveries made it possible for Paul Ehrlich to find a 'magic bullet' to aim at syphilis. In 1905 in Berlin, Professors Fritz Schaudinn and Erich Hoffmann discovered the cause of syphilis, the spirochaete *Treponema pallidum*. They isolated this pale, corkscrew-shaped organism in serum from a lesion of secondary syphilis. In addition, Schaudinn and Hoffmann believed there was a relationship between spirochaetes and *trypanasomes*, the microorganism that causes sleeping sickness (an inflammation of the brain causing extreme weakness and drowsiness).[9] The following year the first serologic procedure for diagnosing syphilis (a laboratory test carried out on blood serum to detect antibodies associated with a disease) was invented by a group of researchers that included August von Wasserman, Albert Neisser and Carl Bruck.[10]

By the beginning of the twentieth century syphilis and the symptoms associated with the various stages of the disease were better understood. While sexually transmitted, it can also pass from mother to child in utero, in which case it is called congenital syphilis. The course of the disease is long. With primary syphilis, the chancres form at the point of contact, usually on the genitals, but they can appear almost anywhere on the body. Some can be so small that they may go unnoticed. If the chancres do not become infected, they heal without treatment within a month or two. Primary syphilis lasts for ten to 50 days.

While the chancres are healing, the second stage begins. Secondary syphilis starts with the appearance of a rash at six weeks to six months after infection. Bones and joints often become painful and the circulatory system can be affected, causing heart palpitations. These symptoms can be accompanied by fevers, indigestion and headaches. Sometimes lesions develop into moist ulcers (including open sores in the mouth) that are actually teeming with the spirochaetes.

People suffering from syphilis experience a period of latency that lasts anywhere from a few weeks to 30 years. During that time all symptoms disappear until the third stage, tertiary syphilis, begins. Tumours, which are characteristic of late syphilis, begin to appear because of the concentration of spirochaetes in the body's tissues. This is the most acute stage of the disease which can lead to death because the cardiovascular and central nervous systems are compromised. At this stage the disease can also cause a softening of brain tissue resulting in progressive paralysis and insanity.[11]

Syphilis was a dreaded disease, one of many that had wrought immeasurable damage and brought misery to the human race for centuries, virtually unchecked by any drug or therapy. It was via a circuitous route, however, that syphilis came under the scrutiny of Paul Ehrlich. Although his initial intention was to find a cure for sleeping sickness, what transpired was not uncommon when it came to early medical breakthroughs. While following a pre-determined path to find a cure for one disease, the seeker would take a sudden and unintended detour.

Paul Ehrlich was born into a prosperous Jewish family on 14 March 1854 at Strehlen in Upper Silesia in German East Prussia, an area now in Poland.

He was the only son of Ismar Ehrlich, a lottery-office keeper, and Rosa Weigert. Paul's parents were keen for their son to be well educated and when he was ten Paul was sent to preparatory school at Breslau and went on to attend a number of universities between 1872 and 1878.

At eighteen Paul Ehrlich entered the University of Breslau to study natural sciences but soon transferred to Strasbourg University to study medicine. He also spent some time at Freiburg University.[12] As a young student Ehrlich already had interests that he wished to pursue and he began to conduct experiments to test the concept that certain cells seemed to have an affinity for certain chemicals. This was Paul Ehrlich's particular preoccupation.

At Breslau University, Ehrlich studied under the physiologist Heidenhain and the pathologist Cohnheim. Cohnheim's assistant was Ehrlich's older cousin, Karl Weigert, and it was Weigert who introduced Ehrlich to aniline dyes.[13] At the time that Ehrlich was a student, the German dye industry was thriving and new aniline dyes, which had been discovered in 1853, were being used by researchers for tissue staining to enhance the normally colourless tissue sections. Joseph von Gehrlach had shown that nerve tissues could be stained with natural dyes and had used gold chloride or carmine to stain his tissue samples, popularising the method among his contemporaries. With the invention of chemical dyes a greater array of stains became available.[14]

Ehrlich continued his medical studies at the University of Leipzig where he was able to expand the range of his research with aniline dyes. Ehrlich had also developed an interest in the body's reaction to chemicals. He found that different cells held different dyes and he used this knowledge to develop effective staining techniques to study bacterial and other tissues. Amongst his fellow students Ehrlich enjoyed a certain notoriety and he was remembered as the man with blue, yellow, red and green fingers.[15]

At the age of 24 Ehrlich was awarded his medical degree and as was to be expected his dissertation was on the theory and practice of staining animal tissues, with the title being, 'Contributions to the Theory and Practice of Histological Staining'. In it he laid down a basic principle that was to pervade his work: that pharmacological activity is based on the affinity of molecules of living matter for various chemical substances when brought into relationship with them.[16] This assumption would come to underpin the foundation of chemotherapy.

After graduating in 1878 Ehrlich was appointed as an assistant to Professor Friedrich von Frerichs at the medical clinic of Charité Hospital in Berlin. Frerichs recognised Ehrlich's talent and made it possible for him to continue his work with dyes and tissue staining rather than practise clinical medicine even though he was given the position of Senior House Physician. In his research on the reactions of dyes on living cells, Ehrlich gradually developed the fundamental concept that to understand biological processes it would be necessary to describe them in chemical terms.

While still a student, Ehrlich had begun to prepare papers for publication on the morphology of blood, an extension of his work with tissue staining, and had published his first paper on the effects of aniline dyes on living cells. Ehrlich was able to differentiate the elements of blood by colour analysis and this work on the staining of granules in blood cells laid the foundation for another medical discipline, haematology. We tend to forget or are unaware that there are so many specialist areas within medicine that once did not exist because the requisite knowledge was unknown. The discoveries were cumulative. Without an understanding of blood, how much less medicine would be able to do for humans today.

In 1882, after being present at the Physiological Society in Berlin where Robert Koch announced that he had isolated the tubercle bacillus, Ehrlich developed his new method of staining it which Koch then adopted. The method proved to be of decisive importance in finding a way to diagnose tuberculosis. Subsequent modifications to Ehrlich's method were introduced by two scientists who gave their names to the Ziehl–Neelson (ZN) stain which is used today to detect *Mycobacterium tuberculosis*.[17] An even more sensitive diagnostic test was announced in South Africa in 2002 at the Medical Research Council's Molecular and Cellular Biology Centre. Less time-consuming than the ZN stain, the new test can pick up the disease in patients who have very low counts of bacilli which are not detectable with a ZN stain. It was the work of Ehrlich that made possible the development of Gram's method by Danish scientist Hans Christian Gram (see Chapter Five).

Ehlich's scientific output for such a young man was phenomenal but in the midst of this, in 1883, not long before he turned 30, Paul Ehrlich married nineteen-year-old Hedwig Pinkus. It was apparently a happy marriage during which the couple had two daughters, Stephanie and Marianne.[18] They were a close family, which no doubt helped Ehrlich in his frenetic and sometimes troubled and insecure career.

The year after his marriage Ehrlich received an appointment to the University of Berlin as Titular Professor, later becoming Associate Professor. His doctoral thesis, 'The Need of the Organism for Oxygen', was published in 1887. In it he established that oxygen consumption varies with different types of tissue and that these variations constitute a measure of the intensity of vital cell processes.[19] In the course of ten years, Ehrlich had published more than 40 articles on various aspects of his work, but he considered this to be one of the most important.

Ehrlich's early interest was in dyes and how they had a selectivity for specific organs, tissues and cells. He had shown that dyes react specifically with various components of blood cells and the cells of other tissues. Considering the scientific climate of the 1880s and the feverish search for cures, it was probably a natural progression that Ehrlich would begin to test dyes for their therapeutic properties, to determine whether they could kill pathogenic, or disease-producing, microbes.

The end of the first phase of Ehrlich's frenzied scientific research coincided with a change in policy at the medical clinic at the Charité following the death of Frerichs in 1885. Ehrlich was a non-conformist and his position was in jeopardy because he did not enjoy the support of the new administration. He confided in Hedwig that he wanted to quit but this would put them in financial jeopardy.[20] When Ehrlich suddenly became ill with pulmonary tuberculosis, he tested himself with Robert Koch's new diagnostic tuberculin. The test was positive and suddenly circumstances were out of his and Hedwig's control and permanent work was no longer an option. Because of its mild climate Paul Ehrlich spent periods of time during 1888 and 1889 recuperating in Egypt in the hope that his lungs would heal. Hedwig went with him. It has been suggested that this brush with a deadly disease at such an early stage in his scientific career, and the knowledge that he carried the tuberculosis bacteria within him, may have prompted Ehrlich to turn to the study of immunity and to develop his unique chemical approach to the treatment of disease.[21]

When Paul Ehrlich returned to Berlin in 1889 he was free of tuberculosis but was unable to get work. Undeterred, like Koch and Jenner before him, Ehrlich set up his own laboratory where, despite the primitive conditions, he worked out methods for assaying toxins and antitoxins and for determining their correct physiological doses.[22] In 1890 he was approached by Robert Koch, who was then directing the newly established Institute for Infectious Diseases, and Ehrlich was invited to work with him as an assistant.

Ehrlich thus entered a new phase of his research and soon began his trademark immunological studies. It was while working on Blood Serum Therapy with Emil von Behring that Ehrlich solved the puzzle of why Behring was experiencing inconsistencies in the serum and then he devised the procedures for standardising the antitoxin content. Despite the success these two men enjoyed while working together, they were fundamentally different and the rift that developed between them was never breached.

Paul Ehrlich's skill as a researcher at the Berlin institute was acknowledged when, in 1896, he was asked to head the new Royal Institute for Serum Research and Testing, which was established in Steglitz, a suburb in Berlin. Behring could not help but feel resentful, even though the building where Ehrlich was to carry out his work was small and run down and the facilities quite basic compared to what Ehrlich had been used to at the Berlin institute. Such conditions did not phase Ehrlich, who plunged headlong into his work on immunology. He was heard to say that he could work in a barn as long as he had a water tap, a flame and some blotting paper.[23]

Through the efforts of the Lord Mayor of Frankfurt am Main, the Royal Institute for Serum Research and Testing was transferred there in 1899 and Ehrlich accepted an invitation to become its director. For the first time, he was in control of modern, well-equipped laboratories. In Frankfurt, Ehrlich was required to conduct cancer research and evaluate serums for the government, but this was his opportunity to follow his heart. His mind was already investigating chemical therapies.

Ehrlich was indefatigable in his laboratory work, but was surrounded by what appeared to be disorder. He now had his own team of capable assistants and, almost fanatical in the way he ran the laboratory, he assigned daily tasks scrawled on small coloured cards to each person. His instructions were to be carried out to the letter and every team member was required to give a daily progress report. Although described as kindly and verging on shy, Ehrlich was capable of flying into a rage if his directions were not adhered to. Researchers who did not comply soon left the institute. To many Ehrlich was an enigma but no one doubted his genius; a person with the capacity to visualise chemical structures in his mind, even before they had been synthesised, is unlikely to be pedestrian.[24] Those who worked closely with Ehrlich saw him as original and daring in his approach to science.

EHRLICH DEVELOPS A LANDMARK THEORY

Along with the many other things he did, from very early in his career Ehrlich began to develop a chemical structure theory to explain the immune response. At a time when very little was understood about toxins and antitoxins he deduced that they were chemical substances. Chemical knowledge was limited even among scientists who were synthesising therapeutic agents, and very few hypotheses had been put forward about how the therapeutic agents that had been created actually interacted with living systems.[25]

From around 1897, informed by his immunological work with Behring and other research he had undertaken at the Berlin institute, Ehrlich began to formulate his famous Side-chain Theory of Immunity, *Seitenkettentheorie*, in which he sought to explain immunity and how antibodies are formed. Although some of the concepts have since been proven to be incorrect, this theory allowed Ehrlich to achieve new breakthroughs while providing the groundwork for later researchers in the immunological field.

When presenting his Side-chain Theory to the Royal Society in London in March 1900, Ehrlich summarised the science that had led him to his theory and acknowledged the work of those who had paved the way. A century had passed since Jenner had made his great discovery of the protective action of vaccinia against smallpox and, in that time, Ehrlich said, the 'terrible scourge of mankind' had been almost completely eradicated from the civilised world. However, Ehrlich lamented that Jenner's discovery of inducing artificial immunity had stood almost alone in all that time. [26]

Jenner had shown that by the use of an attenuated virus, which itself caused no injury, it was possible to ward off the disease caused by the virulent virus. Jenner had also established that vaccination with the weakened poison produced not only immediate, but also enduring protection. Ehrlich believed that Jenner's discovery remained so isolated because the theoretical conceptions of the cause and nature of infectious diseases had not advanced in the decades after the introduction of the smallpox vaccine. And that was indeed the case.

It was under Pasteur, Ehrlich claimed, that investigation into the cause of infectious disease reached its zenith. Ehrlich was referring to Pasteur's Germ Theory of Disease and he saw the revolution in wound treatment that was led by Joseph Lister as the most significant outcome of Pasteur's fundamental work. This was followed by what Erhlich called Koch's profound investigations on anthrax and the pure cultivation of the most important pathogenic bacteria. Therefore, Ehrlich explained, it was the work of Pasteur and Koch that provided the basis on which the study of artificial immunity could again be undertaken. Because of their work the possibility existed for producing a number of the most important infectious diseases of men and animals, and of modifying pure cultivations of bacteria, either by Jenner's method or in artificial culture media.[27] As a result further advances were at last possible.

After Jenner, Pasteur had been the first to produce an artificial immunity by using an attenuated virus, but even so, asserted Ehrlich, theoretical explanations lagged far behind the practical effects. Behring's remarkable discovery that the blood serum of animals that had been immunised against diphtheria and tetanus contained bodies which were able to specifically protect other animals against the toxins of these diseases, opened the door to new possibilities for protecting humankind against even more diseases.

This, in fact, is what occurred as the twentieth century progressed, but in the short term Ehrlich was disappointed when the success of the diphtheria antitoxic serum that he had worked on with Behring did not lead to a rapid succession of similar achievements. Ehrlich believed that success would only come through an accurate knowledge of the theoretical considerations underlying the question of immunity. To find an answer to that question, he explained to the Royal Society, he had laboured for years trying to 'shed some light into the darkness' that shrouded the subject, and the result was his Side-chain Theory.[28]

Ehrlich then went on to explain. His theory was that every cell has various special receptors, which he called side-chains, similar to the side-chains in dye molecules that he had studied. A side-chain in organic chemistry and biochemistry is a part of a molecule that is attached to a core structure. According to Ehrlich the side-chain receptors work like gatekeepers or locks for the cell, their primary function being to absorb nutrients for the cell.[29] However the receptors also allow many toxic substances to enter. When a cell is attacked by a toxin, it produces excess side-chains matching the toxin which are then released, flooding the body and neutralising toxins by attaching to them. The toxin is wiped out by these 'magic bullets' as Ehrlich called them, immunity is induced and the remaining healthy cells are protected.[30]

Ehrlich's concept was that Blood Serum Therapy was an excellent method of contending with infectious diseases, of providing immunity by stimulating side-chains to act against toxins, but in cases where effective serums could not be discovered, new chemicals could be synthesised to do the same thing. Instead of serum therapies, the magic bullets would be chemical therapies, or 'chemotherapies', a term that Ehrlich coined.[31] As Ehrlich saw it, he would create new substances that would have a specific affinity for pathogens such as bacteria and the chemotherapies would act only on these, and possessing no affinity for any other cells in the body would therefore cause no harm.

With his Side-chain Theory of Immunity and his magic bullet vision of chemotherapy, the chemical understanding of disease and its treatment became possible. Ehrlich's key insight was to think of the specific molecular structure of a substance as leading to specific biological effects.[32] Ehrlich eschewed orthodoxy and to make his vision of magic bullets a reality, against the advice of his colleagues he left the potentially profitable field of serum therapy to immerse himself in developing chemical antitoxins and vaccines that would stimulate the body to fight disease. Ehrlich was motivated by the science and the possibilities for curing disease, never profit.

And so began the third phase of Ehrlich's eclectic research. In the thesis that he had written as a young man he had foreshadowed the direction he would eventually take. Ehrlich had written that the chemical constitution of drugs must be studied in relation to their mode of action and their affinity for the cells of the organisms against which they were directed.[33] Now the time had come. Paul Ehrlich's aim was, as he put it, to find the chemical substances that would naturally go to, or seek out, pathogenic organisms because they are specifically related, in the same way that antitoxins go to toxins. In lay terms he would shoot chemical magic bullets at disease-causing organisms.

Paul Ehrlich began conducting his chemotherapeutic research in earnest at the Institute of Experimental Therapy but he faced opposition from Emil von Behring and his ally the Under-Secretary of Education and Cultural Affairs, Friedrich Althoff. Pressure was applied on Ehrlich to give up his chemical research. Another powerful opponent was Dr Hans Wolfert, the head of the Medical Board who like many doubters amongst the medical profession saw Ehrlich's project as a pipe-dream and a waste of money. Opposition to Ehrlich was also tinged with an undercurrent of anti-Semitic feeling in Germany at the time. Undaunted Ehrlich carried on regardless even when, without warning, his funding was cut in half.

In 1906 fortune smiled on the beleaguered Ehrlich. A benefactor, Frau Franziska Speyer, founded Georg Speyer Haus, a research institute dedicated to chemotherapy. Built next to Ehrlich's institute it had its own staff directed by Ehrlich. In another windfall, the Hoechst and Cassella chemical companies, confident that Ehrlich's project would be a commercial success, entered an agreement with Georg Speyer Haus giving the company the right to patent, manufacture and market preparations discovered by Ehrlich and his colleagues. The companies further agreed to supply the chemical substances that were needed for the chemical synthesis.[34]

Paul Ehrlich decided to find a magic bullet to aim at *trypanosomiasis*, human sleeping sickness, the disease which Robert Koch had spent time researching in Central Africa. He targeted *trypanosomes*, the protozoa that were known to be responsible for a number of diseases including sleeping sickness, with coal-tar dyes, but he had no success. An arsenical compound, Atoxyl, had been discovered in England in 1906 and had proven to be effective with some *trypanosomes* but it caused damage to the optic nerve. Ehrlich became embroiled in a debate with other chemists about the chemical structure of Atoxyl but his preliminary work proved that he was correct.[35]

The exhaustive and obsessive search for an arsenical compound began. Setting a punishing schedule Ehrlich and his assistants began creating chemical variants, seeking one that would possess maximum killing power against the *trypanosomes* while at the same time cause minimum damage to other cells. Ehrlich and his team created 417 separate compounds and tested each thoroughly on laboratory animals before Number 418, arsenophenylglycine, proved somewhat effective against tropical diseases caused by *trypanosomes*. The repetitive research continued. In 1907, compound 606 was created, the hydrochloride of dioxydiaminoarsenobenzene.[36] The compulsive and patient Ehrlich was optimistic about this compound but an assistant erroneously reported that it had no effect whatsoever on *trypanosomes*, and so it was put aside.

It was at this point that Ehrlich changed tack. He decided to pursue the spirochaete *Treponema pallidum*, the micro-organism that causes syphilis and which had been isolated in 1905. While engrossed in this research, in 1908, Paul Ehrlich's remarkable contribution to science was recognised when he was awarded the Nobel Prize in Medicine or Physiology for his scientific work in the field of immunity. He shared this honour with Elie Metchnikov. Ehrlich's work on serums and antitoxins had provided the key concept that the body produces substances that fight disease-causing micro-organisms, which we now call antibodies. Metchnikov, for his part, had discovered that certain body cells, white blood corpuscles, which he called phagocytes, could destroy pathogens by simply engulfing or eating them. Because of the discoveries made by Ehrlich and Metchnikov it is now known that the incredibly complex human immune system mounts attacks in both of these ways.[37] When Ehrlich received the Nobel Prize, however, some of his finest work was still ahead of him.

COMPOUND 606, THE WONDER DRUG

An event that proved critical to finding a cure for syphilis was the arrival at the institute of Dr Sahachiro Hata from Tokyo. The scientific world was somewhat incestuous. Hata was a pupil of Professor Shibasaburo Kitasato who had worked with Emil von Behring on tetanus twenty years earlier, at the time that Ehrlich had joined Robert Koch's team. In Japan Sahachiro Hata had been experimenting with syphilis in rabbits and was sent to Frankfurt for further study.[38] His first assignment after joining Ehrlich was to test every arsenical compound that the team had developed thus far in their search for a cure for sleeping sickness, on animals infected with syphilis. This was a daunting task but also a prime example of Ehrlich's rigour and the commitment he expected from those who worked with him.

Hata set about the task in a thorough and logical way and the break-through came in 1909 when he tested compound 606, which had been discarded in 1907 as being ineffective against sleeping sickness. Hata reported to Ehrlich that it was by far the most effective against syphilis and also the least toxic of all the compounds.[39] Here was a magic bullet that destroyed the micro-organism *Treponema pallidum*. It had been three years of painstaking work for Erhlich and his team, testing over 900 different com-pounds. Compound 606, a cure for syphilis, would soon be marketed under the more manageable name, Salvarsan. The name was chosen by Ehrlich and its meaning, 'that which saves by arsenic', is inherently paradoxical.[40]

Ehrlich was pleased, but true to his nature he demanded further tests, hundreds more tests, to determine effective and safe doses of the com-pound and to establish whether cures were permanent or whether relapses would occur. Hata tested compound 606 over and over again, on mice, on guinea pigs and on rabbits. All had been infected with syphilis and all were completely cured within three weeks. Testing then commenced on humans. Patients at nearby hospitals who were suffering with dementia associated with the final stages of syphilis were treated by physicians willing to cooperate in the trials. Astonishingly, several of these terminal patients recovered after treatment. When hundreds of experiments had repeatedly proved that Salvarsan cured syphilis, Ehrlich announced its release.

Paul Ehrlich and Sahachiro Hata reported on the development of com-pound 606 and the success of their experiments at the Congress for Internal Medicine at Wiesbaden on 19 April 1910. Dr Schreiber of Magdeburg Hospital, who had been involved in the trials, gave an account of the first successful treatment of syphilitic patients at his hospital. When Ehrlich published his seminal paper, 'Experimental Chemotherapy of Spirochaetal Diseases', the medical world went into a frenzy. What Ehrlich had achieved was unprecedented and he was immediately bombarded with requests for the wonder drug.

Salvarsan was registered with the patent office. Facilities at Georg Speyer Haus were geared up in order to make large quantities of the drug. The Hoechst Chemical Works began to build facilities for its manufacture but nevertheless for some time demand far exceeded supply. The success of this revolutionary drug spurred the expansion of the German pharmaceutical industry and Germany soon led the world in chemical and drug production. Within no time Salvarsan was being sold all over the world. Ehrlich received reports from as far away as the St Petersburg Hospital for Men in Russia that Salvarsan had completely cured patients and not one had relapsed.[41]

In 1910 Salvarsan was heralded as a miracle cure for syphilis but Ehrlich insisted on keeping a close check on any irregularity that might arise from its use. It soon became apparent that the magic bullet was not as wondrous as first thought. The treatment was both expensive and painful. Initially Salvarsan was administered by injection but if the injection was not confined to the vein severe local pain resulted. Even when the drug was administered properly, it often caused necrosis, or tissue death, at the injection site. In some cases blood clots caused a swelling of the vein that could result in life-threatening infections. The side-effects were so severe for some patients that they died. Even worse, within a year, some patients who appeared to have been cured had relapsed.[42] The early elation had to be tempered and once again Ehrlich found himself facing powerful opponents, some of whom mounted a legal challenge to have Salvarsan banned.

A court found in Salvarsan's favour and Ehrlich was vindicated. The stress from the trial and the setbacks with his magic bullet left Ehrlich deeply troubled. Determined to find a safer and more effective compound than Salvarsan he returned to the laboratory and began testing again. The 914th arsenical substance, which was given the name Neosalvarsan, was found to be safer, more easily manufactured and, being more soluble, much less difficult for physicians to administer. Although it was not quite as active against the spirochaete, and therefore had less curative effect, it was still preferable to Salvarsan as a treatment.[43] Ehrlich, once again revealing the depths of his enormous intellectual talent and his commitment then devised a method of intravenous injection so that tissue damage and the danger of infection could be minimised and he ensured that the medical profession was instructed on its use.

Paul Ehrlich had created his magic bullet, winning him praise and honours, but fame also put him in the firing line. He had to battle opposition and criticism before Salvarsan and Neosalvarsan were accepted, but opposition was not new to him. There were attacks from crackpots who accused him of trying to poison people, his reputation was sullied by his contemporaries who were motivated by professional jealousy and he also endured slurs that were anti-Semitic in nature.

Salvarsan and Neosalvarsan were a first step only in a cure for syphilis, but they were miraculous compared to what had been on offer for syphilis sufferers in the past, and they gave hope for the discovery of better chemotherapeutic drugs in the future. In 1913 a doctor in the United States, Henry Pulsford, reported on the side-effects of Salvarsan and Neosalvarsan. Within six to eight hours of an injection, patients suffered nausea, vomiting, abdominal pain and diarrhoea. He attributed this reaction to the toxic effects of arsenic and the susceptibility of patients to varying doses of Salvarsan.[44] Pulsford warned about the risk of unnecessary deaths.

Henry Wallhauser, another US physician, elaborated on Pulsford's conclusion and recommended that Salvarsan be administered like other 'dangerous remedies' by giving small, repeated doses at varying intervals.[45] In 1914, Wallhauser grouped the deaths resulting from treatment with Salvarsan into two categories: degenerative and sudden. The latter category perplexed doctors. Patients would fall into a coma on the third or fourth day following injection. Wallhauser came to the conclusion that Salvarsan was safe in the early stages of syphilis, but as the disease progressed and damaged organs, patients could not cope with the toxicity of the arsenic.

In Paris, Ernest Fourneau at the Pasteur Institute applied Ehrlich's techniques to bismuth and created several antisyphilitic compounds to supplement the arsenicals. Some physicians used applications of mercury or bismuth ointments in conjunction with Salvarsan and Neosalvarsan.[46] It was trial and error and prior to World War II the medical profession accepted that while syphilis could be cured, it was a slow, painful and expensive process. Twenty to 40 injections over the course of a year were necessary. However, there was still optimism that the disease would eventually be eradicated.

Salvarsan and Neosalvarsan remained the most effective drugs for treating syphilis until the advent of antibiotics in the 1940s. Without the discovery of Salvarsan the development of antibiotics and also sulfa drugs may not have happened when they did or perhaps not at all. Ehrlich's work inspired other researchers including Alexander Fleming, the discoverer of penicillin. Fleming was one of the first doctors to administer Salvarsan in England and did so using Ehrlich's new intravenous method.[47] Its success encouraged him to search for drugs that would treat and cure bacterial disease even though the consensus amongst the establishment was that vaccination research was the only way forward in the battle against micro-organisms.

Paul Ehrlich lived for five years after the release of Salvarsan. In his personal life he was content despite what seemed to be recurrent turmoil in his professional life. Hedwig had supported him during the good times and the most trying. When World War I broke out Ehrlich was very distressed by the carnage, in the same way that his one-time friend, Emil von Behring, was. Neither of them lived to see the end of the war. Ehrlich never overcame nor did he understand the barrage of unwarranted and unscientific attacks that he endured over Salvarsan. The actions of his critics perturbed him and like-behaviour was not in his nature. Ehrlich's motives were altruistic, his primary motivation being to advance science in order to cure disease. Ehrlich's long career had revealed that, apart from diseases of the body there were also diseases of the soul — greed, hate and ignorance — which humankind seemed incapable of curing.

Late in 1914 Paul Ehrlich suffered a stroke but recovered quickly. Apart from the bout of tuberculosis early in his life, he had enjoyed excellent health. However, at the age of 61 while on a holiday in Bad Homburg, he suffered a second, fatal stroke and died on 20 August 1915. Ehrlich had continued his research almost to the end of his life with his last project being an investigation of tumours. He was buried in the Jewish Cemetery in Frankfurt. An obituary in *The Times* in England acknowledged Ehrlich's scientific and medical achievements, affirming that 'the whole world is in his debt'.[48]

Ehrlich's indefatigable and obsessive nature, his kindness and modesty, his lifelong habit of eating little and smoking cigars incessantly, his insistence on repeating experiments before publishing results, and the respect and dedication of those who worked with him have been vividly captured in a biography entitled *Paul Ehrlich als Mensch und Arbeiter*, written by his secretary, Martha Marquardt.

Paul Ehrlich's place in the history of medicine rests not only on his cure for syphilis. His methods for staining bacteria were of great importance to the development of bacteriology. Through his demonstrations of the chemical reactions of dyes with living cells, haematology and later histology came into their own as sciences. Likewise his methods of assaying and standardising antitoxins are still the basis of immunology. He is credited with conceptualising the cell membrane receptor and was the first person to produce a chemical substance that had measurable chemotherapeutic effects, thus launching the age of chemotherapy. Ahead of his time, Ehrlich also theorised about a concept that he called '*horror autotoxicus*', which is what we now know as auto-immunity.[49] Paul Ehrlich's was an extraordinary mind.

Renowned and revered, Ehrlich was a member of no less than 81 academies and other learned bodies worldwide. His work was honoured with the bestowing of Orders in Germany, Russia, Japan, Spain, Romania, Serbia, Venezuela, Denmark and Norway. He won a plethora of prizes apart from the ultimate, the Nobel Prize. The Prussian government elected him to the highest rank of the Privy Medical Counsel in 1911 which came with the title of Excellency. As recently as 1996 a 200 Deutsche Mark banknote showing Paul Ehrlich was released into German currency. Hedwig Ehrlich also honoured her husband publicly when in 1929 she established the Paul Ehrlich Foundation in association with the Johann Wolfgang Goethe University in Frankfurt am Main. Each year the foundation awards the Paul Ehrlich and Ludwig Darmstaedter Prize, the most distinguished award for biomedical research in Germany.

In 2001 members of the Nobel Foundation looked back over the previous century at the list of people who were considered to have brought the greatest benefit to humankind. Rolf Luft, a physician and scientist who had been chair of the Nobel Committee for Medicine and Physiology, placed Paul Ehrlich at the very top because of what he had achieved both through experimentation and because of his creativity as a theorist.[50]

The Institute for Experimental Therapy in Frankfurt which Ehrlich set up and directed, now bears his name, the Paul Ehrlich Institute, and the address is Paul Ehrlich Strasse. When the Jewish persecution by the Nazis began in the 1930s, the name was removed but has since been restored. The institute, now operated by the Ministry of Health, oversees the control and testing of vaccines. Strehlen, Ehrlich's birthplace, was renamed Ehrlichstadt by the Polish authorities after World War II.

EHRLICH'S INFLUENCE EXTENDS TO CANCER TREATMENT

Paul Ehrlich's legacy is perpetual. A scientific symposium to commemorate the 150th anniversary of his birth and to honour his historic contribution to medical research was held in March 2004 in Frankfurt. Among the institutions that organised the symposium, *Combating Pathogens and Cancer*, were the Paul Ehrlich Institute, Georg Speyer Haus, the Paul Ehrlich Foundation and the Paul Ehrlich Society for Chemotherapy.

The title of the symposium reflects the fact that the human species is in a constant tug-of-war for survival with micro-organisms and disease. In 1945, when penicillin became widely available as an accepted treatment for syphilis coupled with public health measures, the fight against the 'great pockes' appeared to have been won. As it transpired, however, new strains of the spirochaete *Treponema pallidum* developed resistance to penicillin and other antibiotics, as have other diseases, due to the overuse of these drugs. Since the 1950s the incidence of sexually transmitted diseases has been on the rise.

The World Health Organization reports approximately 12 million cases of syphilis each year. In the same way that AIDS is having an impact on other re-emerging diseases, there is a two- to five-fold increased risk of acquiring HIV infection if syphilis is present. It is to be lamented that in the 21st century approximately 500,000 infants, most of them in the developing world, are being born each year with congenital syphilis.

New campaigns against syphilis are ongoing and although Ehrlich may have hoped for more with Salvarsan, he may never have envisioned just how far-reaching the repercussions of his discovery of 'magic bullets' would be. For most of us living in economically advanced countries, because of the phenomenal developments in medicine that took place in the twentieth century, the fear of catching and dying from infectious diseases has diminished. Smallpox, bubonic plague, polio, diphtheria and their ilk are no longer the threat they once were and the names of the diseases themselves are hardly ever spoken in non-medical circles. Today, the diagnosis which engenders most fear is cancer. Since vaccination has been used to control the contagious diseases that were once universal scourges, cancer has taken their place and is now one of the leading causes of death in developed countries.

Again Paul Ehrlich's legacy can be seen around us in the 21st century. He developed the first chemotherapeutic drug and one of the main treatments for cancer remains chemotherapy. Cancer can be viewed either as the collective name of more than 100 different conditions, or one condition with many different target sites in the body. It is the uncontrolled growth and spread of cells that can affect almost any tissue.[51] Lung, colorectal and stomach cancer are among the five most common cancers in the world for both men and women. Among men, lung and stomach cancer are the most common cancers, and for women it is breast and cervical cancer. More than 11 million people are diagnosed with cancer every year and cancer kills 7 million people annually, amounting to 12.5 per cent of all deaths worldwide. It is estimated that there will be 16 million new cases every year by 2020.[52]

New magic bullets have extended the reach of Paul Ehrlich's imagination, most particularly in the realm of chemotherapy. Behind the chemotheraperutic revolution was Ehrlich's seminal idea that scientists could make chemical compounds that could target specific disease agents and that a toxin for that organism could then be delivered along with the agent of selectivity without harming the person afflicted with the disease. This conviction guided many scientists to follow Ehrlich's creativity in chemistry in their search for new chemical therapies such as antimalarials, sulfonamides, antihistamines and ataraxic drugs (drugs that relieve anxiety), and drugs that they would eventually aim directly at cancer.[53] The discovery that certain toxic chemicals are able to cure specific cancers ranks as one of the greatest in modern medicine.

Cancer has always been with us. Over the centuries there have been many theories about its cause. One theory was that cancer was a poison that spread slowly through the body. Cancer was also once believed to be contagious. With the widespread use of the microscope in the eighteenth century, it was discovered that the 'cancer poison' spread from the primary tumour through the lymph nodes to other sites. In the late 1800s the knowledge that the body was made up of various tissues that in turn were made up of millions of cells marked the beginning of cellular pathology and put an end to old theories about chemical imbalances in the body causing cancer.

Before Joseph Lister introduced his methods of asepsis, the use of surgery to treat cancer had poor results due to problems with infection.

With improved surgical hygiene in the nineteenth century the survival statistics went up and surgical removal of tumours became the primary treatment for cancer. Soon after, however, as medical advances began to accelerate, multi-disciplinary approaches to cancer treatment were introduced. The first effective non-surgical cancer treatment became available soon after Marie Curie discovered radiation in 1898.

The era of chemotherapy began in earnest in the 1940s. In the United States, Gertrude Elion and George Hitchings introduced 'rational drug design' to target specific cancers, a new version of the magic bullet.[54] Early spectacular successes in the 1960s made it seem that cancer would be curable with a new range of chemotherapeutic drugs. Not so, and the cancer puzzle is still being solved one piece at a time and chemotherapy is one piece in that puzzle.

In Ehrlich's time, chemotherapy meant the use of chemical substances to treat disease. Today, chemotherapy refers primarily to cytoxic (literally 'cell destroying') drugs that are used to destroy cancer cells by interfering with cell division in various ways, such as the duplication of DNA or the separation of newly formed chromosomes. Most forms of chemotherapy target all rapidly dividing cells and are not specific for cancer cells, which means that chemotherapy has the potential to harm healthy tissue. Nowadays, in addition to surgery, radiotherapy and chemotherapy, cancer can be treated with immunotherapy, or a combination of all these methods.

The concept of a magic bullet as Paul Ehrlich envisioned it was fully realised according to the scientific world with the invention of monoclonal antibodies. These work by targeting tumour-specific antigens, thus enhancing the host's immune response to tumour cells to which the agent attaches itself. The process of producing monoclonal antibodies was invented by Georges Köhler, César Milstein and Niels Kaj Jerne in 1975.

It is difficult to get one's mind around the complexity of cell structure, DNA, auto-immunity and chemical compounds. The research that has gone into discovering and understanding the complexities of cancer cells, then developing drugs to stop them from reproducing, is almost unfathomable to the scientifically untrained and the science behind the development of cancer-curing, chemotherapeutic drugs is becoming increasingly more complex. By understanding the mechanism of a cancer at the genetic level, the most basic inner workings of the cell, scientists are endeavouring to tailor new medicines to inhibit a cancer growth with a precision not previously possible.[55] And beyond this, the aim is to replace abnormal genes with normal ones, so cells regain their normal function. The quest to find 'magic bullets' continues.

Medical breakthroughs are reported on an almost daily basis in the print and visual media. Only time will tell if these breakthroughs will be significantly measurable and eventually change the world. At the beginning of September 2006 a vaccine to protect women against cervical cancer was launched in Australia. It was developed in the 1990s by a Scottish-born Australian, Professor Ian Frazer, a contemporary medical pioneer, his research partner Dr Jian Zhou and their colleagues at the University of Queensland. Final trials of the vaccine, known as Gardasil, showed it to be 100 per cent effective against the most common strains of human papilloma virus (HPV) which causes an estimated 70 per cent of cervical cancers.[56] Around 300,000 women die from cervical cancer annually, the second-biggest cancer killer of women.

Dr Frazer began his research twenty years ago working in a basement at Brisbane's Princess Alexandra Hospital. Two decades on, his research is likely to revolutionise women's health worldwide. The vaccine is based on Dr Frazer's 1991 discovery of a way to create artificial HPV in the test tube, minus any infectious material. The vaccine works by provoking an immune response to HPV. The researchers made the skin or shell of the virus without the insides so that to the immune system it looks like the virus but is not infectious. The vaccine is now in use in many countries.

On 1 September 2006 it was widely reported that, for the first time, gene manipulations had been shown to cause tumour regression in humans in research carried out by Dr Steven Rosenberg and his colleagues at the US National Cancer Institute. According to the research, two out of seventeen patients with a deadly form of skin cancer, metastatic melanoma, had their tumours wiped out by genetically altered immune cells.[57] Some scientists are hailing the findings as evidence that the troubled field of gene therapy can successfully treat cancer, while other experts say the results are disappointing. As with all great medical breakthroughs, only time will tell.

There may never be one single cure for cancer but over the past century since Paul Ehrlich produced the first magic bullet, a cure for syphilis, there have been many significant breakthroughs. In universities and pharmaceutical laboratories all over the world the hunt goes on for miracle cures.

POSTSCRIPT

In 1940, during World War II, a Hollywood movie, Dr Ehrlich's Magic Bullet was released. The film was particularly timely considering the treatment the Jewish intelligentsia endured during the Nazi regime in Germany and the horrors that would take place during the war. The film was made at the very time that the development of penicillin, the new weapon against syphilis, was occurring in war-torn Britain. It tells the story of a great scientist and benefactor of humanity who went against convention to search for a drug that would cure syphilis. At the time the film was made the full legacy of Paul Ehrlich's humanitarianism and genius could not have been imagined.

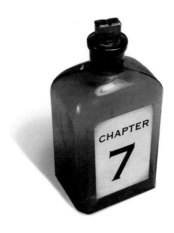

A EUREKA MOMENT
THE DISCOVERY OF INSULIN

Insulin is not a cure for diabetes; it is a treatment. It
enables the diabetic to burn sufficient carbohy-
drates, so that proteins and fats may be added to
the diet in sufficient quantities to provide energy
for the economic burdens of life.[1]

Frederick Banting

At the beginning of the twentieth century, if you were feeling particularly
unwell, had the urge to drink and eat incessantly, felt extremely lethar-
gic, were losing weight and passing urine far too frequently, you would
probably have sought advice from your doctor. Given these symptoms,
the doctor would have immediately tested your urine, and if a high
amount of grape sugar was found, the doctor would probably have diagnosed diabetes.

As to the treatment, the doctor would have suggested that you take a
daily alkaline-sponge bath, prescribed sugar of lead to restrict the flow of
urine and, if that didn't work, suggested you take creosote in two-drop
doses, or even clear opium. You would have been instructed to avoid any
foods that contained sugar and eat only fresh meats. The doctor would also

have told you that your thirst would continue but would have strongly encouraged you to suppress this urge and drink very little.

The prognosis would have been even harder to swallow. In all probability, in a matter of days you would have lapsed into a coma and death would soon have followed.

In 1950, if you presented with the same symptoms, the doctor's examination and explanation would have been much more thorough and detailed. The doctor would have noticed a cloudiness around your retinal arteries and when checking your carotid arteries and the arteries in your feet, would have felt a weaker than normal pulse. Your urine sample would have shown a high level of glucose. The diagnosis: diabetes mellitus, caused by the pancreas not producing enough insulin and therefore preventing the body from absorbing the glucose in your blood. Treatment would have begun immediately with the first and most critical step being to stabilise your blood sugar with insulin. You would have been shown how to test your urine and how to inject insulin and you would have been placed on a special diet. The prognosis would certainly have been better than 50 years earlier. The doctor would regularly monitor the early stages of your disease and give you advice on how to manage the other health issues associated with diabetes — but you would have lived.

What made the difference between life and death for those who develop diabetes was the discovery of insulin. In 1900, many people who were diagnosed with what is now called Type I diabetes died within days of finding out they had the disease, and those with Type II diabetes became ill and deteriorated over a matter of months to years. To say that the discovery of insulin revolutionised treatment for diabetics is an understatement. It saved lives. Although insulin may not be a 'cure' for diabetes — indeed, that search continues today — it has had a profound effect on morbidity and has literally brought salvation to millions of diabetics since it was first used in Canada in 1922.

The discovery in 1921 that insulin, a pancreatic hormone, could be used to treat diabetes was one of the most amazing advances in medicine in the twentieth century. The story has its own subplots of false starts, serendipity, personal and professional rivalry and creative teamwork. The four names most closely associated with the discovery at the University of Toronto are Frederick Banting, a doctor who had been in private practice; Charles Best, a student who had just finished his medical degree; John Macleod, head of the physiology department at the University of Toronto; and James Collip, a gifted biochemist.

UNCOVERING INSULIN

Progress towards the discovery of insulin was cumulative during the late 1800s and early 1900s and was taking place in laboratories all over Europe. Paul Langerhans, a German medical student, was studying the pancreas while writing his MD dissertation in Berlin in 1869. He observed small collections of 'clear cells' within the pancreas that appeared distinct from the surrounding pancreatic tissue. It was known that the pancreas produced digestive enzymes, but Langerhans was puzzled about the function of these isolated cells. The cells now bear his name and are called the 'islets of Langerhans'.

The French physiologist Etienne Lancereaux suggested in 1887 that the pancreas might be related to diabetes. While studying a dog pancreas in 1889, German scientists Joseph von Mering and Oscar Minkowski noticed that flies (not the most sterile of conditions) were swarming around the dog's urine and discovered it contained high levels of glucose. This led them to believe that the pancreas played a role in diabetes but their research took them no further. In 1893 it was the French scientist Gustave-Eduard Láguesse who first referred to the 'islets of Langerhans' and suggested that they made a substance that prevented excess blood glucose.[2]

The research was disparate. In 1901 Eugene L. Opie, an American pathologist studying at Johns Hopkins University, demonstrated the association between the degeneration of segments of the pancreas and diabetes.[3] In 1906 Lydia de Witt, an American experimental pathologist who researched the anatomy of the pancreas, made an extract from the pancreas of cats that produced a significant drop in blood sugar levels. In Germany in 1908, Dr G. Zuelzer produced a pancreatic extract (from whole pancreas) using alcohol as the extractive. When it was given to patients dying from diabetes they experienced a definite fall in blood sugar but the toxic effects were so great that Zuelzer ceased his experiments.[4] In 1912 Aldo Massaglia demonstrated that the destruction of pancreatic segments resulted in glycosuria, the condition in diabetics that causes excretion of glucose in the urine.

The discovery at the beginning of the twentieth century of hormones, which act as 'chemical messengers', was an important step forward. In England in 1916, Edward Sharpey-Schäfer armed with this new knowledge made a discovery, the significance of which was overlooked at the time. He found that the islets of Langerhans remained intact when the pancreatic duct was tied off. It was then that he concluded that these cells manufactured what he referred to as 'insuline', a hormone responsible for regulating blood sugar.[5] Independently in 1916, Nicolas Paulesco, a Romanian physiologist, observed that when pancreatic extract was given intravenously to a diabetic dog it experienced rapid but short-lived symptomatic relief. Paulesco was hampered in his work because he could only produce limited quantities of the extract. His experiments came to an abrupt halt when Bucharest was occupied in 1916 during World War I but he finally published his work in June 1921 when Frederick Banting and Charles Best were conducting groundbreaking experiments in Toronto.[6] They were aware of the article but thought that Paulesco's results showed no significant success. Today, however, Paulesco is credited with being the first person to describe the actions of what is now called insulin. He demonstrated that it was a hormone that acts on all aspects of metabolism.

Ironically, in 1911 Ernest L. Scott, a graduate student at the University of Chicago, experimented with diabetic dogs and was successful in significantly decreasing their blood sugar. His dissertation was later printed in the *American Journal of Physiology*, but apparently a change to the text made his research seem inconclusive. Later, when the Toronto team was having difficulties purifying their pancreatic extracts Scott explained the method he had used to his supervisor, Professor Macleod.[7] When Banting and Best published their results in 1922, they acknowledged the use of Scott's techniques.

What this shows is that in more recent times medical breakthroughs are often the result of many individual, discrete discoveries that finally come together. The breakthrough comes when the picture is complete, like putting the last pieces into a jigsaw puzzle. And by the 1920s the body of scientific knowledge surrounding diabetes was formidable enough to enable a major discovery to be made.

Louis Pasteur's adage that 'Chance favours the prepared mind' is certainly apt in this instance. Late one night in October 1920, the Canadian doctor Frederick Banting chanced to read an article that had been written in 1919 by Moses Barron, a researcher at the University of Minnesota. The content of the article left Banting unable to sleep. It concerned an autopsy that Barron had carried out on a patient who had an obstructed pancreatic duct. Barron found that although the pancreas itself was shrivelled, the islets of Langerhans were not. The blockage of the duct connecting the two major parts of the pancreas caused shrivelling of a second cell type, the acinar. Barron thought his findings suggested the patient had not been diabetic.[8] The paper that he wrote and that Banting read in October 1920 suggested that the islets of Langerhans played some part in blood sugar metabolism. When Banting read this, he immediately conceptualised that by tying off the pancreatic duct to destroy the acinar cells, he could preserve the hormone and extract it from islet cells and that he may be able to extract the hormone in an experiment which involved tying off the pancreatic ducts in dogs. And there it was! In the early hours of that fateful morning Banting put his thoughts down on paper in his diary: 'Ligate pancreatic ducts of dog. Keep dog alive till acini degenerate leaving islets. Try to isolate the internal secretion of these to reduce glycosurea [sic].'[9]

Without delay Frederick Banting approached the head of the University of Toronto's Physiology Department, Professor John Macleod, a Scottish scientist who had moved to Canada in 1918 to take up the position.

Macleod doubted Banting's proposal but diabetes was a hugely important area of research so almost grudgingly he supplied Banting with laboratory space, ten dogs and an assistant. The assistant was the medical student Charles Best. What followed was to have monumental consequences. Their discovery of insulin has been described as one of the spectacular triumphs of medical science.

Insulin is a hormone that humans cannot do without. It is produced by the islets of Langerhans cells in the pancreas, which regulates the amount of glucose (sugar) in the blood and is required for the body to function normally. The pancreas is an organ that sits behind the stomach and has many functions in addition to insulin production; it also produces digestive enzymes and other hormones. The islet cells in the pancreas continuously release a small amount of insulin into the body, but also release surges of insulin in response to a rise in the blood glucose level.[10]

Certain cells in the body change the food that we ingest into energy, or blood glucose, that can be used by cells. Every time you eat, the blood glucose rises. Raised blood glucose triggers the cells in the islets of Langerhans to release the required amount of insulin which allows blood glucose to be transported from the blood into the cells. The cell's membrane controls what enters and exits the cell. Insulin binds to receptors on the cell's membrane and this activates a set of transport molecules so that glucose and proteins can enter the cell. The cells can then use the glucose as energy to carry out their functions. Once transported into the cell, the blood glucose level is returned to normal within hours.

Without insulin, the blood glucose builds up in the blood and the cells are starved of their energy source, which means that diabetics can eat a large amount of food and actually be in a state of starvation because cells cannot access the calories contained in the glucose.[11] Symptoms suffered by diabetics include fatigue, constant infections, blurred eyesight, numbness, tingling in the hands or legs, increased thirst and slow healing of bruises or cuts. The cells will also begin to use fat that the body has stored as an emergency energy source. If this process happens for an extended time, the liver produces chemicals called ketones which can poison and kill cells. When ketones build up in the body the result is serious illness and coma.

Because of the discovery of insulin it became possible for researchers to study diabetes more effectively and two principal types were distinguished. Type I diabetes is caused when the pancreas stops producing insulin altogether. Type II diabetes occurs when the pancreas does not produce sufficient insulin and the body does not respond to insulin properly. Ten to 15 per cent of people who develop diabetes have Type I, which is also called juvenile-onset diabetes. [12]

Diabetes is an auto-immune condition, meaning that the body's immune system turns on its own tissue — in the case of diabetes it is the insulin-producing cells that are destroyed. Type I diabetes occurs in a small number of people who have the genes that confer susceptibility to this form of the disease, and research is still being conducted to find what triggers diabetes in some people. The triggers could be a virus or some other toxin. Type I diabetics must have insulin shots to sustain life. On average they have three to four injections a day.

The majority of people with diabetes have Type II. Insulin is still produced by the pancreas but it is less effective than normal. Type II diabetics respond sluggishly to the insulin they make, which can be in similar or even higher amounts than normal. The problem is that their cells do not absorb the sugar molecules efficiently which leads to blood sugar levels that are higher than in non-diabetic people. This insulin resistance is an inherited characteristic made worse by lifestyle factors such as excess weight or a lack of exercise and is more common in middle-aged or older people. Occasionally Type II diabetics will need insulin shots but most of the time other methods of treatment will work including a regulated diet. A form of diabetes that occurs during pregnancy is called gestational diabetes, and affects approximately 1 in 20 pregnant women. It is usually detected when a woman is around 26 to 28 weeks pregnant and disappears after pregnancy but there is a 2 in 3 chance that it will return in future pregnancies.

People who suffer from diabetes often develop other serious health issues. Diabetic retinopathy causes blindness and occurs as a result of long-term accumulated damage to the small blood vessels in the retina. After fifteen years of diabetes, approximately 2 per cent of people become blind and about 10 per cent develop severe visual impairment. Diabetes is among the leading causes of kidney failure, with approximately 10 to 20 per cent of people with diabetes dying as a result. Diabetes also increases the risk of heart disease and stroke; 50 per cent of people with diabetes die of cardiovascular disease.[13]

There is a misconception today that diabetes is a lifestyle disease, but this is not at all the case with Type I diabetes. Like many of the other life-threatening diseases it has a long history in many countries and cultures. Medical historians believe that diabetes has been known for well over three millennia. In written texts from India dating back to 800 BC there are descriptions of diabetic symptoms. Arataeus of Cappadocia, an eclectic medical philosopher who lived in Alexandria some time between 30 and 150 AD described the condition as 'a melting down of the flesh and limbs into urine', reflecting the weight loss and excess passing of urine that occurs in acute diabetes.[14]

The name of the disease, diabetes mellitus, is derived from the Greek word *diabetes*, meaning 'to siphon' or 'to pass through', and the Latin *mellitus*, meaning 'honeyed' or 'sweet'. This latter word refers to a major symptom of diabetes, sugar in the urine, and was first used in the eighteenth century when it was recognised that this is a symptom of diabetes. In 1670 the British physician Thomas Willis discovered that people 'labouring with this disease piss a great deal more than they drink' and that the urine of diabetics was 'very much sweet, loaded with sugar or honey'.[15]

Willis knew this because he dipped his finger in chamber pots and tasted the urine. It was soon confirmed that the sugar was glucose and the standard way for physicians to test for its presence in urine was the somewhat unscientific and unsavoury taste method. In the seventeenth century the disease had been commonly known as the 'pissing evil', certainly a less acceptable name than diabetes mellitus — but far more descriptive.

By the nineteenth century knowledge of digestion and metabolic processes had expanded markedly and this provided a basis for understanding diabetes. Many scientists had made their contributions and their discoveries were a series of dots, but it required someone with an incisive mind to join them up. It needed Frederick Banting to act on his 'Eureka!' moment.

BANTING AND BEST, COLLIP AND MACLEOD

The son of a farmer, Frederick Grant Banting was born in Ontario in Canada, on 14 November 1891. At school Banting was an all-rounder excelling in the classroom and on the sports field. He went on to study medicine at the University of Toronto and as part of his course worked as an intern at Toronto's Hospital for Sick Children. When World War I broke out in August 1914, Banting immediately attempted to enlist in the Canadian army but was not accepted because of his poor eyesight; however, the following spring he enlisted in the Canadian Army Medical Service.

Banting was quickly promoted to the rank of sergeant. So that he could complete his medical school program, the university condensed his fifth and final year, which in effect cut his training short, something he later regretted. Banting sat his final exams in October 1916 and graduated on 9 December. The following day he reported for active duty and as Lieutenant Banting sailed for Britain to his first overseas posting at the Granville Canadian Special Hospital in Ramsgate. Banting had recently become engaged to Edith Roach, a young woman from his hometown of Alliston and like many young soldiers he left his fiancée behind wondering if he would ever return.

Banting was promoted again to the rank of captain and saw active service in France where he treated the wounded and served with distinction. Frederick Banting was awarded the Military Cross for bravery during events that took place on 28 September 1918 and in 'recognition of gallant and meritorious' service. According to the citation:

> ... when the medical officer of the 46th Canadian Battalion was wounded, he immediately proceeded forward through intense shell fire to reach the battalion. Several of his men were wounded and he, neglecting his own safety, stopped to attend to them. While doing this he was wounded himself [severed artery in his right arm] and was sent out notwithstanding his plea to be left at the front. His energy and pluck were of a very high order.[16]

Apparently Banting had continued to tend the injuries of others for nearly seventeen hours, despite his own wound.

After the war Banting returned to Canada but was unable to secure a staff position at Toronto's Hospital for Sick Children where he had trained. A close friend suggested that he set up a private practice in London, a large city in Ontario that had an established medical school. A classmate of Banting's had already started a practice there. Another compelling reason to move to London was that Edith Roach was teaching at the Ingersoll District Collegiate Institute which was nearby. Banting took the only option open to him, left Toronto and began practising medicine in London in July 1920.

In his biography, written in 1940, Banting looked back on his experience in London as a time of misery and failure — he was unhappy, he was a newcomer, his practice was slow to develop and he was devastated when his engagement to Edith was broken off, but he also reflected that had he not gone to London he might never have started his research. It was here, he said, that, 'I obtained the idea that was to alter every plan that I had ever made. The idea which was to change my future and possibly the future of others.'[17] The house in which Banting suffered such misery and where he read the article that would reveal the secret to saving so many lives is now called Banting House and is a national historic site.

When Frederick Banting approached Professor John Macleod at the University of Toronto in 1921 seeking research assistance for his plan to extract insulin from a dog pancreas he knew that he did not have substantial credentials or a proven track record in research. He was grateful that Macleod, who openly expressed his misgivings, was prepared to give him the opportunity. In May 1921, Frederick Banting was ready to begin his history-making experiments and he had Charles Best to assist him. Best had only just completed his university degree and had been working in Macleod's laboratory during the summer as a research assistant in preparation for enrolling in a Master's program.

Charles Best was born on 27 February 1899 in West Pembroke in the United States but he was a Canadian citizen because his father, Dr Herbert Best, was Canadian. Herbert Best had been born in 1871 in Nova Scotia and six generations of his family had lived there before him.[18]

Charles had attended high school in West Pembroke but continued his education in Canada at the Harbord Collegiate School in Toronto and in 1916 entered the University of Toronto. But it was wartime. At the end of his first year Charles enlisted in the Canadian army and served in the artillery in Canada and England. After the war he resumed his studies and in 1921, a few weeks after receiving an Honours Baccalaureate in Physiology and Chemistry, Charles Best found himself working with Dr Frederick Banting.[19] It would prove to be a very hot and very exciting summer. The young researcher was in the right place at the right time, and in less than three months the names Banting and Best would be echoing throughout the medical world.

Best was engaged to be married when he began his association with Frederick Banting. He met his fiancée, Margaret Mahon, in February 1919 at a dance in Rosedale and they married in 1924. During the period from 1914 to 1984 Margaret wrote and kept 80 volumes of diaries as well as keeping thousands of letters and many scrapbooks and photo albums, which are mirrors into much more than family life and her long and successful marriage.[20] Apparently in her last years Margaret threatened to destroy the love letters from her husband, but fortunately she did not. The memorabilia that she left behind are an incredible archive of historical documents providing insight into the years surrounding the discovery of insulin.

During the summer of 1921, while Margaret was away visiting relatives, Charles Best wrote letters to his fiancée which contained candid comments about what was going on in the medical building at Toronto University as Banting and Best began their research.

After a few setbacks, Banting and Best had developed a suitable experimental regime for the ten dogs that they had been given for their experiments. In some dogs they tied off the pancreatic ducts so the acinar cells would atrophy, but they left the islets of Langerhans in place. From other dogs they removed the pancreas entirely; these dogs developed diabetes. Some weeks later they removed the degenerated pancreases from the first group of dogs. In order to extract fluid from the islet cells in these organs, they placed the pancreases in solution, ground them up with a mortar and pestle and then filtered them through cheesecloth. The islet cell fluid was then injected into the sick dogs that had previously had their pancreases removed.[21] Within hours the blood glucose levels of these dogs improved markedly.

In a letter to Margaret on 8 August 1921, Charles Best wrote, 'I went back to the lab at eleven p.m. and we worked all through the night and today until two. We got fine results.' He mentioned that he was becoming an insomniac, unable to sleep even when he had the chance.

Charles wrote the following on 10 August:

> We have mailed our report to Dr. Macleod. He will have food for
> thought for a little while at least ... We are doing identical

operations on the dogs. We are going to give one the extract and the other none and study the condition of each — how long each lives, etc. It will be quite a crucial test for our 'isletin'. I am glad you asked to hear about the dogs, dear. I know you are not interested in them apart from my work.[22]

While this work had been going on in Toronto, Macleod was away in Scotland on a fishing trip. When he received the report he was not convinced, but even though he raised questions about the procedures Banting and Best had used, he acquiesced to Banting's request for a dedicated laboratory and more staff. At this point James Collip, considered to be one of the great minds of Canadian biochemistry, came on board.

James Bertram Collip was born in Belleville in Ontario in 1892. In 1907, when he was only fifteen he enrolled in an honours physiology and chemistry program at Trinity College at the University of Toronto. Collip completed his doctorate in biochemistry in 1916 and accepted a position as a lecturer at the University of Alberta where he began his outstanding career in biochemical research. He worked in a somewhat primitive laboratory but within a year had produced important work in the relatively new field of internal secretions.[23] In 1921 when Collip was on a Rockefeller Travelling Fellowship he was invited by Professor Macleod to join the Banting team to assist them on the insulin project.

When Collip arrived at the Toronto laboratory Banting and Best had already produced a crude pancreatic extract. Soon the laboratory was set up with the equipment needed for the next phase of the work. Banting did the surgical work, Best carried out the chemical assays and Collip worked on methods for the purification of the chemical extracts and in a remarkably short time had refined the technique of insulin extraction and purification (eventually the process was patented in the names of the three principal researchers, Banting, Best and Macleod, and given to the University of Toronto).[24] Professor Macleod became involved in the project on his return from his trip and from that time on directed the work.

As the experiments continued Banting began to use cow foetuses as the source of insulin when he realised that the islets of Langerhans cells were more numerous in developing animals than in mature ones. While Collip began work in his laboratory, Banting and Best, during the week of 12–16 December, continued work on their pancreas extract. On the first day an alcoholic extraction of whole pancreas seemed to work on the laboratory dogs when administered through a stomach tube, apparently causing a blood sugar reduction from 0.42 to 0.28 in four hours.[25] They found that whole cow pancreas injected intravenously also seemed effective.

On 14 December Banting and Best administered extracts of liver, spleen, thyroid and thymus to the dogs, all prepared the same way as the pancreatic extracts, but none of them had any effect. To make the pancreatic extract purer they then experimented with dialysis and chemicals. An injection of a piece of dried extract that had been washed twice in toluene (a colourless, liquid hydrocarbon) and redissolved in saline when administered to one of the dogs resulted in a decrease in its blood sugar from 0.37 to 0.06 over a period of four hours. Following this extraordinary moment the work became tedious and did not go well over the next week. The men varied the way they prepared batches of extract and some had no potency at all when administered to the test dog.

According to Michael Bliss in his book *The Discovery of Insulin*, at this point Banting and Best decided, without revealing their plans to anyone, to try the extract that had been successful on the dog on a human diabetic. One of Banting's classmates, Joe Gilchrist, had become diabetic in early 1917, a few months after they had graduated. In 1921 his condition was deteriorating rapidly. An index card is apparently the only record of the actual 'first' clinical trial and it notes that Joe Gilchrist was contacted by phone on 20 December. He obviously agreed to be a 'guinea pig', or 'dog' in this case, and was given the extract by mouth. The index card records that on 21 December there had been 'no beneficial result'. Bliss makes the point that the extract may have worked on Gilchrist, as it had for the dog, if it had been given intravenously but the risk was too great for Banting and

Best to inject something so experimental into a human. When Banting and Best reported on their findings at a meeting of the American Physiological Society on 28 December 1921 Joe Gilchrist was not mentioned.

Frederick Banting knew that the real test of his extract would be success with a human patient. When a clinical trial was arranged at Toronto General Hospital, the university's teaching hospital, Macleod gave James Collip the job of preparing the extract that would be used. According to Bliss, at this point Banting began urging Macleod to let him try the extract he and Best had successfully used on the test dog and unbeknown to Macleod, unsuccessfully on one human. Because Banting had no professional association with the university's teaching hospital, and no doubt wanting to conduct the trial himself without discussing his plans, he applied to Duncan Graham, the Eaton Professor of Medicine at the Toronto Department of Medicine for a temporary appointment. Graham dismissed Banting's request and condescendingly pointed out that he was not currently practising medicine and was not qualified to experiment on patients or to treat diabetics. Although the relationship between Banting and Macleod had never progressed beyond tense, Macleod agreed to intercede with Graham, who was a personal friend. As a result a clinical trial of the extract prepared by Banting and Best proceeded.

The patient chosen for the trial was fourteen-year-old Leonard Thompson, a diabetic who was a public ward patient. Leonard had been admitted to the diabetic clinic at Toronto General Hospital rather than the Hospital for Sick Children so that he could receive the extract. His diabetes had been diagnosed in 1919 and Allen therapy (during which patients are required to eat a low-calorie diet) had been tried on the boy without success. [26]

By December 1921 when Leonard was admitted to hospital he was emaciated, pale and listless, his hair was falling out, his abdomen was distended and he was too ill to get out of bed. 'All of us knew that he was doomed,' a senior medical student in the hospital recalled.[27] Leonard's distressed father gave permission for Banting and Best's new extract to be administered because he knew it was his son's only hope.

Best prepared the extract of whole cow pancreas using the same process that had worked on the dog early in December, and tested it again. What they delivered to the clinic was described as very thick and brown.[28] On the afternoon of 11 January, a young house physician, Ed Jeffrey, injected 15 cubic centimetres of the extract into Leonard Thompson, half the dose it was thought would be effective on a dog of the same weight. Banting and Best, who were treated like interlopers, waited in the corridor on tenterhooks hoping to get a sample of the boy's urine to test. After being told that all samples were the property of the hospital they returned to their laboratory having been given no information at all.

The results of the first trial were reported later in a joint publication by Banting, Best, Collip and Walter Campbell, another member of the laboratory team. Leonard Thompson's blood sugar dropped from 0.44 to 0.32. The 24-hour excretion of glucose fell from 91.5 grams in 3625 cubic centimetres of urine to 84 grams in 4060 cubic centimetres and his ketones count continued to be strongly positive.[29] The only evident side-effect was a sterile abscess at the site of one of the injections on Leonard's buttock. Despite the general opinion that this constituted a success the decision was made by the doctors at Toronto General not to give Leonard further injections of Banting and Best's extract.

Collip had continued working on the problem of purifying insulin to remove the harmful impurities and only a few days after the first trial had produced a batch of extract made from purified ox pancreas. On 23 January 1922 Collip's extract was administered to Leonard. The almost immediate and dramatic improvement in the boy's condition was convincing proof that the Toronto team had made a life-saving discovery. Banting and Best had made insulin, Collip had purified it and the hospital records show that Leonard Thompson received 'Macleod's serum'.[30] This is not untoward considering Macleod was the head of the team and of the laboratory where insulin had been produced.

Word of the latest medical marvel spread quickly, circling the globe and giving immediate hope to thousands of diabetic people who were near death. A frenzied quest for insulin followed and appeals arrived daily in Toronto from parents desperate to save their children. As the use of insulin spread it lived up to its reputation and even patients who had lapsed into diabetic comas were making miraculous recoveries.

Although the relationship between Banting and Macleod had always been strained, the underlying hostilities at the laboratory were becoming more obvious. The heady nature of success can sometimes do strange things to scientists. In February 1922 Macleod publicly announced the discovery, and the patent for manufacturing the pancreatic extract was approved. All financial proceeds from the patent went to the British Medical Research Council and the discoverers were given nothing. Amidst the excitement and the tension Banting and Best published a summary of their work in April 1922. The title of their joint paper was, 'The Effect Produced on Diabetes by Extracts of Pancreas'.[31]

It was at this time that Banting picked up on several clues and became suspicious that Macleod wanted credit for the discovery that Banting believed was his and Best's. As head of department, however, Macleod could expect some acknowledgment. Tension escalated when James Collip refused to reveal to Banting the method he had used to purify the insulin in the second trial. Banting was disappointed and hurt. However, rage is the emotion he is said to have exhibited when he and Macleod, not Best, were jointly named as the recipients of the 1923 Nobel Prize for Physiology or Medicine. Collip, who accepted a share of the Nobel Prize money from Professor Macleod, wrote somewhat bitterly in 1923 that the extract that Banting and Best had prepared was absolutely useless for a human subject.

What actually happened between these four men has been debated in scientific and lay circles for decades. One of Charles Best's two sons, Henry Best, a professional historian, threw some light on those frenetic and troubled times from his father's perspective in a speech he delivered to the Academy of Medicine in Toronto on 24 April 1996 during the celebrations for the 75th anniversary of the discovery of insulin. Henry Best had abandoned his medical career to study history and at the time he gave the speech was in the process of writing a biography of his famous father. According to Henry, Frederick Banting and Charles Best both believed that there was a demarcation line between the discovery of insulin and its early development. They were the discoverers. John Macleod, James Collip and other members of the team made very important contributions, but at another level. Banting and Best were involved in both the discovery and the development of insulin. Banting had been motivated by Barron's article about the islets of Langerhans, had hypothesised how insulin might be extracted, and from that moment it became Frederick Banting's goal to convert his theory into a cure for diabetes. Banting brought his proposal to Macleod. The initial work, without which the rest would not have been possible, was carried out by Frederick Banting and Charles Best.[32] There can be no doubt about who connected all the dots.

'In my father's view, as in Fred Banting's,' Henry Best said, 'the Nobel Prize should have gone to Banting and Best, rather than to Banting and Macleod.'[33] He said that his father rarely talked about this but he had no doubt that the issue played on his father's mind later in his life. It is probably a matter of opinion as to whether Charles Best was simply overlooked or deliberately sidelined.

There have been many people who felt that they or others should have received credit for the discovery of insulin, aside from those in Toronto. There was Ernest Scott in the United States, whom the Toronto team had acknowledged; and Nicolas Paulesco in Romania, whom they had not. However, surely this goes to the nature of what constitutes a discovery? As medical research has become more sophisticated and complex, scientists increasingly base new research on earlier discoveries and more and more people have a hand in each new development. It was perhaps different centuries ago when Edward Jenner discovered a vaccine for smallpox, but even then Jenner had been aware of folklore and earlier procedures such as variolation, all of which informed his research.

At the 1991 Meeting of the International Diabetes Federation in Washington DC, Henry Best spoke with Professor Rolf Luft of Stockholm's Karolinska Institute, the body that awards the Nobel Prizes. Following the meeting Professor Luft wrote to Best to say that after the passing of so many years and so much debate, with reservations, he thought that it might have been fair to have awarded the Nobel Prize to Banting, Best and Paulesco.[34] The method of selecting Nobel laureates is complex and the choices do not always meet the approval of individuals or their supporters. When one person is pushed forward the role of others might be negated. Banting and Macleod were each nominated separately by American proposers and then jointly by Professor August Krogh, a Danish Nobel laureate.

During his speech to the Academy of Medicine in 1996 Henry Best read out a Resolution passed by the Council of the Academy on 23 March 1923 in regard to the discovery of insulin. It stated that:

> ... in view of the importance of the discovery and isolation of a substance purporting to be the internal secretion of the pancreas controlling carbohydrate metabolism, and consequently of great value in the science of Physiology and Biochemistry, and possibly, in practical medicine by reason of its presumed ability to control Diabetes Mellitus, the Council of the Academy of Medicine, after careful investigation, believes that conclusive evidence has been furnished of: FIRST the isolation of such a substance from the pancreas of various animals and termed 'insulin' by Dr. F.G. Banting and Dr. C.H. Best in the summer of 1921 at the University of Toronto.[35]

Although the significance of the discovery is qualified there is no uncertainty about who the discoverers were. However, Charles Best was referred to as Dr Best, a title he did not actually have until 1925. Henry

Best felt that the council's statement was possibly a reflection of the sub-liminal belief that someone who was not yet a medical doctor or did not have a PhD could not really have been a co-discoverer of insulin and therefore could hardly be a contender for the Nobel Prize. As with all medical breakthroughs, when fame and money are at stake emotions can be extraordinarily volatile.

From various accounts it would seem that Charles Best had a reasonable relationship with John Macleod, always referring to him with deference as his professor. Macleod had taught him the physiology he used in his insulin work. Best, according to his son, believed that Macleod was influenced by his European experience of the way discoveries were recognised and that the possibility of fame may have affected his judgment. It was not that Macleod had promoted his own claim unfairly, but that he had neglected to present the case for Best. The relationship between these two men was not severed, and although later in life Best was concerned about how things had turned out, he saw Professor Macleod during trips overseas after the older man returned home in 1928 to Aberdeen in Scotland.

As for Best and Collip, they had a cordial working relationship but were never close friends and there were always underlying tensions. Charles Best was uncomfortable talking in public about the discovery of insulin when Collip was present and carried with him the memory of an incident in January 1922 when an argument between Banting and Collip about the purification of insulin had apparently become physical. Charles Best wrote to his father on 10 May 1922 that there had been 'a lot of trouble, quarrels etc., but we are getting on'. Collip left the laboratory at that time and Best told his father in the letter, 'I am now in charge of making the dope.'[36] He was only 22 years old.

James Collip went on to become a distinguished researcher and administrator at a number of Canadian universities as well as the National Research Council and was a leading endocrinologist and worldwide authority on the properties of insulin. He accepted the Chair of Biochemistry at McGill University, where he conducted extensive studies on hormones. In 1941, he became Chairman of McGill's new Institute of Endocrinology and capped off a brilliant career as Dean of Medicine at the University of Western Ontario.[37]

In recalling the events of 1921 and 1922, at the request of Sir Henry Dale, a distinguished scientist, Nobel laureate and President of the Royal Society who became Charles Best's greatest mentor, Best wrote on 22 February 1954:

> *I have to confess that even after all these years, the revival of the memory that Professor Macleod and later Collip, instead of being grateful for the privilege of helping to develop a great advance, used their superior experience and skill, with considerable success, in the attempt to appropriate some of the credit for a discovery which was not truly theirs, still makes me warm with resentment. I must state, also that I have only to think of the understanding and fairness of scientific colleagues in many countries who have read our reports carefully, to replace resentment with a much better feeling.*[38]

Charles Best was not the first or the last scientist to feel such resentment. Frederick Banting's reaction to the announcement that Macleod, not Best, was to share the Nobel Prize is probably best shown by the telegram he sent to a colleague in Boston where Best was about to make a speech. The telegram said:

> *At any meeting or dinner, please read the following stop I ascribe to Best equal share in the Discovery stop hurt that he is not so acknowledged by Nobel trustees stop will share with him stop.*[39]

As for Professor Macleod, there are those who feel he was treated unfairly in the insulin wash-up. It was a period of frantic activity before and after the discovery. Macleod worked to promote the distribution of insulin around the world and co-authored a series of papers on its use and actions. The pro-Macleod camp feels that the bitter infighting that followed the great discovery was the result of Banting forcefully promoting his own role in the discovery. Banting is accused of lacking the scientific background to appreciate the value of the advice and contributions that Macleod and Collip made to the work. Macleod has been described as a reserved and modest man who was not equipped to stand up to the campaign waged against him — but that may be selling Macleod short in one way.[40] He was actively involved in the research program and, according to some, provided the conclusive demonstration that insulin comes from the pancreatic islets.

John Macleod left Toronto in 1928 (it is said with some relief) to become Regius Professor of Physiology at Aberdeen University, a post he held until his death. His published output was phenomenal, although his final years were marred by ill health from progressive rheumatoid arthritis. He died at his home on 16 March 1935, aged just 58. His supporters say the accusations that he stole the credit for work done by his juniors did lasting harm to his reputation and his contributions to the discovery of insulin were largely forgotten following his death.

In more recent times the debate was in evidence again when a disagreement arose about changed wording on a plaque outside the medical sciences building at the University of Toronto. It commemorates the work done in the old medical building in 1921. On the original plaque Banting and Best were acknowledged as the co-discoverers of insulin. At the beginning of the 1990s this was changed to Banting, Best, Collip and Macleod.

When asked about his reaction to a Canadian TV program about the discovery of insulin — the theme of which is obvious from its name, *Glory Enough for All* — Charles Best's son said that some of the characters and events had been fictionalised but, as is the case with extraordinary breakthroughs in science and medicine, the real story is dramatic enough without invention.[41] It is no wonder that humans, being the flawed creatures that we are, with our vanities and foibles, are reluctant to share fame and fortune and so often there is not 'glory enough for all'.

After the discovery of insulin in 1921 Frederick Banting became a popular hero and a force in medicine in Canada. When his work on insulin was complete he undertook research into heart disease and cancer. Banting's broken relationship early in his career had left him free to devote himself to research. His fame after the award of the Nobel Prize in 1923, combined with his charming personality and sense of humour, made him a sought-after marriage prospect and in 1924 Frederick Banting married Marion Robertson. They had one child but the marriage ended unhappily in divorce.

Both Banting and Best received offers to leave Canada to carry out research in the United States, but neither did. There was a continuous shower of glory, awards and honorary degrees for Banting, and an institute bearing his name, the Banting Institute, was opened in 1930. In 1934 Frederick Banting was knighted, some years before Charles Best. Frederick Banting married again in 1939. His second wife was Henrietta Ball but the marriage was destined to be a short one, this time for a different reason. Sir Frederick Banting met with a tragic early death. He had joined the army and was serving as a major with the Medical Corps when in February 1941, on one of many flights that he made from Canada to England, the plane crashed into a lake at Gander in Newfoundland. Frederick Banting had not reached his 50th birthday. His memory is perpetuated, however, as the lake is now known as Banting Lake.

Henry Best surmised that Charles Best probably received more honours than would have come his way if Banting had lived. Best's was a long and illustrious career. When visiting Toronto in 1922, Sir Henry Dale asked Best to come to the National Institute for Medical Research in London but he stayed in Canada and continued working with Banting at the Banting and Best Department of Medical Research at the university and completed doctorates in both medicine and physiology. Best did spend time abroad between 1925 and 1928 while doing postdoctoral work at the University of Freiburg in Germany and the University of London in England.

By 1929 Charles Best had been appointed head of the University of

Toronto's physiology department. He returned to Canada to take up the position and resumed his work as research associate in the Banting and Best Department of Medical Research. As time progressed, Frederick Banting and Charles Best developed different research interests. Best's work had a high public profile. He successfully isolated and purified heparin, an effective anti-coagulant for the treatment of thrombosis, investigated histamine and conducted research into the vitamin choline.[42]

According to his son, Charles Best's ambition possibly irritated Banting. Those who knew Best describe him as ambitious, not just professionally but for his family, his colleagues and his students. However, in 1933 Best turned down an offer to succeed Sir Edward Sharpey-Schäfer to the Chair of Physiology in Edinburgh. Best's ambition did not override his loyalty to the University of Toronto.

During World War II Charles Best joined the Royal Canadian Navy and directed the Medical Research Unit. Working with the Red Cross and the Canadian government he was involved in wartime projects developing night lighting, remedies for seasickness, and the design and equipping of survival rafts. He also collaborated on devising a method for transforming human blood into dried blood serum (plasma) that could be stored indefinitely.[43] Research took on a different focus in wartime but it was still about survival. In 1941 Best found himself taking over the role of director of the Banting and Best Department of Medical Research but it was not a cause for celebration, coming as a result of Banting's unexpected and tragic death.

In 1949 the post of secretary of the Medical Research Council of Great Britain was offered to Best followed by another offer in 1951, the Chair of Physiology at Cambridge. But Charles Best could not be tempted to leave the University of Toronto. He had been promised his own building, where he could combine the two departments he headed, Physiology and the Banting and Best Department of Medical Research. That building, the Charles Best Institute, was finally opened in 1953 and became a centre of further outstanding research.

Honours and awards came later to Best than to the older scientists involved in the discovery of insulin. The four main contenders became Fellows of the Royal Society of London: Professor Macleod in 1923, James Collip in 1933, Frederick Banting in 1935 and Charles Best in 1938. James Collip received the CBE (Commander of the British Empire) in 1943 and Best received the same award in 1944. The first of Best's 30 honorary degrees was presented at the 50th Anniversary Convocation of the University of Chicago on 29 September 1941. Charles Best was also awarded the Companion of the Order of Canada in 1967 and the Companion of Honour in 1971.

Charles Best had a sense of humour. He was awarded Membership in the Papal Academy of Sciences. The parchment accompanying the gold medallion stated that henceforth Charles Herbert Best should be addressed as 'Your Excellency' and he often quipped at home that he should be addressed by his full title. When giving lectures and talks to audiences which included a number of Roman Catholics he would say that the Holy Father, the Pope, was getting good advice on matters such as birth control from the nephew of an Anglican Bishop and the son-in-law of a Presbyterian Minister.[44]

Best enjoyed the life that success and fame brought him but he also enjoyed simpler pleasures and retained an affinity with the small village of West Pembroke where he grew up. Horses had been a part of his childhood and he never lost his love of riding and kept his father's horses on a farm that he bought close to West Pembroke. Interestingly, both Charles Best and Frederick Banting had a deep interest in painting (shades of Louis Pasteur) which Best found totally absorbing and relaxing, a foil to the pressures of his medical life.

The inexhaustible energy and enthusiasm for life that Best had always exhibited began to wane in 1953 when he suffered a series of heart attacks. He made a good recovery but a decade later in 1964 he experienced the onset of a sudden and severe depression from which he never quite recovered. Charles Best did, however, enthusiastically take part in the celebrations surrounding the 50th anniversary of the discovery of insulin in 1971. During that and the following year he and Margaret travelled extensively, having been invited to events in Brazil, England, Israel and many countries in Europe. On 3 September 1974, the devoted couple celebrated their 50th wedding anniversary.[45] Margaret had always exercised a degree of influence in the relationship. She travelled everywhere with Charles, except during World War II when his trips overseas caused her great anxiety. Margaret was afraid her husband might meet the same fate as Frederick Banting.

On Easter Sunday, 1978, Charles Best suffered an aneurysm of the aorta the day after one of his sons, Sandy, died of a massive heart attack at the age of only 46. Five days later Charles Best, aged 79, was also dead. For Margaret Best, it was a terrible double blow.

Posthumously Charles Best was inducted into the Canadian Medical Hall of Fame in 1994 and in 2004 he was inducted into the National Inventors Hall of Fame. He has been honoured on stamps in his own country and in Belgium, Croatia and Uruguay. In 1971 Kuwait issued a set of two stamps showing portraits of Frederick Banting and Charles Best and featuring a syringe. This is a reminder of just how far-reaching and significant the work of the co-discoverers of insulin has been to humankind. Although not a cure for diabetes, insulin has saved the lives of millions and today most sufferers lead relatively normal lives. Each day diabetics all over the world hold in their hands the physical evidence of the gift given to them by two exceptional scientists. Theirs is a daily dose of salvation.

DEVELOPMENTS IN INSULIN AND DIABETES RESEARCH

The production of insulin has changed a great deal since 1922 when Frederick Banting and Charles Best first successfully extracted it from a dog's pancreas. In May 1922 Eli Lilly and Company and the University of Toronto entered into an agreement for the mass production of insulin in North America.[46] In the first successful commercial insulin preparations from cows and later pigs — the chemical structure of insulin in these animals is only slightly different to human insulin — the pancreatic islets and the insulin protein contained within them were extracted from animals slaughtered for food in a similar but more complex process than was used by Banting and Best.[47] Bovine and porcine insulin still work well for many people although some people are allergic to foreign or non-human protein.

In 1936 researchers found a way to make insulin with a slower release in the blood. They added a protein found in fish sperm, protamine, which the body breaks down slowly.[48] One injection lasted 36 hours. Professor Macleod was involved in research associated with this development. Another breakthrough came in 1950 when a type of insulin was produced that acted slightly faster and did not remain in the bloodstream as long. In the 1970s research began on producing insulin that better mimicked how the body's natural insulin worked, releasing a small amount all day with surges occurring at mealtimes.

The science becomes more complex and the technology more breathtaking. By 1977 a research team had spliced a rat insulin gene into a bacterium that then produced insulin. By the 1980s due to the development of recombinant DNA techniques it became possible to make human insulin.[49] In simple terms (one hopes) the human gene which codes for the insulin protein was cloned and then put inside common bacteria. A number of tricks were performed on the gene to make the bacteria want to use it to constantly make insulin. In 1982 the Eli Lilly Corporation produced human insulin, the first approved genetically engineered pharmaceutical product.

Pharmaceutical companies no longer needed animals and could produce genetically engineered insulin in unlimited supplies. Big vats of bacteria now make tons of human insulin. *Escherichia coli* is the most widely used type of bacterium, but yeast is also used. Using human insulin has eliminated concerns about the potential for transferring animal diseases. While companies still sell a small amount of insulin produced from animals, mostly porcine, from the 1980s onwards diabetics have increasingly moved to human insulin created through recombinant DNA technology. In 2001 it was estimated that around 95 per cent of insulin users in most parts of the world took some form of human insulin. In keeping with these developments, in the 1980s researchers began providing alternate drug delivery systems to the syringe, which had been used since the 1920s. Insulin pens, jet injectors and pumps are now available.

In the mid 1990s researchers began to improve the way human insulin works in the body by changing its amino acid sequence and creating an analogue, a chemical substance that mimics another substance so well that it fools the cell. Analogue insulin disperses more readily into the blood, allowing the insulin to start working in the body minutes after an injection. The work to produce better insulin goes on. Researchers have taken up the challenge to produce edible insulin, experimenting with a plastic coating that is only the width of a few human hairs that would protect the drug from stomach acid. Since 2000 there have been promising tests on inhaled insulin devices.[50]

Of course much of the research that is conducted today is focused on seeking a cure for diabetes so that in the future there would be no need for synthesised insulin and state-of the-art, easy-to-use delivery methods. In 2005 a national genetic study was launched by Professor Grant Morahan, head of the Western Australian Institute of Medical Research's Diabetes Research Centre and discoverer of the gene IL12B which is implicated in Type I diabetes. DNA from 3000 Australian families with diabetic children will be collected and studied. The aim of the project is to determine the precise genetic causes of both Type I and Type II diabetes, both of which are on the increase. [51]

The World Health Organization estimates that more than 180 million people worldwide have diabetes and it is predicted that this number will more than double by 2030. In 2005, an estimated 1.1 million people died from diabetes. Almost 80 per cent of diabetes deaths currently occur in low- and middle-income countries but there is an alarming trend: diabetes deaths are projected to increase by over 80 per cent in upper-middle income countries between 2006 and 2015.[52]

Frederick Banting in his eureka moment solved the insulin puzzle. Today because of his legacy researchers are working on creating the cells that produce insulin in the laboratory in the hope that, one day, non-working pancreas cells can be replaced with insulin-producing cells. Another hope for diabetics is gene therapy. Scientists are focusing research on correcting the insulin gene's mutation so that diabetics would be able to produce insulin on their own. In a worldwide breakthrough, reported in the May 2005 issue of the science journal *Nature*, researchers at the John Curtin School of Medical Research at the Australian National University in Canberra discovered a gene that if mutated in a person might be responsible for the development of juvenile diabetes.

One technique that has been pioneered in an attempt to restore normal blood glucose levels in people with Type I diabetes is islet transplantation. Transplantation as a treatment has become possible because of the development of the science of immunology, which began with Paul Ehrlich. Since the 1970s, transplantation of islets has been investigated as an alternative to whole-pancreas transplants, the first of which was carried out in 1966. Islet transplantation involves transplanting only the islet cells that contain the critical insulin-producing beta cells.[53] Compared to whole-pancreas transplantation it is a simpler and less invasive procedure. Following the transplant, patients must take immunosuppressive drugs to keep their bodies from rejecting the new islets. Islet transplantation is limited, however, because very few donor pancreases are available each year.

For decades, success rates for this procedure remained under 10 per cent. However, in 2000 the introduction of the Edmonton Protocol — a new set of procedures for conducting islet transplants — raised success rates to 80 per cent.[54] Research is underway to answer questions about safety and effectiveness, such as how long the transplanted islets will survive and whether the success rate can be sustained and thus be considered a 'cure'. In October

2006 the Mayo Clinic reported on a study of 36 islet cell transplant recipients. More than 40 per cent were off insulin therapy completely within one year of the transplant. By two years, however, less than 14 per cent of transplant recipients remained free of insulin therapy.[55]

Today, things have almost come full circle with what is called xenotransplantation, the transfer of living cells or tissues from one species to another.[56] For 60 years, before synthetic insulin was available, people with Type I diabetes injected pig insulin, and now researchers are investigating whether islets from pigs can be successfully transplanted into humans. Another exciting possibility is stimulating stem cells to become beta cells that could then be transplanted. This approach would overcome the risks of immune reaction to foreign tissues and problems associated with the transfer of tissue from donor to patient.

With such a shortage of islet cells available for transplantation, news of the world's first successful transplant of *living* human donor islet cells in 2005 raised exciting possibilities for the treatment of diabetes. A medical team that included Japanese doctors and the US surgeon Dr James Shapiro, who developed the Edmonton Protocol, removed part of a 56-year-old woman's pancreas and transplanted the insulin-producing cells into the woman's 27-year-old diabetic daughter.[57] The transplanted islets began producing insulin within minutes. The recipient was able to stop using insulin after 22 days; she had been on daily injections for twelve years. Both women were well three months after the operation and doctors predicted that the transplant could last up to five years.

Research scientists associated with the Juvenile Diabetes Research Foundation Islet Transplantation Centres in North America and Europe are investigating new therapies that can achieve 'selective immune tolerance' by targeting the cells that destroy islets while leaving the beneficial, disease-fighting immune responses untouched.[58] Another approach is to re-engineer islet cells so that they escape recognition by the immune system, or encapsulate islets in protective membranes to protect them from immune attack. The scope of this type of research is truly breathtaking.

In April 2007 it was widely reported that researchers had come closer than ever before to finding a cure for diabetes. A pilot study of fifteen people newly diagnosed with Type I diabetes found that stem cell therapy eliminated the need for insulin therapy for varying periods of time. Patients were treated with a high dose of immune-suppression drugs followed by an intravenous injection of their own blood stem cells, in a procedure called autologous nonmyeloablative hematopoietic stem cell transplantation (AHST). The new study was conducted by scientists in São Paulo in Brazil and in Chicago under the direction of Julio C. Voltarelli from the University of São Paulo. It was the first trial to look at stem cell therapy in humans with Type I diabetes. Richard Burt, the senior author of the study, said that he believed that the treatment helped the body regenerate its immune system.[59]

During a three-year follow-up it was found that patients had become insulin free for varying periods, the longest of which was 35 months, and there were few adverse side-effects. Experts stressed, however, that the research is preliminary and urged caution when interpreting the results, which were published in the 11 April issue of the *Journal of the American Medical Association*. The gene therapy intervention took place within six weeks of the onset of Type 1 diabetes and the question remains as to whether intervention later would be as successful. Further biological studies are now necessary to confirm the role of the treatment in changing the natural history of Type I diabetes and to evaluate the contribution of adult stem cells to this change.

Time will tell. Perhaps when the cause of diabetes is finally understood, then not long after a cure will at last be found. That will be another medical breakthrough, and like Frederick Banting's and Charles Best's discovery of insulin, it will change the world. Until then, there are many great minds on the job.

Postscript

Leonard Thompson, the fourteen-year-old boy who was the first diabetic to be treated with insulin, lived for thirteen years after receiving the pancreatic extracts prepared by Frederick Banting and Charles Best, and James Collip. But Leonard did not die from diabetes. In a cruel twist of fate he died tragically, as too many young people do, in a motorcycle accident. At the time of his death Leonard Thompson's pancreas was preserved and it is displayed as item 3030 in the anatomical museum at the Banting Institute.

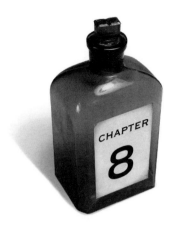

MAKING A MIRACLE
OUT OF A MOULD
THE DISCOVERY OF PENICILLIN

I became interested — immediately — in
Fleming's paper, not because I hoped to discover
a miraculous drug for the treatment of bacterial
infection which for some reason had been overlooked, but because I thought it had great scientific
interest. In fact, if I had been working at that time in
aim-directed scientific surroundings, say in the laboratory of a pharmaceutical firm, it is my belief that
I would never have obtained the agreement of my
bosses to proceed with my project to work with
penicillin.[1]

Ernst Chain

Before the second half of the twentieth century infections engendered the
same kind of fear that cancer creates today. Even a thorn or needle prick
could lead to infection. Glands would swell, ulcers would form and require
lancing to release pus, amputations were common, and very often a gruesome and painful death would result. The infectious wards in hospitals

were crammed with people suffering from puerperal fever, scarlet fever, meningitis, osteomyelitis, heart disease and pneumonia, and one in three cases ended in death. This was the nightmare of wound infections and many infectious diseases before penicillin.

The discovery of penicillin dramatically changed the world and has been interpreted as the pinnacle of medical achievement, but the story of penicillin is set against a backdrop of rivalry, hardship and disappointment. It begins in 1928 with a stroke of luck, when Alexander Fleming, a Scottish bacteriologist, noticed mould had prevented the growth of bacteria on a Petri dish in his laboratory. But the main plot of the story is the rediscovery of penicillin ten years later by an Australian pharmacologist, Howard Florey, and his dedicated team at Oxford University. Their systematic work transformed the antibiotic ingredient in the mould, *Penicillium notatum*, into penicillin, a drug that has since saved millions of lives. The story is even more dramatic and astonishing because these history-changing events took place in Britain during the dark days of World War II.

A decade after Alexander Fleming abandoned penicillin and went back to working on lysozyme, an enzyme in bodily secretions, he became an international *cause célèbre*. So widespread was his fame that it extended beyond Earth. After the Americans landed on the moon in 1969, a crater was named after Fleming, the discoverer of penicillin.[2] But had it not been for Howard Florey; Ernst Chain, a German-born biochemist; and Norman Heatley, a biochemist whose background was in the natural sciences; and their colleagues at the Dunn School at Oxford University, the world might not have had penicillin.

Fleming — a small, neat man with a mild Scottish accent, who sported a bow tie — discovered penicillin, and Florey — his opposite, tall, testy and a chain smoker — developed it. However, the controversy and confusion about who did what continues. In 1998, Professor Sir Henry Harris, who succeeded Florey as Professor of Pathology at Oxford, succinctly summed up the situation: 'Without Fleming, no Chain or Florey; without Chain, no Florey; without Florey, no Heatley; without Heatley, no penicillin.'[3]

FLEMING'S ACCIDENTAL DISCOVERY

Alexander Fleming was born into a Scottish sheep-farming family in 1881, the seventh of eight children. His family worked an 800-acre farm in a remote part of Scotland and their nearest neighbours were a mile away. The Fleming children spent much of their time roaming the streams, valleys and moors of the surrounding countryside, and this, Fleming said, was where he learnt a great deal from nature.[4]

After their father's death, Alexander's eldest brother inherited the farm and another brother who had studied medicine opened a practice in London. At fourteen Alexander followed his siblings to London and attended the Polytechnic School in Regent Street after which he found employment in a shipping firm, but the job provided little satisfaction. In 1900, when the Boer War broke out between the United Kingdom and its colonies in southern Africa, Fleming and two of his brothers joined a Scottish regiment. Their training was not onerous, consisting mostly of shooting practice and swimming. All three remained in England and did not see active service. After leaving the army Alexander was encouraged by his brothers to study medicine, something he could afford to do after inheriting money from an uncle. Alexander topped the qualifying examinations and had his choice of medical schools. It is said that his decision to go to St Mary's in London was influenced by the fact that he had played water polo against their team. Perhaps this was an indication that Fleming was not imbued with lofty ideals.

In 1905 circumstances led Fleming to specialise as a surgeon, but to take up a position in the specialty would require leaving St Mary's. The story goes that the captain of the rifle club did all he could to keep Fleming at St Mary's because Fleming was an expert marksman. He also convinced Fleming to work in his department, the Inoculation Service. Fleming made a surprising switch to bacteriology, joined the rifle club and remained at St Mary's for what was a lengthy career.

In 1909 after developing Salvarsan, his chemical treatment for syphilis, Paul Ehrlich went to London to discuss his findings. Fleming, in addition to his hospital commitments, had established a successful private practice treating syphilis patients, many from the artistic fringe. An expert in this field, he was one of very few physicians in London to administer the 'magic bullet' and he also adopted Ehrlich's pioneering intravenous injection method. Because of the success of Salvarsan, Fleming's practice boomed and he was given the nickname 'Private 606', an allusion to both the disease and to Salvarsan, called 606 because it was the 606th arsenical compound that Ehrlich had tested.[5]

When World War I broke out in 1914, many of the staff of the St Mary's bacteriology department went to France to set up a battlefield hospital laboratory. Soldiers suffered horrendous infections even from insignificant wounds. Fleming, inspired by Ehrlich, believed that there must be a chemical like Salvarsan that could help fight microbial infection even in wounds caused by shrapnel. During the course of the war, Fleming made many innovations in treatment of the wounded, and because of his battlefront experience he was determined to find a substance that could stop bacterial infection. Ironically, without knowing it had happened, he did find one.

Back in his St Mary's laboratory in the 1920s, Fleming had searched for an effective antiseptic. He was conducting an experiment with bacteria when a tear fell from his eye into a culture plate. Later he noticed that a substance in his tear killed the bacteria but was harmless to the body's white blood cells. Fleming had discovered an enzyme that occurs in many human body fluids, and in animals and plants. He named the enzyme lysozyme and although it had a natural antibacterial effect it did not work against strongly infectious agents so Fleming continued his search.[6]

There are various stories about how Fleming actually discovered penicillin, but whether any are entirely correct is perhaps debatable. In 1928, Fleming was doing research into influenza and one detail that does not seem to vary is that Fleming was away from his laboratory on a holiday for two weeks. During his absence a fungus spore entered the laboratory by some means and ended up on a Petri dish on which bacteria had been growing. Some accounts say that the spore drifted into Fleming's laboratory through a window he left open when he went away. The more accepted version now is that the spore had drifted up the stairs from a mycology laboratory one floor below.[7] What the spore did when it got into Fleming's laboratory is also up for debate: the spore landed on a Petri dish of staphylococcus Fleming had cultured as part of the research he was doing for the chapter in a book on bacteriology; Fleming hadn't properly disinfected the Petri dish; it was on top of a pile of others in a tray of disinfectant, ready to be cleaned; the Petri dishes were in a messy pile that Fleming was straightening and the telltale mould escaped being washed away to oblivion by a matter of centimetres. Take your pick.

What is important is what Alexander Fleming saw. When he came back from his holiday he noticed a clear patch, a halo surrounding a yellow-green mould that was growing on the Petri dish of staphylococci bacteria and supposedly said, 'That's funny.' The halo indicated that the bacteria around the mould had been killed. Or according to another account he didn't notice it at all. When he came back from his holiday the mould on the Petri dish was about the size of a 20-cent coin and, around it, the bacteria had died, but as it wasn't very noticeable he threw it in a bucket. His friend and colleague Professor Hare came in to talk about some subject, noticed it, pulled it out and said, 'That's interesting.'[8] Again, take your pick.

It was all a matter of luck. Fleming had decided not to store his culture in a warm incubator (and why would he if he had put it in the washing pile?), and London was then hit by a cold spell, giving the mould a chance to grow. Later, as the temperature rose (London experienced unusually warm weather), the staphylococcus bacteria flourished until it covered the entire plate, except for the area surrounding the mouldy contaminant — the mysterious spore. In short, while Fleming was out of the lab, London experienced ideal conditions for bacteria and mould growth.

So was this Fleming's 'Eureka!' moment, an instant of great personal insight and deductive reasoning? Some biographers see it in this light. Whatever the truth of the matter, Fleming took a sample of the mould and found that it was the somewhat rare *Penicillium notatum*. His discovery started a chain of events that would literally change the world — but the world had to wait ten years before Florey and his Oxford team got on the case. Fleming's notes reveal that he did not consider his discovery to be momentous. He merely concluded that the mould was producing an antibiotic substance, which he named penicillin.[9]

Fleming worked on penicillin for four years, but refining it and growing it was a difficult process for him. Every attempt he made to isolate the active ingredient from the broth used to cultivate the mould failed because he lacked the chemical expertise to extract the bacteria-killing substance. Consequently he was unable to test its efficacy against general infections and did not try it against syphilis. In 1929 Fleming published a report describing his initial work on penicillin and its potential uses in the *British Journal of Experimental Pathology* but it raised little interest.[10] There were other researchers who experienced similar frustration with penicillin in the early 1930s. Fleming had willingly provided them with samples of his mould in order to safeguard the unusual strain of *Penicillium notatum*. This unselfish act was to prove critical ten years down the track when penicillin finally emerged from obscurity.

By 1932 Fleming had put penicillin aside and was not involved in any way in its later development nor did he discover any other 'magic bullet'. Fleming would later say that his only merit was that he did not neglect the observation he had made when he found the mould and that he pursued it as a bacteriologist.[11] But while Alexander Fleming did not pursue penicillin any further, he would eventually pursue the glory for discovering it.

BEFORE FLEMING

Three thousand years before penicillin, moulds and fermented materials had been used to cure various skin infections, even though why or how they worked was not understood. Traditional healing practice in many cultures included the application of fungi to wounds or cuts. The Chinese had used mouldy soybeans, the Greeks had used mouldy cheese and the

Australian Aboriginals took mouldy bark from the shaded side of trees to make bandages.

It was not until the late 1800s that scientific studies of antibiotics began, made possible after Pasteur had established his Germ Theory of Disease which proved that infectious diseases are spread by micro-organisms. When carrying out his work on anthrax, Pasteur had observed that mould inhibited the growth of anthrax; that when more than one bacterial pathogen is living in the same space, including on human tissue, there is a microscopic struggle for existence. One life form produces an 'antibiotic', meaning 'against life', to vanquish others.

British surgeon Joseph Lister, a proponent and beneficiary of Pasteur's work, was aware that bacteria did not grow in urine contaminated with mould but he was unable to identify the active substance in the mould. In 1875, long before Fleming's observations, John Tyndall, an English physician had discovered that *Penicillium* killed bacteria. He published his findings in *Transaction of the Royal Society*, but did no further work on the mould because before Germ Theory was established it was not known that most common infections are caused by bacteria. In 1912 Ernest Duchesne, a French medical student, successfully tested a substance from mould that inhibited bacterial growth in animals.[12] Duchesne died not long after and so never saw the impact of what he had discovered.

In 1925 the Belgian researcher André Gratia, while researching ways to kill bacteria, discovered bacteriocins. These are toxins produced by bacteria to inhibit the growth of similar or closely related bacterial strains. He called the bacteriocin a *colicine* because it killed *E. coli*. He was also one of the first to discover bacteriophage, often referred to as phage, which is any virus that attacks bacteria. Smaller than bacteria, a phage infects bacteria by attaching itself to the cell wall of bacterium and injecting genetic material into it.[13] Gratia developed selection techniques that were adopted by other antibiotic hunters. Today there are hospitals in Russia where phage are used to treat infections.

Penicillin G was the first naturally occurring antibiotic to be discovered, the same one that killed bacteria during Duchesne's work in 1896 and that both Fleming in 1928 and Florey in 1939 experimented with. Today it is the most widely used form of penicillin and is obtained in a number of forms from *Penicillium* moulds. There are now more than 60 antibiotics, which work by preventing bacteria from reproducing. Bacteria reproduce by dividing to form two new cells. They enlarge to about twice their size before the DNA chromosome is copied. The two new chromosomes move apart and a cell wall forms between them. But penicillin prevents the new cell wall from forming so the bacteria cannot reproduce and the wonderful consequence is that the disease cannot spread.[14] Under a microscope you can see bacteria growing in the presence of penicillin. They look like thin jellybeans and as they extend they eventually rupture because they are unable to divide. Before penicillin they just kept dividing and dividing inside the unfortunates who had been infected.

ENTER HOWARD FLOREY

The scene was set for the development of penicillin in 1935 when Howard Florey, considered an outsider because he was Australian, was appointed Professor of Pathology at Oxford University, the youngest person ever to hold that position. It was a long way from the modest stone cottage in Malvern, a suburb of Adelaide, South Australia, where Florey was born on 24 September 1898. He was the only son of Joseph and Bertha Florey and was doted on by four older sisters. Joseph's first wife died of tuberculosis soon after they migrated from England in search of a warmer climate and Joseph remarried. An ambitious man, he started a shoe business in Adelaide and quickly established factories across the Australian continent.

By the time Howard was eight, his father was wealthy and the family moved to a sandstone mansion in the Adelaide Hills. Howard was a happy, energetic child who spent time roaming the green fields around his home in much the same way that Alexander Fleming roamed the Scottish countryside, both developing an interest in nature. Brilliant at schoolwork and outstanding at sport, Howard's commitment to study and his natural talents earned him bursaries which helped to fund his education. When he was thirteen, Howard attended St Peter's Collegiate School in Adelaide.

Florey later recalled that at about the age of twelve, although he was not very good at mathematics, he was interested in chemistry and already had some idea of doing research. When he told one of his sisters about his ambition she asked him if he wanted to be a 'sort of Pasteur'.[15] It was the ultimate irony. Florey admitted that he did not know what she meant. And yet, in the not too distant future Howard Florey would advance both the work and the ideals of Louis Pasteur. Fortunately, his interest was nurtured during his school years by an inspired chemistry teacher.

When World War I broke out in 1914 many students from St Peter's Collegiate School went into the armed forces. Australia, although it had recently become a nation, still had strong colonial bonds and supported the British in their fight against Germany. Howard, who was about to turn eighteen, wanted to join the war effort but his parents were bitterly opposed. It was not a good time for the family. Joseph Florey's health and his businesses were failing. In an attempt to persuade his father, Howard wrote a letter in which he said that he believed he should enlist:

> ... not because of a lot of balderdash that's talked about king and country, and other patriotic rubbish, but because it's the right thing to do ... When I hear a chap saying he'd like to go to the war, I feel like calling him a liar or a damn fool. I don't want to go, but I ought to.[16]

The Floreys refused their consent despite Howard's entreaties and so Howard entered medical school at Adelaide University instead of the armed forces. It was here that he met his future wife, Ethel Reed, a fellow medical student. The two were destined to make history together but their marriage would suffer as a result. Ethel was spirited and intelligent, they both had an interest in sport and, according to those who knew them, both were extremely strong-willed.[17]

Mary Ethel Hayter Reed was born in 1900. Ethel's father was the manager of the Bank of Australasia in Adelaide and her mother was proud of her aristocratic French ancestry. The family home was large and elegant. Called 'The Red House', it overlooked a park in North Adelaide. Mr Reed gave a tenth of his income to charity but this generosity did not extend to his family. Although his four children were well educated they were constantly reminded of the cost. In 1919, against her parents' wishes, Ethel began studying medicine at the University of Adelaide and was the only woman in her year. Ethel was ambitious, a trait that would have been necessary at the time for a woman to achieve success in the degree and career she had chosen.

Friends and fellow students from that time described Ethel variously as popular, pretty, vivacious and fond of parties, dancing and tennis. Because she was one of the few women studying medicine, in January 1920, when Howard Florey was the editor of the Adelaide Medical Students' Society's publication, *The Review*, he wrote to Ethel asking her to contribute an article on 'Women in Medicine'.[18] Over the next six years Howard wrote 153 letters and Ethel kept every one. In December that year Ethel contracted the first of many bouts of pleurisy and in May 1921, when it was feared she had tuberculosis, she was advised to spend a year in the mountains recuperating.

While Ethel was coping with illness, Howard Florey was sailing to England to take up a Rhodes scholarship at Oxford University. Late in 1921, aged 23, Florey left Australia wondering if he would ever return as there was a dearth of opportunities for researchers in the discipline of physiology.[19] As Florey made the long sea voyage to England as a ship's doctor, unbeknown to him, the research that Alexander Fleming was engaged in at St Mary's Hospital would influence the course of his own research and indeed his life. Fleming and Florey would share a Nobel Prize, but would never work together and would never be friends; ironically, however, their individual contributions to the discovery of penicillin would often be confused.

At the time that Florey arrived in England, Australians had a fairly mixed reputation because of the stigma of their colonial background. Florey was the archetypal Australian, somewhat brash and he never wore a collar and tie in the laboratory. There are various descriptions of him as a rough, tough Australian, energetic, tense like a coiled spring and completely uncompromising. By his own account, however, Florey was well treated at Oxford, social faux pas often being excused because he was 'just one of these rough colonials'.[20] His acceptance had much to do with his outstanding intellect, which earned him enormous respect in the academic sphere.

After completing his Bachelor of Science in the Honours School in Physiology at Oxford Florey came under the attention of Sir Charles Sherrington, whom Florey considered to be one of the greatest physiologists of all time, while doing research in his department. Sherrington, who had been asked to recommend someone for a studentship at Cambridge, approached Florey and enquired if he was interested in experimental pathology. Sherrington believed that if the right person could combine physiology and pathology then science had a lot to gain and that Florey was that person.[21] Florey's name was put forward and he took up the position at Cambridge where, as was expected, he excelled.

According to biographers, Florey did not make friends easily and was lonely at times but in his correspondence with Ethel in Australia he said that he particularly liked London, that it pulsated with life. He was scathing of the upper classes, whom he said squandered their 'infinite educational advantages'.[22] The letters went back and forth and in one Howard asked Ethel to join him in England. They had not seen each other for five years.

Ethel had graduated in 1924 as a Bachelor of Medicine and a Bachelor of Surgery and worked as a house surgeon at the Royal Adelaide Hospital where she was highly regarded. But her health problems persisted. In 1926 while Ethel and Howard were debating the possibility of marriage in the exchange of letters, Ethel was becoming increasingly deaf after having developed otosclerosis, an abnormal bone growth in the middle ear that causes hearing loss. The decision to be together was made and in 1927 Ethel completed a six-month residency at Adelaide Children's Hospital but just before setting sail for England she had another health scare and had some enlarged tuberculous glands surgically removed from her neck. Despite the setback, Ethel Reed arrived in England on 24 September 1927.

It had been a long and distant engagement and although there seems to have been some doubt on both sides, Howard and Ethel married less than a month later on 19 October at Holy Trinity Church in Paddington. The couple settled into life in Cambridge although by all accounts the marriage did not start well. Ethel and Howard had their first child, a daughter, Paquita Mary Joanna, on 26 September 1929. In 1930 Florey was appointed as a very young professor to Sheffield University where the family stayed for five years. A second child, Charles, was born on 11 September 1934. By this time the relationship had deteriorated further as Ethel's deafness worsened. Both Ethel and Howard, however, were devoted to their children, and despite the growing barrier between them — which they tried to bridge by communicating through notes — they stayed together.

In 1935 Howard Florey was appointed Professor of Pathology at the Sir William Dunn School at Oxford. He was just 37, younger than anyone who had previously held this position. The scene was set. Florey would remain at the Dunn School for the next 30 years providing exceptional leadership and guiding inspired research programs. Being head of the laboratory when he arrived was a daunting task in the economically straitened late Depression years. Florey inherited an impressive laboratory building, a façade really, because he soon found that the Dunn School was not engaged in cutting-edge research, was under-financed, and as a result morale amongst the staff was low.

From the start, Florey had to fight for funds, a task that irritated him because it monopolised his time. In a letter he wrote to the Medical Research Council he expressed his feelings in his blunt Australian style: 'It seems to me that I have acquired a reputation of being some sort of academic highway robber, because I have to make such frequent applications for grants.' When he found out that the university planned to cut his grant because of the cost of a new heating plant he wrote, 'You may gather that I am fed up.'[23]

Despite these economic constraints Florey was determined to turn things around and improve the department's scientific output. To achieve this Florey adopted an approach that was uncommon in the 1930s. He gathered together a group of researchers who had talent in different fields, an interdisciplinary team where chemists, pathologists, bacteriologists and physiologists could share expertise. Florey realised that science had reached a point where any research project was too big for one person. Gone were the days of Robert Koch beavering away in his own laboratory, carrying out every aspect of his work quietly, secretly and alone.

After Fleming's discovery of the antibiotic lysozyme Florey and other researchers had turned their attention from chemical drugs to biologically created ones produced by the human body or by moulds and animals. This led to a search in the late 1930s for similar compounds which could kill invading bacteria. After arriving at the Dunn School, Florey made the decision to investigate lysozyme and its properties and began gathering his team. He applied to Cambridge for a biochemist with the appropriate skills to assist him. Many Jewish scientists and intellectuals had been driven out of Germany after the rise of Adolf Hitler and the implementation of anti-Semitic policies. Ernst Chain, a gifted biochemist with a difficult personality, was one of them. He joined Florey at Oxford in 1935, appointed as a demonstrator and lecturer in chemical pathology.

Chain had fled Nazi Germany in 1933, some years before the transportation of Jews to concentration camps began, leaving his mother and sister behind in the belief that Hitler was a one-day wonder. He had been pursued by the Gestapo and kept a wanted poster on the wall in his laboratory at the Dunn School.[24] Chain had an incisive mind and from 1935 to 1939 worked on snake venoms, tumour metabolism and the invention and development of methods for biochemical microanalysis. Chain's innovative approach to a biological problem was to reduce it to its chemical components. It was relationships that were difficult for Chain. His relationship with Florey fluctuated and on occasion he clashed with others on the Oxford team and with university administrators. Because of his background, Chain may also have had to cope with covert discrimination and was perhaps at times treated unfairly.

Working together, Florey and Chain set out to understand the actions of lysozyme. In 1938 Chain solved the biochemical riddle surrounding it. This success led Chain and Florey to the search for other naturally produced antibiotics, a decision which was not regarded as either startling or significant at the time, just a natural extension of their work. It was the confluence of circumstances that led to the penicillin project. Because Florey had somehow wangled some funding from the Rockefeller Foundation in the United States, the two scientists were now sufficiently funded and set out to systematically identify and isolate substances from moulds that could kill bacteria.

Fleming's work had provided impetus but Florey and Chain were also inspired by the earlier work of Gerhard Domagk, a German pathologist and bacteriologist who, inspired himself by Paul Ehrlich, showed in 1935 that the injection of a simple compound, the sulfonamide Prontosil, cured systemic streptococcal infections. It was the first drug to be effective against bacterial infections. Domagk treated his own daughter and saved her from having her arm amputated. The discovery of Prontosil earned Domagk the Nobel Prize in 1939 but he was unable to accept the award until 1947 because of opposition from the Nazi regime.

Florey and Chain had different explanations for why they decided to pursue antibacterial substances. According to Florey, while they were working on lysozyme it was Chain who suggested it and he agreed to go along with it. Chain's explanation was that the project evolved, that in science there is no blueprint and each discovery is as individual as art. The scientist looks for interesting biological phenomena which it might be possible to explain in chemical terms. Again we are reminded of Pasteur's adage, that chance favours the prepared mind.

Chain began enthusiastically conducting a thorough review of related scientific literature. In 1938, while looking at old articles written about lysozyme, including those written by Fleming in the 1920s, Chain happened across the one Fleming had written on *Penicillium notatum* in 1929. While Chain was reading Fleming's paper, the memory of a woman walking along a corridor in the Dunn School with a dish of mould in her hand came to him. Chain sought her out and when he questioned her about the mould she told him it was *Penicillium notatum*. Ernst Chain exclaimed that this was the species of mould that Fleming found in 1928. The woman confirmed this. Among the various samples that Fleming had given out at the time, one had gone to the Dunn School and the mould had been kept alive ever since.[25] How often do science and serendipity go hand in hand.

Chain approached Florey, who gave the go-ahead to investigate penicillin. Over the course of the penicillin project individual members of the team concentrated their attention on areas in which they had the most knowledge, but they often met to exchange ideas. Norman Heatley, whom Florey had invited to join the Dunn School interdisciplinary team in 1936, devoted his energies to the production of penicillin by improvising methods for extraction, his specialty being microchemical methods. The team grew with Arthur Gardner taking up the bacteriological investigations, assisted by Jena Orr-Ewing for the studies on the anaerobic bacteria. Dr Margaret Jennings (an Oxford-educated doctor who joined the team as a junior research assistant, and whom Florey would eventually marry after Ethel's death) was responsible for some bacteriological work and assisted in the pharmacological and biological investigations into the impact of penicillin on animals. The group was joined by A.G. Sanders, who later set up and operated one of the large-scale extraction plants, and by E.P. Abraham, who collaborated with Ernst Chain on the chemical and biochemical aspects of the work. Ethel Florey joined the team to work with her husband and Charles Fletcher on the clinical trials. There were also a number of devoted technical assistants who saw the project through.

Initially Chain and Florey worked to identify the active ingredient in the penicillin. It then took Chain almost two years to extract it because it is so unstable. In early 1940 he delivered the first tiny amount of yellow powder. Florey's team was ready to perform one of the most important medical experiments in history on 25 May 1940. The team was so eager that everyone came into the laboratory on a Saturday morning to test penicillin for the first time.[26] Eight mice were injected with a lethal dose of a virulent strain of streptococci bacteria — 110 million of them, more than enough to kill the mice within a day. After an hour four of the mice were injected with a penicillin solution and the other four were used as controls. Norman Heatley kept an hour-by-hour vigil.[27]

By late afternoon the four control mice were sick and they began to die soon after midnight. By 3.30 a.m., sixteen and a half hours after being injected with the bacteria, all four were dead. The four treated with penicillin exhibited no symptoms whatsoever. Heatley cycled back to his rooms through wartime, blacked-out Oxford to sleep for a couple of hours before returning to the lab. Howard Florey, when told of the success, uttered what must have been the understatement of the century: that things looked quite promising.[28] The results were in fact phenomenal because by the end of World War II there was enough penicillin to treat every soldier who needed it.

Four small mice had provided the proof that Howard Florey, Ernst Chain and Norman Heatley needed. Chain apparently was almost dancing with delight and the usually laconic Florey telephoned Margaret Jennings and with a little more exuberance said that the outcome looked like a miracle. The results of the mouse experiment were published in *The Lancet* on 24 August 1940, including a stated claim that the team members were the discoverers of penicillin. The names included were Florey, Chain, Heatley, Gardner, Orr-Ewing, Jennings and Ethel Florey.[29] This article was considered to be the most important ever published in medical history.

The next major hurdle as Florey saw it was to prepare penicillin for a human trial. It had taken two years to produce enough for the mice and they now needed 3000 times that amount. Factories were on a war footing and military needs took precedence, so Florey decided to set up a clandestine mould factory at the Dunn School. First they needed containers in which to grow the fungus, so anything that was functional was used: laboratory glass, biscuit tins, trays and enamelled bedpans. Every warm spot was located (mould grows at around 24°C). Heatley then worked in a cold room when the mould was ready, as ice was needed for the extraction process. Throughout the Dunn School there were dangerous machines full of highly flammable substances and bedpans filled with mould.

Progress was slow and large quantities of mould produced only minuscule amounts of penicillin. Production had to be scaled up. Funding would help. After a surprise visit by Sir Edward Mellanby from the Medical Research Council in London, Florey wrote and asked for £600 but was awarded only £25.

During a meeting between Florey, Chain and Heatley to discuss their progress, or lack thereof, in March 1940, Heatley listened as Chain and Florey hotly debated why penicillin vanished. In his modest way Heatley put forward what he later called a 'laughably simple' idea, which involved extracting penicillin from a neutral buffer of water into ether and then transferring it out of the ether into water made alkaline by passing the mould broth back and forth between acid and alkaline to purify it.[30] Florey accepted Heatley's idea but it led to vehement argument between Florey and Ernst Chain, who felt his control over the chemical work had been usurped. From that time on Chain was suspicious of Florey and the incident created difficulties between Chain and Heatley as well.

It was largely due to the technical ingenuity of the unassuming Norman Heatley that enough penicillin was produced for the first hospital tests. On leaving university, having completed a PhD in biochemistry, Heatley's aim had been to set up his own commercial analytical service, but when Florey offered him the job at Oxford University he changed his plans. Heatley had an inventive mind and engineering skills that he now put to work in March 1940 to make his automated extraction apparatus. Because of war shortages

Heatley improvised: the frame was made from a discarded oak bookcase from the historic Bodleian Library and was about 6 feet (1.8 metres) high and 3 feet (0.9 metres) wide. He used glass tubing, assorted pumps, laboratory bottles, an old doorbell to signal when a bottle was about to become empty or full, coloured warning lights, nozzles and copper cooling coils.[31] This ingenious continuous reverse extraction contraption was ready for use early in 1941.

In one hour 12 litres of crude penicillin broth could be extracted and it was ten times more powerful than any previously produced. Chain admitted that he had been wrong but relationships were never really restored. The machine did not survive either.[32] The early industrial producers of penicillin used Heatley's extraction and purification process for several years but they spent thousands of pounds building their apparatus.

Heatley had also turned his resourceful mind to finding the best way to grow the most penicillin in the shortest time. He meticulously recorded the details of every ingredient in his lab notebook, jotting pertinent notes in red. In something akin to Paul Ehrlich's testing of 900 arsenical compounds, Heatley added substance after substance to the penicillin broth: nitrate, sodium, aluminum salts; he put in glucose, sucrose and lactate; a reduction of cow and horse muscle; extracts of malt and various meats; greater and lesser amounts of phosphate, glycerol, peptone, oxygen, carbon dioxide; he even added Marmite.[33] But to no avail. Finally the addition of yeast halved the growing time to ten days but did nothing to increase the yield.

The Blitz also thwarted Florey's plans. The sustained bombing of the United Kingdom by Nazi Germany began in September 1940 and continued until May 1941. Although the main attacks were focused on London, the Luftwaffe carried out air raids on towns and cities all over Britain, night after night, killing 43,000 people and destroying more than a million houses. It came as no surprise to Florey that pharmaceutical companies that had the equipment to culture mould in the amount he needed were unwilling to divert vital resources from the war effort into producing an untested drug.

Professor Gus Fraenkel, the founding Dean of the School of Medicine at Flinders University in Australia, was a medical student at the Dunn School during World War II. He later recalled those strange times for medical students who were studying with Florey. One of Fraenkel's duties was to patrol around the School of Pathology. Students were equipped with a tin hat, a civilian gas mask and a wooden cudgel inscribed 'Oxford University Police' which may not have been that effective against the Luftwaffe and German parachutists. [34]

As it was highly likely that Oxford would be bombed, the team interrupted their work to dig air-raid shelters. Highly flammable liquids used for the extraction process were buried in the grounds. Florey, concerned for the survival of the mould rubbed some into his, Chain's and Heatley's coats. Stocks could then be destroyed if the Nazis invaded. [35] Penicillin could be a valuable weapon and there were rumours that the Germans had tried to acquire *Penicillium* mould through neutral Switzerland.

The fact, however, remained: more penicillin was needed. The make-do containers that were used as fermentation vessels were now completely inadequate for the teams' needs. Unable to find an alternative, Heatley designed his own, based on the bedpan and shaped so that they could be stacked in the department's small autoclaves for sterilisation. They were to hold 1 litre of culture medium at a depth of 1.7 centimetres, the optimum for fungal growth and penicillin yield. [36] The Pyrex Glass Company was approached but was unable to produce them because of war commitments, and another firm that could wanted an up-front fee of £500 to prepare a special mould, plus there was a waiting time of six months.

The team was frustrated, production was held up. It was Heatley to the rescue again, suggesting ceramic vessels glazed only on the inside would be easier to handle. Florey sent Heatley's designs to a contact in an area called the Potteries located in the English Midlands, where fine tableware had been made for hundreds of years. The firm of James MacIntyre and Co. agreed to make the vessels at a very reasonable cost and gloom immediately lifted at the Dunn School. Just before Christmas in 1940 Heatley borrowed a van and brought back the first batch of 174 vessels to Oxford, one of which Heatley kept in his home for years afterwards.[37]

On Christmas Eve everyone at the Dunn School pitched in washing, sterilising and filling the new fermentation vessels. On Christmas Day Heatley seeded them with the spores of the fungus *Penicillium notatum* and stacked them for their ten-day incubation period, at the end of which time Florey's team hoped the liquid on which the fungus was growing would contain enough penicillin to begin tests on humans. Assisting the team with the mass-production were three women who were dubbed the 'Penicillin Girls'. Although they were not formally trained, they quickly became efficient at setting up the cultures and harvesting the penicillin fluid. Within a month there were 80 litres of crude penicillin solution, with around 1–2 units of penicillin per millilitre. Later developments in commercial production would increase the yield of penicillin to an astonishing 40,000 units per millilitre.[38]

By February 1941 Howard Florey had enough penicillin to conduct a human trial. It was thought unwise to inject this unknown substance into a healthy member of the team. Florey, however, gargled with some liquid penicillin to see if it would have an effect on his sore throat but there was no noticeable improvement. A young doctor at the Radcliffe Infirmary, Charles Fletcher, was asked to select a patient. In the septic ward (a ward which no longer exists in hospitals) was a 43-year-old policeman, Albert Alexander, who had been injured in a bombing raid two months earlier and was near death with a staphylococcal and streptococcal infection. Alexander's face and scalp were swollen, his head was covered with suppurating abscesses, one of his eyes had been removed and the other had to be lanced to relieve the pain of the swelling. Abscesses on Alexander's arm had to be drained and his lung was also abscessed.[39] He had been treated with sulfonamides but these are ineffective once a patient is saturated with pus.

Given Alexander's desperate situation, Florey and his team had nothing to lose yet everyone had something to gain. On 12 February Charles Fletcher administered the first dose of penicillin and Alexander immediately started to improve. More penicillin followed with more improvement. But Florey had no idea how much penicillin would be needed, and for how long, for the patient to make a full recovery. Despite the production efforts there was precious little of the wonder drug. After the first day, Fletcher collected the patient's urine so that the penicillin could be extracted and reused. Staff members from the Dunn School took turns in riding their bicycles to the laboratory to deliver the urine to Florey and Chain as quickly as possible. Someone was available every two hours to take their turn on what had been christened the 'pee patrol'.[40] This included Ethel Florey, who ironically had been able to return to her medical career because of the war.

The circumstances under which Ethel was able to resume work were not ideal for a mother. In 1938 she had begun to help organise teams of doctors for the new blood transfusion service in Oxford which was essential because of the war. Late in 1940, she and Howard and other Oxford academic families had taken the decision to evacuate their children and send them to the safety of America; 127 children were accompanied by 27 mothers.[41] Fortunately the Floreys had friends in the United States with whom their children could stay, but it was a wrench and Ethel was devastated. The children were so young — Paquita was ten and Charles only just five.

By 19 February Albert Alexander was well on the way to recovery — his temperature had come down and he was sitting up in bed — but each day a little less penicillin could be retrieved from his urine. When the supply was exhausted and the injections ceased, the bacteria began to regain their hold. Alexander relapsed and died on 15 March. It had been harrowing for the Oxford team and they were deeply affected by Alexander's death. A necessary decision was made to concentrate their efforts on sick children, who would not require such large quantities of penicillin.

Their second patient was a boy, fourteen-year-old Johnny Cox who had a staphylococcus infection in his eye socket. He was not expected to live.

Within hours of his first injection Johnny improved. The next day the boy was well enough to play and the penicillin was stopped. Totally unexpectedly, four days later Johnny went into convulsions and died. The team was devastated, heartbroken. Florey convinced Johnny's parents to agree to an autopsy. No bacteria were found but the infection had weakened one of Johnny's vital arteries, which had consequently burst.

And then success! A fifteen-year-old boy, Arthur Jones, whose wound had become septic after a hip operation to insert a pin, had not responded to sulfonamides. His temperature had been over 100°F (37.8°C) for two weeks. He was given penicillin, and within two days his temperature was normal. Four weeks later, Arthur was fit enough to undergo another operation to remove the pin.[42] Four more patients were then successfully treated and the results were described in a landmark paper modestly entitled, 'Further observations on penicillin', which was published in *The Lancet* in August 1941.

Success with the trials meant the Oxford team had to find some way to get adequate funding to ensure that penicillin production progressed from the manufacture of a scarce, impure brown powder manufactured at the Dunn School to the commercial production of a purified and powerful antibiotic that could have widespread benefits. Heatley was still trying to improve the yield and with each batch he set aside a few vessels, varying the culture medium or the conditions, but his efforts were in vain.

Florey first approached British firms to take up the production of penicillin but heavy bombing closed that avenue even though the need for an antibacterial was more critical than ever. British people were living in dangerous times and suffering great privation. A two-fold plan was adopted. The Oxford team helped the government set up a network of 'minifactories' for penicillin production while their leader, urged to do so by contacts he had established at the Rockefeller Foundation, travelled to the United

States to try to interest pharmaceutical companies there to take on large-scale production of penicillin. Accompanied by Norman Heatley, Florey left England in July 1941 and flew to neutral Portugal while battles were being waged all over Europe. From there the two flew to New York on the Pan-Am Clipper seaplane. The windows were blacked out as the plane crossed the dangerous Atlantic Ocean.

Even though Ernst Chain opposed the trip, believing that they should first patent penicillin in Britain, he felt that *he* should have accompanied Florey, not Heatley. Chain and Florey had argued bitterly about seeking a patent for penicillin. Chain understood the importance of patenting and put his suggestion to Sir Edward Mellanby in London. His entreaty met with severe criticism and he was accused of wanting to profit personally. Ernst Chain was told that in England patenting medical discoveries was unethical and not the British way. [43] But it was the American way.

Oxford University was never to receive the financial rewards that were its due. It was US companies and individuals who eventually enjoyed the astronomical profits generated by penicillin. The ultimate irony was that for 25 years after World War II the British, along with everyone else, had to pay royalties to the United States on the wonder drug that had been discovered, researched and developed in Britain. Ernst Chain had been right.

When Florey and Heatley arrived in the United States a friend of Florey's, in what was a million-to-one chance, suggested he visit an obscure agricultural research centre in Peoria in Illinois, the middle of the American wheat belt. The Department of Agriculture's North Region Research Laboratories had developed a fermentation process that would be suitable for penicillin. The director of the laboratories, Dr May, and the head of the Fermentation Division, Dr Coghill, agreed to take on the task of increasing the yield of penicillin.

While Florey visited US drug companies, initially without success — although some began their own experiments — Heatley stayed in Peoria and worked at the research laboratory with an American scientist, Dr A.J. Moyer, who suggested adding corn-steep liquor, a by-product of starch extraction, to the growth medium. With this and other subtle changes, such as using lactose in place of glucose, Moyer and Heatley were able to push up yields of penicillin from 1–2 units per millilitre to 20 units per millilitre.[44] In the midst of this success Heatley began to notice that his working relationship with Moyer, who seemed decidedly anti-British, had become one-sided with Moyer no longer sharing information.

In December 1941, Pearl Harbor was bombed by the Japanese, and America entered the war. This event changed everything. Self-interest now meant the United States government considered penicillin of national importance. Its production soon took second place only to the Manhattan Project, the development of the atomic bomb.[45] Funding was no longer an issue. At Peoria yields had improved but not in sufficient quantities to meet military demand and certainly not for civilian needs. What was needed was a new strain of the mould that would be more suited to the deep fermentation processes that had been developed to increase production.

Military personnel around the world collected handfuls of soil containing moulds that were flown to Peoria and analysed. Local people collected mould. Even the tea lady at the laboratory rummaged through rubbish bins collecting old socks, soggy newspapers and rotting food. One day she brought in a decaying piece of cantaloupe (rockmelon) that she had found in a Peoria market. The mould growing on it produced penicillin 3000 times more effective than Fleming's original mould.[46] The local mouldy melon was the answer and the tea lady earned the honourable nickname 'Mouldy Mary'.

Florey returned to Oxford in September 1941 but Heatley stayed in Peoria until December and then spent six months working for Merck & Co. Inc. pharmaceutical company in New Jersey. After returning to Oxford in July 1942, Heatley soon learnt why Moyer had become so secretive. Despite an original contract stipulating that any publications should be jointly authored, when Moyer published the results of their collective research he omitted Heatley's name. In so doing, Moyer was able to apply for patents naming himself as the sole inventor.[47] This was not the last time Heatley would not be acknowledged for his work.

In 1942 Norman Heatley's contract with the Dunn School expired and he sought employment elsewhere. The possible loss of one of his most productive researchers came as a total surprise to Howard Florey. It is reported that Florey berated Heatley for wanting to leave, dumbfounded that he would want to do so. For his part, Heatley had no idea that Florey would simply have expected him to stay on. Heatley himself said that when the dust cleared on what had been a mutual misunderstanding he was delighted to remain with Florey. In fact, Norman Heatley stayed at Oxford for the rest of his career, continuing his research on antibiotics and writing or co-authoring 65 scientific papers.

It was also in 1942, when he was busier than ever, that Florey unexpectedly and for the second time in his life heard from Alexander Fleming. Fleming had visited the Oxford team only once in August 1940 when he became aware of their work on penicillin. He had made very little comment and left as abruptly as he came. This time, when a close friend of Fleming's was dying of bacterial meningitis and Fleming had tried unsuccessfully for more than a week to cure him with sulfa drugs, the 'discoverer' of penicillin, in a panic, on a Sunday morning, telephoned the man who had developed penicillin and pleaded for some.[48]

Generously but unwisely, Florey travelled to London and gave Fleming powdered penicillin with instructions on dosage and how to inject it. Fleming treated his friend and saved his life. It was revolutionary. Hospital administrators at St Mary's invited the press to the hospital to announce a modern miracle. Fleming was ready in his white coat to claim his place in history. In August 1942, Alexander Fleming, the man who had returned to studying nasal secretions after putting penicillin aside, found himself, some would say not unwittingly, the centre of international media attention.

When journalists went to Oxford to get the other side of the story, because there certainly was one, Florey refused to be interviewed. Later he explained that he believed publicity would have had a detrimental effect by creating a huge demand for a drug that was in scarce supply.[49] So the man who was available to the media was the man the media sought. Florey did in fact receive no end of entreaties for penicillin from desperate people. At times Florey wrote replies himself, often getting Margaret Jennings to edit them and soften his somewhat abrupt and seemingly unsympathetic style.

Fleming happily took the limelight that Florey eschewed. As the number of deaths caused by bacterial infections plummeted, penicillin was being hailed all over the world and Fleming travelled to America where he met Ann Miller, the first person to have been successfully treated with penicillin in the United States. She was cured literally overnight and her temperature chart is now preserved in the Smithsonian Institute in Washington. Fleming had not been involved in her case in any way but when he met her he claimed, 'this is my most important patient'.[50] It would seem that Fleming was an early master of spin and not averse to self-aggrandisement. Ann Miller died in 1999, 57 years after being treated with penicillin.

In the United States the government had wasted no time, recruiting more than twenty chemical companies to produce penicillin. Between January and May 1943, only 400 million units of penicillin were made. Then researchers at Pfizer devised a method for growing penicillin in three dimensions, like brewing beer, which exponentially increased the yield.[51] Mass production went into full swing by the end of 1943. There was enough penicillin to meet the demand of Allied casualties when the Allied Forces invaded Normandy on D-day, June 1944, the offensive that turned the tide against the Germans in Europe. By the time the war ended in 1945, only four years after the first mouse experiments, US companies were making 650 billion units of penicillin a month.[52]

Florey's part in the penicillin story continued. In 1943, with Hugh Cairns, a professor of surgery at Oxford and a fellow Rhodes scholar from Adelaide, Florey flew to the North African battle zone to test penicillin on wounded soldiers. He wrote to Ethel describing the carnage and the horrendous wounds and infections some soldiers had endured for months without receiving proper treatment, and in some cases no treatment at all.[53] The trials were an unmitigated success. Florey revolutionised the treatment of war wounds. Instead of amputating wounded limbs or leaving wounds open to minimise the risk of infection, as was common practice, wounds were cleaned, sewn up and penicillin injected into the site. As is usual with anything new, field surgeons were furious and vociferously ridiculed the procedure, but not for long.

It was during the war that penicillin also became the method for curing the venereal disease gonorrhoea, which was rife amongst the troops. Military commanders were astonished that one or two injections of penicillin cured the disease. Thousands of troops who were due to take part in the invasion of Sicily in July 1943 were infected with gonorrhoea and the commanders appealed for penicillin to treat their soldiers so that they could return to their units. Florey and Cairns felt that penicillin should be reserved for battle casualties, but when one of the generals referred the matter to Winston Churchill, Churchill sent back a somewhat ambiguous note saying that the drug should not be wasted but must be used 'to the best military advantage'.[54] The generals determined that the best military advantage was to use penicillin so that their soldiers could be soldiers.

The benefits of penicillin were enormous and the world was indebted to Howard Florey but he continued to shun publicity and his vital role was not widely known. This was in keeping with his personality. Florey was humble about his achievements, describing the development of penicillin in an interview in 1967 as a 'terrible amount of luck' that 'involved many others'.[55] He was a quiet man in an assertive way, sure of himself and his direction. His scientific enthusiasm, exceptional skill, his total honesty and lack of pretentiousness inspired those around him. Professor Gwyn McFarlane, who first met Florey in 1938, wrote in her biography of him that Florey's extraordinary dedication and enthusiasm was very infectious, and the commitment of the Oxford team was evidence of that.

The relationship between Ernst Chain and Howard Florey, however, became increasingly difficult and their difference of opinion over patenting penicillin sounded the death knell. Chain was eventually vindicated. By not taking out the patent Florey had failed to acquire funds and prestige that would have provided equipment and autonomy on the scale that Chain thought he and Florey should have at Oxford. Whatever Chain's motives had been, the loss of the patent had a detrimental effect on the team and the university and, in fact, on the entire pharmaceutical industry in Britain.

AFTER THE WAR

In 1945, when Florey, Chain, and Fleming equally shared the Nobel Prize for Physiology or Medicine 'for the discovery of penicillin and its curative effect in various infectious diseases', the man who had made the trials possible, Norman Heatley, remained in the background. Florey led the work, Chain's contribution to determining penicillin's chemical make-up was critical, and Fleming had given them a starting point when he 'discovered' penicillin in 1928. But the 1945 Nobel Prize, so the story goes, was very nearly given solely to Alexander Fleming because of the public perception that he alone had discovered the magic penicillin and turned it into a miracle drug.

Ernst Chain left the Oxford team in 1948 when he was appointed Scientific Director of the International Research Centre for Chemical Microbiology at the Istituto Superiore di Sanità in Rome. In the same year he married Dr Anne Beloff and they had two sons, Benjamin and Daniel, and one daughter, Judith. After 1948 Chain's research interests continued to be varied and throughout his long career he co-authored many scientific papers. In 1961 Chain returned to England and joined the faculty of Imperial College University of London, where he held various positions including Professor of Biochemistry, professor emeritus and senior research fellow, remaining a fellow until his death on 12 August 1979.[56]

Ernst Chain's list of honours is extremely long. He held honorary degrees from innumerable universities and was a member or fellow of many learned societies in several countries. In addition to the Nobel Prize he was awarded, among others, the Paul Ehrlich Centenary Prize in 1954. Ernst Chain received a knighthood in 1969 from the Queen of England, the country in which he and Howard Florey had laboured under the most difficult of conditions to ensure the successful development of penicillin.

Awards and accolades came to Fleming in rapid succession, including a knighthood in 1944. On 6 June 1954, the 25th anniversary of the discovery of penicillin was celebrated at St Mary's Hospital Medical School in the presence of Prince Philip, the Duke of Edinburgh. Sir Alexander Fleming presented the duke with a culture plate with a specimen of penicillin mould.[57] Fleming's death after a heart attack in 1955 was broadcast around the world and he was buried as a national hero in the crypt of St Paul's Cathedral in London. Although Fleming's scientific oeuvre may not have reached greatness, his singular contribution, discovering penicillin, changed the practice of medicine and deserves recognition, but not at the expense of those who developed it. Alexander Fleming once said: 'One sometimes finds what one is not looking for.'[58] In this instance he was probably not referring to fame and publicity.

Sir Robert Menzies, the Australian prime minister during the first three years of World War II, said of Howard Florey that he had more effect on the welfare of the world than any other Australian. But Florey did not ascribe any altruistic motives to himself. In an interview recorded by the National Library of Australia in 1967 Florey said that there are many misconceptions when it comes to medical research.

> *People sometimes think that I and the others worked on penicillin because we were interested in suffering humanity. I don't think it ever crossed our minds about suffering humanity. This was an interesting scientific exercise, and because it was of some use in medicine was very gratifying, but this was not the reason that we started working on it.[59]*

Howard Florey's scientific contributions were not limited to penicillin. Like Louis Pasteur, Robert Koch and Alexandre Yersin before him, his work was eclectic. Florey also studied the role of white cells in the fight against viruses and bacteria. Another branch of his research involved the lining of the stomach and why it is not eroded by acid and bodily secretions. Gus Fraenkel explained that the motivation for this research was personal, beginning when Florey, because he was plagued with indigestion, had examined the contents of his own stomach and found that it contained no acid. Florey's subsequent published research on mucous secretion in the gut forms a theoretical base for an outstanding and more recent medical break-through: the cure for stomach ulcers. In the 1980s another Australian scientist, Professor Barry Marshall, like Florey, literally studied his own gut. Using the Haffkine technique — try it on yourself first — Marshall gave himself stomach ulcers by drinking a Petri dish of bacteria. He wanted to prove to a sceptical world that ulcers were not caused by stress or smoking, but by the bacteria *Helicobacter pylori*. This gung-ho approach eventually changed stomach ulcer treatment worldwide. But there is a recurring theme: in 1982, when Barry Marshall and pathologist Robin Warren cultured *Helicobacter pylori* and developed their hypothesis on the bacterial cause of peptic ulcers and gastric cancer, the theory was immediately ridiculed by the members of the medical and scientific establishment. They dismissed totally the idea that any bacteria could live in the acidic stomach.

Marshall and Warren proved them wrong and in 1984, applying Koch's postulates, showed that the *Helicobacter pylori* are the cause of stomach ulcers and gastritis.[60] To kill the bacteria they used different kinds of penicillin. Marshall believes that without Howard Florey's discovery theirs would not have been possible but also, and paradoxically, the discovery of antibiotics and penicillin may have put a stop to research on *Helicobacter pylori*.[61] In the first half of the twentieth century scientists like Florey and Fleming were researching bacteria in the stomach but then lost interest because of a plethora of new discoveries such as penicillin and other antibiotics. As Ernst Chain had done, Marshall and Warren resurrected some of the old ideas they found in reports of *Helicobacter pylori* going back over 100 years. In 2005 Marshall and Warren won a Nobel Prize for their work. In medical science one path certainly leads on to another.

Because of his prodigious scientific output, by the early 1940s Howard Florey was elected to the Royal Society, the oldest and most famous scientific establishment in the world. For his role as the leader of the team of scientists that developed penicillin and its influence on the outcome of World War II he was honoured and decorated around the world. In 1960, twenty years after being elected to the Royal Society, Florey became its president, the first pathologist and the first Australian to hold this prestigious position. He became affectionately known as 'the Bushranger President'.[62]

Ethel Florey's contribution was recognised in her home country in 1950 when Adelaide University honoured her with an MD, Doctor of Medicine. The separation from her children had given Ethel the opportunity to throw herself into the clinical work on penicillin throughout the war and afterwards. Once the trials had begun in earnest she was involved in the selection of patients, control of treatment, organisation of tests and record keeping and was on call 24 hours a day, seven days a week. Ethel and Howard published the results of 187 cases of septic infection treated with penicillin in an article in *The Lancet* on 27 March 1943. This was the first of the series of clinical trials that Ethel conducted.[63] However, she was never given a bona fide hospital appointment and officials came to regard her simply as Howard's assistant.

Ethel Florey published the results of her clinical work in two volumes, the first in 1952 and the second in 1957. She and her husband left Oxford for three years in 1957 while they built a house in Old Marston, a picture-postcard village a few miles north of Oxford. Ethel's health continued to become more precarious. She had recurrent respiratory illnesses and developed hypertension and heart problems and an operation to relieve her deafness was unsuccessful. Ethel's youthful determination remained with her and after suffering a myocardial infarct she travelled alone to America in 1965 to lecture, and then to Australia to visit friends and relatives.

That year was a busy one for Howard Florey as well. He was elevated to the peerage by the Queen of England and was made Baron Lord Florey of Adelaide and Marston. He also accepted the inaugural Chancellorship of the Australian National University, which he helped to establish. In the midst of all this, Ethel's health was rapidly deteriorating. In the spring of 1966 she went to America for her son's wedding and not long after her return died on 10 October at Marston. A long marriage that had been far from happy came to an end.

The year after Ethel's death, on 6 June 1967, Howard Florey and Margaret Jennings married in London. Those who knew them, like Gus Fraenkel, believe that Florey had found happiness late in life.[64] A discreet affair between the two during the early Oxford years had not been as secretive as they thought. After the war in 1946 Margaret and her first husband divorced but she continued to work with Florey for another two decades, publishing over 30 joint scientific papers with Florey and other authors. Sadly, the marriage was very short. Florey was in a very poor state of health and the couple had just over a year together before he died of a heart attack at the age of 69. After Lord Florey's death in 1968 Lady Margaret Florey remained at the family home in Old Marston, until she passed away in 1994.

And what of Norman Heatley? He had devised the improved extraction process, designed the ceramic vessels that facilitated the successful production of penicillin and his work in the United States was invaluable in ensuring penicillin was manufactured on an industrial scale. By the end of the war other countries were beginning to produce penicillin. Florey's own country, Australia, was the first to make the drug available for civilian use. Norman Heatley did not share the 1945 Nobel Prize nor did he receive a knighthood. Finally, in 1978, when Heatley retired from Oxford University, he was honoured with an Order of the British Empire.

Patience had always been one of Heatley's virtues. In 1990, on the 50th anniversary of the Oxford team's success in producing penicillin, the University of Oxford bestowed on Norman Heatley the first honorary

Doctor of Medicine degree in its 800-year history. Heatley was still living in the same country cottage that he and his wife, Mercy, bought in 1948 in Old Marston and where they had raised their family. As one would expect he accepted the belated honour humbly: 'This is an enormous privilege since I am not medically qualified … I was a third-rate scientist whose only merit was to be in the right place at the right time.'[65] Norman Heatley died on 5 January 2004.

No matter who received the credit for penicillin, the metamorphosis of penicillin from Alexander Fleming's observation of an 'interesting' mould into a life-saving drug could not have happened without the systematic, detailed work done by the Oxford team under the leadership of the unusual, urbane and circumspect Howard Florey. He recognised the potential of penicillin, something which Alexander Fleming had failed to do, during the violence and carnage of World War II. As Pasteur had said, humans were always finding new and barbaric means of destruction while, at the same time, evolving new ways for delivering humanity from the scourge of disease.

Sixty years on the story of the Oxford team remains a fascinating one and their collective achievements have made the world a better and healthier place. But even as penicillin was being hailed as 'the miracle drug' in the 1950s, reports began trickling in of patients failing to respond to treatment, of allergic reactions and improper use. In 1946 Alexander Fleming wrote, somewhat scathingly, that if the time came when patients could indulge in self-medication by buying penicillin over the counter and large enough doses were not administered, then the microbes would not be killed and there would be a danger that they would be educated to resist penicillin, resulting in the development of resistant strains of bacteria.[66] It was a bleak but incisive prophecy.

Despite the early, galloping success of penicillin, as Fleming predicted several strains of bacteria became resistant to penicillin after a few years through mutation. Resistant bacteria multiply when non-resistant bacteria die. To overcome this problem, scientists in the 1950s made artificial penicillin by chemically changing natural penicillin.[67] In recent years ever more powerful antibiotics have been produced to fight an increasingly broad spectrum of microbes and they have been provided to billions of people worldwide.

It is hard for us nowadays to imagine the world before antibiotics. However, the overuse of antibiotics has continued, creating a frightening new phenomenon: the adaptation through natural selection of genes for resistance to antibiotics by virtually every bacterial pathogen. Hospitals are particularly vulnerable to a new onslaught from these antibiotic-resistant bacteria. More than 70 per cent of bacteria that cause hospital-acquired infections are resistant to at least one of the drugs used to treat them.[68]

The microbes are fighting back.

POSTSCRIPT

A woman named Emma Burkervisc was in a German refugee camp after World War II when her life was saved by a new drug called penicillin. Like many displaced people Emma migrated to Australia as a refugee. Years later she had a job as the tea lady at the Australian National University's John Curtin School of Medical Research, which Howard Florey had helped to establish. One day on her rounds of the university, Emma bumped into a man who was striding through the corridor. Emma was overcome when she realised that she had come face to face with a legend. The man was Howard Florey, the genius who made penicillin possible, the benefactor who had saved her life and millions more.

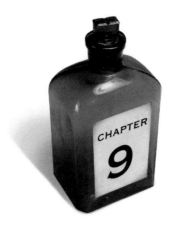

THE MARCH AGAINST POLIO

JONAS SALK, ALBERT SABIN AND
THE RACE TO MAKE A VACCINE

As a child I was not interested in science. I was
merely interested in things human, the human side
of nature if you like, and I continue to be interested
in that. That's what motivates me.[1]

Jonas Salk

It is unusual for a vaccine to take the name of its inventor but in the case
of the Salk vaccine, this probably reflects the iconic status of Jonas Salk —
and also hints at why controversy courted him. Because of the monumental nature of his achievement, the discovery of a vaccine for polio, Jonas
Salk was hailed as the new Pasteur. His is one of the greatest medical
success stories of the twentieth century. History does tend to repeat itself,
however, and so it is not surprising that Salk's fame laid him open to attack
by his colleagues in the biomedical sciences. Nor is it surprising that his
achievements were immediately denigrated and disputed. The sometimes
vicious nature of the campaign that was mounted against him revealed the
petty side of 'things human', in particular the capriciousness of human
nature.

Poliomyelitis has its own modus operandi. Unlike other viral diseases such as smallpox, yellow fever and influenza, polio did not occur in epidemic proportions until relatively recent times, the late nineteenth century. It was an unpredictable and puzzling enemy that seemed to strike out of nowhere and, like diphtheria, many of its victims were children. In the first half of the twentieth century polio epidemics hit many nations and the United States suffered particularly badly. Although polio never killed with the ferocity of other epidemic diseases like smallpox and bubonic plague, it engendered a unique terror. The poliomyelitis epidemics of the 1940s and 1950s inspired dread and panic. Known as infantile paralysis, polio conjured images of children sitting in wheelchairs, walking on crutches and wearing metal leg braces that looked like torture implements from mediaeval times.

The pursuit of a vaccine to eradicate polio is the stuff of legend, complete with presidents, heroes, archrivals, claims and counterclaims, vilification and disappointments. Fuelling it all was a frightening disease that took the lives of countless children and left many others paralysed, crippled or condemned to life in an iron lung. The competition to be first with a cure created animosity between two men who both had the same goal but who espoused different ways of achieving it. Dr Jonas Salk and Dr Albert Sabin became the public faces of two opposing schools of thought on vaccination and became locked in a battle of their own in the race to find a cure for polio.

The word 'poliomyelitis' was formed from two Greek words — *polios*, meaning 'grey', *myelos*, meaning 'marrow' — and the English suffix 'itis', meaning 'inflammation' and together they describe the disease. Polio, as it is more commonly called, causes an inflammation of the 'grey matter' of the spinal cord.[2] Like many other diseases, it has its own list of aliases. Apart from infantile paralysis, it has also been known as Heine-Medin's Disease and spinal paralytic paralysis.

Poliomyelitis is extremely infectious. Spread through human-to-human contact, it usually enters the body through the mouth due to faecally contaminated water or food. The poliovirus is a small ribonucleic acid (RNA) virus. There are three separate strains or immunologic types of the disease: Type I (Brünhilde), Type II (Lansing) and Type III (Leon). The Brünhilde strain was named after a laboratory chimpanzee when this type of polio was isolated in the chimp's spinal cord. Type II was recovered from the brain and spinal cord of a young boy from Lansing in Michigan, and the third strain was recovered from an eleven-year-old boy named Leon.[3]

After entering the body and infecting the intestinal wall the virus makes its way through the blood stream to the central nervous system causing muscle weakness and often paralysis. The onset of paralysis can be frighteningly rapid, occurring within a matter of hours — a moment once feared by hundreds of thousands of families. The incubation period can range from three to 35 days, which means that polio can spread widely and take hold in a community before an outbreak becomes apparent. Most people who are infected initially have no symptoms and are unaware that they have been infected; they can pass the disease on through poor hygiene. In all forms of polio, the early symptoms are fatigue, fever, vomiting, headache and pain in the neck and extremities. Although polio can strike a person at any age, over 50 per cent of cases occur in children between the ages of three and five.

Polio is as tenacious as other scourges that seem determined to survive despite humanity's best efforts to expunge them from the Earth. Egyptian paintings and carvings dated between 1580 and 1350 BC depict young people with withered limbs walking with canes, the cause of which may have been polio. The Roman Emperor Claudius, who walked with a limp, may have been stricken with polio as a child. Medical historians have pointed to the Bible and other early writings in which there are many descriptions of lame and crippled children and of healthy children suddenly becoming paralysed.[4] Polio may very well have been the culprit in some of these cases.

The nature of polio began to be understood in the late eighteenth century. After numerous outbreaks of a disease that caused 'debility of the lower extremities', a British physician, Michael Underwood, wrote the first clinical description. In 1840 a German physician, Jakob Heine, published a medical report which not only described the clinical features of polio but also noted that its symptoms suggested the involvement of the spinal cord. Yet the limited medical knowledge pre-Pasteur's Germ Theory of Disease, and the fact that the virus escaped detection under the microscopes of the time, meant that Heine and others could not understand polio's contagious nature. Even with the relatively large outbreaks of polio in Europe during the second half of the nineteenth century, physicians suggested stomach upset, trauma, teething, overheating and chilling as causes, which in the light of what we now know is ludicrous.[5]

In 1885 the German neurologist Ernst von Strümpell described a cerebral form of poliomyelitis and it was given the name Strümpell's disease II. The Swedish physician Oskar Karl Medin's study of poliomyelitis in 1890 led to an understanding of its epidemic character. Dr Ivar Wickman, a pupil of Medin's, was the first to conclude that polio was transmitted person to person, a realisation he came to because of his experience during the great Swedish epidemic of 1905.[6] It was Oskar Medin and Jacob Heine's names that were joined in polio's alias Heine-Medin's disease.

The actual poliovirus was identified by Karl Landsteiner in 1908. When the Austrian-born American physician became director of the laboratories of the Royal-Imperial Wilhelmina Hospital in Vienna he began an intensive study of poliomyelitis. One day in 1908 the body of a young polio victim was brought in for autopsy and Landsteiner, assisted by the German pathologist Erwin Popper, began a series of experiments. They injected matter from the brain and spinal cord of the dead child into the abdomens of two rabbits, two guinea pigs, two mice and two different species of monkey. On the sixth day following the injections one of the monkeys was ill, showing signs of paralysis similar to that in poliomyelitis patients.[7] It died two days later but the other animals remained well.

When Landsteiner and Popper examined the monkey's central nervous system it appeared similar to that of humans who had died from the disease. Landsteiner could not prove the presence of bacteria in the spinal cord of the child and so concluded that a so-called invisible virus or a virus belonging to the class of protozoa causes the disease. He then transmitted the disease from monkey to monkey and eventually it was possible to transfer a strain of the virus to a rat and a mouse. Thus both the existence and the virulence of the poliovirus were established. In a German publication in 1909 Landsteiner and Popper reported that they had found what they believed to be the cause of the polio epidemics. In the same year, American physician Simon Flexner also successfully induced polio infection in monkeys.

The pace of research was picking up and with each breakthrough came heightened optimism about a cure for polio. However, by 1913 as epidemics burgeoned in Europe and America they were accompanied by a realisation that a cure was not really on the horizon. From 1900 onwards the cycle of epidemics worldwide became more frequent and destructive. In a major outbreak of polio in the United States in 1916 the government reported over 27,000 cases with 6000 deaths nationally. In New York alone there were 8928 cases and 2407 deaths.[8] In desperation all the authorities could do was to implement quarantine measures which proved utterly ineffective in containing the rampant spread of the disease.

As polio cut a swathe through more and more countries during the 1920s, afflicting more and more people and leaving many debilitated and unable to breathe, the infamous 'iron lung' was developed. This piece of medical equipment, which aided respiration, looked like a metal coffin. Polio patients who needed an iron lung as a substitute for their own lungs spent a large part of the rest of their lives imprisoned in it, lying on their backs, immobile. But there was no choice. Hospital wards filled with rows of these massive machines from which tiny heads protruded were the cause of great despair and a further impetus to find a cure.

During the 1920s much of the research into polio focused on what was called convalescent serum, which was made from the blood of monkeys and humans who had recently recovered from polio. Some physicians were convinced that injections of the serum could prevent paralysis, as a similar approach had apparently been successful in treating meningitis. Even serum from horses that had been 'hyperimmunised' (repeatedly injected with convalescent serum in order to increase their immunity) was tried.[9] This harkened back to the work of Emil von Behring and his Blood Serum Therapy for diphtheria and tetanus. As had been the case with variolation in Edward Jenner's day, many physicians, including some from the established medical hierarchy, promoted the value of convalescent serum despite the parlous evidence to support it. In the 1930s several reliable field trials indicated that convalescent serum was neither beneficial nor harmful and after two decades it fell out of favour. Hope of an imminent cure for polio was dashed again.

One of polio's most high-profile victims was struck down in 1921 and, like so many others, was left paralysed from the waist down. Franklin Delano Roosevelt, who had been a US vice-presidential candidate in 1920, was not a typical polio patient by any means. He was 39 years old at the time he became ill and his illness was to have a long-term impact on the attitudes towards and the treatment of people with disabilities. Although there is some debate today about whether FDR, as he was known, was diagnosed correctly, his experience had a profound effect on his outlook and his policies during his four terms in office as president of the United States from 1933 to 1945. The prestige and wealth of the Roosevelt family were also valuable weapons in the fight against polio.

In a letter he wrote in October 1924, FDR described his symptoms as the disease began to manifest itself:

> *I first had a chill which lasted practically all night. The following morning the muscles of the right knee appeared weak and by afternoon I was unable to support my right leg. That evening the left knee began to weaken also and by the following morning, I was unable to stand up. This was accompanied by a continuing*

temperature of 102 [38.8°C], and I felt achy all over. By the end
of the day practically all muscles from the chest down were
involved. Above the chest the only symptom was a weakening of the
two large thumb muscles making it impossible to write. There was
no special pain along the spine and no rigidity of the neck.[10]

Roosevelt helped found the National Foundation for Infantile Paralysis (NFIP) in 1937, which later became known as the March of Dimes. The aim of the organisation was to support the rehabilitation of victims of paralytic polio and to assist in the discovery of a vaccine. The foundation was directed by FDR's friend and former law partner Basil O'Connor. President Roosevelt's premise was that any problem can be solved if people work together. He created a partnership of volunteers and researchers all with the same goal and within seventeen years of taking up the challenge the Salk vaccine had been developed and polio was on the run, a glorious day that FDR would not live to see; he died in 1945 during the last days of World War II.

Polio began to strike the United States every summer and autumn with increasingly virulent epidemics. In 1946, 35,000 cases were reported. By the early 1950s the summer had become a time of fear and anxiety for many parents; it was the season when children by the thousands became infected with the crippling disease. Panic and dread would escalate, and in medical and scientific circles the search for a cure picked up pace. At this crucial moment Jonas Salk took up the challenge.

SALK BEGINS HIS RESEARCH

Jonas Salk, the son of orthodox Jewish immigrants from Russia, was born in New York City on 28 October 1914. Although his parents did not have a formal education they were ambitious for their three sons to succeed and encouraged Jonas, the eldest, in his studies. Jonas' father was a designer in the garment industry and the children were brought up in a cultured environment. Because of the opportunities available in the United States, Jonas was able to take advantage of free public education and was the first member of his family to go to college.

After enrolling at the City College of New York with the intention of studying law, Jonas Salk soon became intrigued by medical science. Salk said that he probably made the right choice because his mother never thought he would make a good lawyer, as he could never win an argument with her. Jonas channelled his interest towards biology and chemistry and decided to go into research rather than medical practice. His ambition, as he saw it, was to be of some help to humankind, not so much on a one-to-one basis but in a larger sense.[11]

In 1938, while attending medical school at New York University, Salk was invited to spend a year studying virology and researching influenza at the University of Michigan. There, Salk worked on an influenza vaccine with the distinguished microbiologist Dr Thomas Francis, a coup for a young researcher, and Francis became Salk's lifelong mentor. The virus that causes influenza had only recently been discovered, but the principles for developing a vaccine were still the same as those established by Edward Jenner. If the body is exposed to a very weak or small amount of the disease virus, it will produce antibodies which can resist and kill the virus when a full-strength version attacks. Each virus, however, requires a custom-made vaccine. Salk experimented, hoping to deprive the influenza virus of its ability to infect while still giving immunity. This was the basis for the influenza vaccine that Francis and Salk developed, the principles of which Salk later applied to developing his polio vaccine. When World War II began in 1939 public health experts feared a repeat of the influenza epidemic that had killed millions in the wake of World War I. Fortunately, the influenza vaccine was a bonanza for the armed forces and was used to successfully control the spread of flu during and after the war.[12] The feared epidemic did not happen and Jonas Salk, as a student, had already done much to advance medical progress.

Salk received his medical degree from New York University in 1939, completed his internship and in 1942 was appointed Assistant Professor of

Epidemiology at the University of Michigan where he resumed his study of influenza. It was around this time, though, that Salk began to realise a career path might not be easy for him. He applied to some of the more prestigious universities, including Columbia University, and was turned down. In an interview he gave later in his life for the Academy of Achievement in Washington DC he revealed that he believed anti-Semitism played a role. Then in 1947 he accepted an appointment to the University of Pittsburgh Medical School as the head of the Virus Research Laboratory. (Despite the earlier setbacks and rejections, Salk would go on to become that university's Research Professor of Bacteriology in 1949, Professor of Preventive Medicine and chairman of the department in 1956, and by 1957 he would hold the position of Professor of Experimental Medicine.) In moving to Pittsburg Salk saw an opportunity to continue his work on influenza and begin work on polio.[13] One can only wonder at the part played by Providence in many of the monumental medical breakthroughs. For the next eight years of his life, Jonas Salk devoted himself to the mission to save children from the horrors of polio.

Within a few months of arriving in Pittsburgh, Salk was visited by Basil O'Connor, the head of the National Foundation for Infantile Paralysis, who asked him if he would be interested in participating in a program on typing polioviruses. (Typing is the process of classifying or distinguishing types and strains within a seemingly homogeneous species of micro-organism.) The push was on to find a cure and a committee had been set up to deal with all aspects of research. Salk accepted and the funding he was given provided laboratory facilities, equipment and staff.[14] According to Wilfrid Sheed, in an article he wrote for *Time* magazine in 1999, Salk had somehow found time to do some basic research on the poliovirus and Basil O'Connor, who was zealous in his quest for a cure (his daughter having been afflicted and left partially paralysed), was impressed with the theoretical papers Salk had written. As a result O'Connor had decided to 'shove some dimes in Salk's direction with instructions to get going'.[15]

Jonas Salk was one of many researchers who were seeking a cure for polio and some had been involved in the quest for much longer. No doubt the seeds of resentment were sown when the apparent newcomer was given funding and hence freedom for his research. As Jonas Salk began his work to combat a disease that had caused untold tragedy to so many families, one of the bitterest rivalries in medical science was beginning and soon the competition between two scientific camps to develop a polio vaccine would begin.

CONTROVERSY AND COMPETITION: SALK AND SABIN

Jonas Salk and Albert Sabin led two competing schools of vaccine research. Sabin favoured producing immunity by creating a mild infection with a live but attenuated virus and this was his methodology for preparing his vaccine. However, virulent viruses could be made into a 'killed', non-infectious vaccine by treatment with a standard disinfectant and preservative such as formaldehyde, as Salk had learnt from his flu-fighting days. The immune system could in fact be triggered without infection — using deactivated, or killed, viruses.[16]

Salk argued that the immune system could be set to work against polioviruses with an injected vaccine without the need to trigger an actual infection. Before Salk's work on influenza, the effective vaccines had been made with weakened viruses but they still had the capacity to infect. Sometimes, as in the case of the smallpox virus, immunisation would cause serious reactions and occasionally fatalities. The principle that Salk tried to establish was that it was not necessary to run the risk of infection and so it seemed safer to proceed with a killed vaccine.

As time was of the essence — every summer the number of children who died or were left paralysed from polio kept rising — a vaccine that could be developed quickly was of critical importance. This made Salk's vaccine more appealing. Sabin, on the other hand, favoured an oral, attenuated vaccine. By the late 1930s it was known that polio entered the body via the mouth and digestive tract, which led Sabin and other virologists to believe that an oral vaccine would be more expedient than a killed vaccine.[17] Conflict and controversy plagued the polio project from this point on.

Albert Sabin had sound credentials and had become interested in polio after graduating in medicine from New York University in 1931. Sabin was an immigrant who had been born in Bialystok in Poland on 26 August 1906. He was one of four children born to Jacob Sabin and his wife Tillie. The family immigrated to the United States in 1921 and settled in Paterson, New Jersey. Like Jonas Salk's father, Albert Sabin's father was in the clothing industry, manufacturing silk, and the two younger men were in the same industry, virology.

In 1941 when the United States entered World War II Sabin enlisted and joined the US Army Epidemiological Board's Virus Committee and took on assignments in various theatres of war — Europe, Africa, the Middle East and the Pacific. Sabin's contribution was outstanding and he was involved in the development of vaccines for mosquito-borne diseases.[18] Over 65,000 military personnel were successfully vaccinated against the mosquito-borne Japanese encephalitis with his new vaccine and he also worked on preventive vaccines for dengue fever and sand-fly fever.

Many of the experiments Sabin conducted during his early research on the poliovirus he reported to the National Foundation of Infantile Paralysis. When he and Salk, who came from opposite sides of the vaccine research divide, were appointed to the committee that was established to discuss issues associated with developing a polio vaccine, a clash arose over typing the virus, a necessary first step. Jonas Salk thought the committee was heading in the wrong direction because they favoured determining a strain's virulence rather than its antigenicity, i.e. how much antibody results from the introduction of the virus. At one meeting when Salk said that a better way forward might be to test an unknown virus's capacity to immunise rather than its capacity to infect, Sabin condescendingly dismissed Salk's suggestion. This clash epitomised their different approaches to developing a vaccine, and led to complex and costly experiments that hampered progress.

Although work at Johns Hopkins and Yale University had established the number of polio types at three — Type I (Brünhilde), Type II (Lansing) and Type III (Leon) — the committee demanded that the 125 strains of the virus that had been identified by various members of the scientific community had to be sorted into these three types. The process took Salk three years: one to sort the strains and two to confirm his findings that they all belonged to one of the three types. Salk later said that the work had been invaluable for him in working towards his vaccine, which to be effective had to contain all three types of the poliovirus.

Sabin had delays of his own. His conclusion after conducting a series of experiments was that the poliovirus grew only in the nerve cells in the spinal cord and brain and invaded the body via the respiratory system. This view was supported by an eminent group of scientists and for that reason the virus was grown for some years in the nerve tissue of expensive laboratory primates, monkeys, which made it difficult to obtain.[19] One of the hardest things about working with the poliovirus was manufacturing enough to experiment with, let alone making large-scale vaccine production practical.

At Harvard in 1948, three researchers — John Enders, Thomas Weller and Frederick Robbins — made a breakthrough that facilitated a solution to this problem. They had been working on growing the cold sore virus and mumps virus in a mixture of human embryonic skin and muscle tissue but had not bothered with the poliovirus because of the prevailing view. In the storage cabinet there just happened to be the Lansing strain of poliomyelitis virus so almost on a whim the decision was made to do with it what they had been doing with the other viruses. Utterly surprised, they succeeded in their first attempt.

Enders, Weller and Robbins immediately realised that given the right conditions the poliovirus could grow in many different sorts of cells. They grew it on scraps of tissue from stillborn human embryos, then chicken embryos and then on other tissue, without needing an intact organism.[20] Bacteria usually contaminated the tissue but Enders and his colleagues, thanks to Howard Florey and the Oxford team, now had access to the new drug penicillin, which prevented the bacterial growth. The Enders team won the 1954 Nobel Prize for Physiology or Medicine 'for their discovery of the ability of poliomyelitis viruses to grow in cultures of various types of tissue'.[21] This was the only Nobel Prize ever awarded for polio research. There were no laurel wreaths for Salk or his rival Sabin.

Perhaps this was a case of déjà vu. Without the Oxford team no Enders, Weller and Robbins; and without them, no Jonas Salk or Sabin producing vaccines for poliomyelitis. Salk had a way forward. Enders and his team had shown that viruses like mumps and polio could now be grown in test tubes in large enough quantities for study. Salk made the necessary adjustments to his laboratory and employed the Enders method, incubating the virus using rhesus monkey kidneys and testicles.[22] In a television interview after he had developed his vaccine Jonas Salk said, 'Enders threw a long forward pass and we happened to be at a place where the ball could be caught.'[23] By examining previous research Salk had also found a way to kill the poliovirus with formaldehyde while it remained intact enough to trigger a response in humans. This enabled him to significantly speed up his research program.

It was this ability to inform his own research with that of others which later told against Salk and led to one of Sabin's vitriolic attacks on him. Sabin was quoted in newspapers in the United States as saying that Salk 'never had an original idea in his life' and that 'you could go into the kitchen and do what he did'.[24] John Enders supported Sabin and his approach to developing a vaccine and he is reported to have referred to Jonas Salk's work as quackery.

The National Foundation for Infantile Paralysis was aware of the antipathy between the two camps but supported research efforts by both. A sea voyage was to prove fateful in determining what would happen next in the race for the polio vaccine. Basil O'Connor and Jonas Salk were returning from the International Polio Congress in Copenhagen in 1951 on the ocean liner the *Queen Mary*. The two men spent some time together and once again O'Connor was impressed by Salk's knowledge. Salk convinced O'Connor that the killed virus vaccine was almost ready for trialling and it was unable to cause the disease, whereas attenuated vaccines could because they were still virulent. O'Connor as head of the March of Dimes gave Salk immediate approval to prepare his vaccine for trial.

The year 1952 was a critical one in the United States. That summer 57,628 cases of paralytic polio were recorded.[25] There were 3000 deaths and 21,000 victims were left paralysed, making it the worst year yet. There was a crescendo of hysteria. Children were kept indoors and whole families left the cities en masse, some even escaping to Europe in the hope of finding sanctuary from this destructive disease. Those who stayed were clamouring for a breakthrough. What had been achieved by 1952 was that both vaccines, the killed and the attenuated, caused a rise in blood antibody levels against the virus but no one was sure what level was needed to provide immunity. The real competition was about to begin.

During his research Jonas Salk had noticed an interesting phenomenon. The pattern of infection and transmission of polio had changed over time. Previously it had struck infants first, hence the name infantile paralysis, but as hygienic conditions improved, the virus spread in the population in a different way. If infants acquired polio in the first six months of life they were protected against paralysis because of maternal antibody. However, after the maternal antibody was lost, if infants were then infected with polio, paralysis would ensue.[26] So as time went on and hygienic conditions improved, many people were contracting the disease later in life. By the early 1950s, about 25 per cent of paralytic cases occurred in those aged 21 and older, which could account for the fact that Franklin Delano Roosevelt became paralysed at the age of 39.[27] The age distribution had changed because polio was now spread less by the water supply or by exposure to faecal contamination but more in a family context or amongst playmates through the secretions of the nose and throat. For these reasons polio was on the increase and unpredictable.

It was against the backdrop of fear and hysteria that on 2 July 1952 Salk tried a refined vaccine for the first time. Children from a crippled children's home near Pittsburgh, polio victims who had recovered, were vaccinated to see how well the vaccine elevated the antibodies of the strain of the disease that they had suffered from. After the vaccination, their antibodies increased. Then the vaccine was tested on children from the Polk State School who had not had polio. About 5000 children in all were involved in the trial.

Scientists often have blind faith or perhaps informed faith in their own work. Jonas Salk then tried his killed vaccine on a number of volunteers who had not had polio, including himself, his wife and their three sons, fortunately without detriment. By the end of the year Salk was convinced that antibody response was real in humans because tests showed that the antibodies in both groups of children in the trial had remained high and none of the children had suffered any worrying side-effects.

News of this early testing leaked into the public domain and there are varying accounts of how this happened. Salk himself said that the leak had occurred via a journalist who had tracked down the story after being present at an advisory committee meeting of the March of Dimes. It had been the intention of the committee to avoid any publicity at this stage but Salk decided to publish his results as soon as possible, hoping to prevent any misconceptions about the trial. He did so the following year in 1953, in the *Journal of the American Medical Association*.

The publicity, which had not been sought, brought both accolades and acrimony for Jonas Salk. He was lauded by the public but accused of being a 'glory hound' by opponents. Accusations were rife that Salk and perhaps even the National Foundation for Infantile Paralysis had entered into a deal with the pharmaceutical company Parke Davis. Salk had always felt like an outsider as far as his colleagues were concerned and now he was being marginalised even more. It seemed he could not take a trick and although

Salk called his vaccine 'the Pittsburgh vaccine' after his university, the newspapers called it the 'Salk vaccine', a name that stuck in the public mind causing further affront to the medical establishment.

Amidst this maelstrom, in 1953 Sabin was persevering with attenuated strains of poliovirus and did not have a vaccine ready for trialling while Salk's vaccine had passed the first test and it seemed safe and effective. Many virologists still agreed with Sabin, however, that an oral attenuated vaccine would in the long term provide greater immunity than a killed vaccine. Salk maintained his objection that, unlike a killed vaccine a weakened vaccine was always potentially dangerous and had to be tested with intense rigour.

The fundamental, scientific principle that Salk followed was to choose the safe option that could be controlled. He believed in trying to work like nature instead of simply imitating it and as a result his killed vaccine had been ready while Sabin's still needed fine-tuning. The Salk team had experimented with dose, quantity, duration and the kind of immunity that might be required but did not have to worry about the virulence of the virus. When the leaders of the rival factions presented and defended their positions on polio vaccines at a major medical conference in Rome in September 1953 there was a palpable absence of collegiality.

At the height of the polio epidemic in 1953, the National Foundation for Infantile Paralysis decided to organise mass trials using Salk's killed vaccine. A pattern had been established, however, and as expected Sabin and his supporters were horrified and publicly challenged the approach. The situation Salk found himself in worsened as criticism of the proposed trials reached a peak in early April 1954. Scare tactics were aimed at parents. Fantastic rumours were spread that the National Foundation had a stock of little white coffins for the children who would die as a result of their involvement in the trial and a well-known radio personality, Walter Winchell, who had spoken to one of Salk's opponents, broadcast that the vaccine could be a killer.[28]

Predictably, problems then arose over who should have control of the large-scale vaccine trials. Jonas Salk's mentor, Thomas Francis, with whom Salk had developed the influenza vaccine, was chosen as the director. Laboratories were adapted in order to produce the huge quantities of the vaccine needed. Five pharmaceutical firms manufactured the Salk vaccine: Parke Davis & Co. in Detroit, Pitman-Moore and Eli Lilly & Co. in Indianapolis, Wyeth Inc. in Philadelphia and the Cutter Laboratories in Berkeley in California.

In April 1954 the national field trials began. It was the largest controlled, double-blind study that had ever been conducted, involving nearly 2 million school children aged between six and nine, this age group having become a primary susceptible group to polio. Without knowing which they received, 440,000 children were vaccinated and 210,000 received a placebo. A massive 1,180,000 served as unvaccinated controls.[29] And the results? A staggering 60 to 70 per cent of the vaccinated children were immune to polio.

On 12 April 1955 the world was informed that a vaccine existed which could put an end to polio's tortures. This monumental news story took on a life of its own. It was the 1950s — the beginning of the media age. Speaking directly to an audience of 500 scientists and physicians, Thomas Francis presented the results in a carefully scripted but detailed one hour and 40 minute talk. Sixteen television and newsreel cameras were recording the event and, in a press room three floors above, over 150 newspaper, television and radio reporters were sending out their stories.

The vaccine was a godsend and Salk came close to achieving the status of a deity. Americans breathed a collective sigh of relief. The Salk vaccine was declared 90 per cent effective against Types II and III poliovirus and 60 to 70 per cent effective against Type I. Within two hours, Salk's inactivated polio vaccine (IPV) was licensed for use.[30] Because of guarantees from the March of Dimes, as the National Foundation for Infantile Paralysis had commonly become known, industrial production facilities were already built and ready to operate. The goal was to have 5 million US children vaccinated by July 1955.

Then, suddenly and unexpectedly, thirteen days after the announcement, on 25 April, an incident was uncovered which was reminiscent of the tragic Lübeck disaster (in which children died as a result of contaminated diphtheria serum in 1930). Some 200 cases of polio were attributed to Salk's vaccine. There were eleven deaths and 150 cases of paralysis. Tremendous publicity was given to these cases and once again optimism was shattered. An investigation revealed that the disease-causing vaccine all came from one poorly made batch at a specific drug company. The incident became known as the Cutter Laboratory disaster. On 27 April the surgeon-general recalled all of the Cutter Laboratory vaccines and on 8 May the entire US vaccination program was cancelled. *The Lancet*, published on 11 June, stated in a leading article that 'the most likely explanation is that some of the vaccine contained live poliomyelitis virus which had not been completely inactivated by the formaldehyde treatment'.[31]

Higher production standards were immediately adopted and, after confidence in the vaccine was restored, the vaccination program was resumed. By August 1955 over 5 million doses of the Salk inactivated polio vaccine had been administered in the United States. The impact was dramatic. In 1955 there were 28,985 cases of polio; in 1956 the number had halved to 14,647; and in 1957 only 5894 cases were reported.[32] Across the Atlantic, some European countries imported the Salk vaccine from the United States whereas others, including Denmark, began vaccine production in their own government facilities. In Denmark it was proposed that everyone up to the age of eighteen should be vaccinated as a matter of course.

Early in 1955 the Pasteur Institute in France put out a statement that an anti-poliomyelitis vaccine, developed by Professor Pierre Lepine, would soon be produced in large quantities. According to *The Lancet* published on 7 May 1955, the Swedish government planned to manufacture a vaccine derived from a virus grown in human tissue in the hope that it would be free from the side-effects that might result from the use of monkey tissue; but in the interim the Swedes ordered 100,000 doses of the American Salk vaccine. By 1959, 90 other countries were using Salk's vaccine.[33]

The first country to be chosen by President Eisenhower to receive the formula of the Salk vaccine was India and the presentation was made on

5 May 1955 to the Indian Health Minister by the US Ambassador. This was in recognition of the contribution made by India in developing the vaccine. A polio research centre in Bombay, financed by the Indian Council of Medical Research, had been working on the problem for several years and was said to have produced valuable data. Also, thousands of rhesus monkeys had been imported into America from India for initial experimentation.

Even though the Indian Health Ministry planned to immediately start manufacturing the vaccine they were still willing to continue exporting monkeys as long as they were transported under humane conditions and would only be used for poliomyelitis research. According to David R. Preston, Director of Scientific Information at the National Foundation for Infantile Paralysis at that time, one monkey's kidneys could provide enough vaccine for 6000 injections, enough for 2000 children if a course of three injections was needed for each child.[34] At that time, when so much vaccine was needed, the demand for monkeys exceeded the supply. When addressing an international conference in Rome on the subject of poliomyelitis in 1954, Jonas Salk said that he had already at that time made use of 15,000 monkeys. The rhesus monkeys, each of which weighs around 2 to 4 kilograms, were trapped in northern India, carried in bamboo cages on shoulder poles to the nearest railway station to be transported to Delhi where they underwent health screening. The monkeys were flown 4000 miles (6400 kilometres) to London and then a further 3000 miles (4800 kilometres) to New York's Idlewild Airport from where they were trucked to Okatie Farms in South Carolina. Monkeys were also transported from the Philippines. An average of 5000 monkeys a month passed through Okatie Farms before being dispersed to four laboratories in Toronto, Pittsburgh, Detroit, and Berkeley.[35] At the laboratories the monkeys were anaesthetised, their kidneys were removed and then they were euthanased. Their kidneys were sliced up, placed in a viable solution and rocked gently in an incubator for about six days to promote kidney cell growth.[36]

The success of the vaccine won Jonas Salk unsought fame. The March of Dimes, hoping to boost publicity and donations to fund the vaccination programs, pushed Salk into the limelight, which succeeded in offending his opponents even more, if that was possible. He was attacked again for 'stealing' his success. Salk had, in fact, applied the findings of others in order to discover a successful preventative vaccine for polio. But those 'others' could have done the same.

Another accusation levelled against Salk was that he took credit for himself only, and this would haunt him for many years. Labelled as selfish, he was accused of possessing an egotism that grew parasitically with his sudden rise to fame. It was said that in his press conference in 1955 he had not acknowledged his colleagues. In Salk's defence, it depends on what one is asked in interviews as to what emerges. Salk did in fact mention the work of the Enders team in interviews and this acknowledgement appears in the *New York Times*' five-page coverage of the 1955 press conference. Other researchers were acknowledged in the print media for their contributions as well.[37] That credit was shared cannot be denied.

Conversely, the timing of Salk's successful vaccine at the peak of polio's devastation in the mid 1950s rendered the public deaf to criticism and Salk was felt to embody all that was good about science. He had refused to patent the vaccine, having no desire to profit from the discovery but wanting merely to see the vaccine disseminated as widely as possible. There is no doubt that he lamented becoming a public figure; his time was no longer his own and he had to struggle to continue with his work. Salk described losing his anonymity as akin to being in the eye of a hurricane.[38]

While the Salk circus was in full swing, Albert Sabin did not give up his quest and continued his work at the University of Cincinnati on an oral vaccine. His view, still shared by others in the field, was that Salk's killed virus vaccine was not strong enough and that during the time in which immunity lasted, the body would not have a chance to build up antibodies from natural exposure. In the long run Salk's vaccine would be a disaster waiting to happen. Only a live vaccine, they continued to argue, had sufficient immunogenicity to provide protection. In contrast, an inactivated vaccine would have to be re-administered regularly and, as time would prove, Salk's vaccine did in fact require booster shots. Although it took Sabin longer to produce his oral, attenuated vaccine, the tortoise would eventually win a victory of sorts.

Undeterred by Salk's popular success, other researchers were engaged in developing attenuated vaccines. At the Lederle Laboratories in New York, a commercial interest that had received some of the millions of dollars of funding the US government had invested in polio research, Herald R. Cox, the director of the laboratory, and Polish-born virologist and immunologist Hilary Koprowski continued working on live attenuated virus preparations. Koprowski had been employed by Cox and they were co-researchers until their professional relationship broke down in 1952 and they became competitors instead. Like Sabin and Salk, each developed a polio vaccine the merits of which they vigorously defended and debated. Apart from the good an effective polio vaccine could do for humankind, success could bring with it untold benefits to a scientist.

The in-fighting remained bitter. Koprowski later claimed that he created the first successful polio vaccine in 1950 but his live attenuated oral vaccine was not ready for use until five years after Jonas Salk's injected vaccine reached the market. He also had issues with Albert Sabin, claiming that Sabin used samples of attenuated virus given to him by Koprowski to develop his oral vaccine. Although their relationship had already been strained, one day when Sabin had visited Koprowski at the Lederle laboratory they had agreed to exchange samples; but according to Koprowski, Sabin welshed on the deal. This gave Koprowski grounds for later asserting that the polio vaccine he discovered had become wrongly known as the Sabin vaccine. Everyone wanted the glory.

In his research, it had been Sabin's aim to mimic the real-life infection of polio as much as possible by using a weakened form of the live virus. By

1956 Sabin had administered his vaccine to approximately 9000 monkeys and 150 chimpanzees and before he experimented on 133 young adults, volunteers from an Ohio prison, he and his associates swallowed avirulent live viruses themselves.[39] The results were a significant rise in antibodies and no signs of polio infection. Sabin was fortunate to have the support of the pharmaceutical company Merck, Sharp and Dohme. The company provided approximately 25 million doses of each selected strain of poliovirus. The stakes were as high for drug companies as they were for individual scientists.

Sabin's oral vaccine then underwent two major trials between 1958 and 1960 in the Belgian Congo and in the Soviet Union and Eastern Europe. Relations between the United States and the Soviets were strained but the Russians were prepared to trial Sabin's vaccine because their plight was so serious. At the same time, 1957 to 1960, Koprowski was testing his vaccine in Ireland and in various areas in Africa. It was necessary to trial outside the United States because widespread immunisation with the Salk vaccine meant that most US children had antibody levels that were too high to enable an evaluation of a second vaccine.

Sabin now had new rivals and in an attack similar to that previously aimed at Jonas Salk, Sabin's vaccine was dubbed the 'communist vaccine'.[40] He was at last getting some of his own medicine. Regardless of what the vaccine may have been called this did not detract from its staggering success. By July 1960 more than 15 million Soviet citizens were said to have received Sabin's oral vaccine while Koprowski's had failed. Kropowski accused Sabin of being unfairly supported by the scientific establishment while he was sidelined as an outsider from private industry.[41]

The rivalry continued. Herald Cox from the Lederle Laboratories, who eschewed the Enders technique of growing the polio virus on monkey tissue because of the danger of contamination with monkey viruses, had reported in October 1952 that he had grown the Lansing strain in fertile hens' eggs.[42] He too was developing a vaccine. However, it was not ready until 1961. By the time Cox tested his vaccine in Latin America, Sabin's vaccine was already well on the way to being accepted. This did not stop Maurice Hilleman, a major figure in vaccine research in America and director of the Merck Institute for Therapeutic Research, referring to Sabin as a self-pronounced genius who had taken over Cox's and Koprowski's ideas.[43] The sniping seemed endless.

The tide, however, was turning rapidly in Sabin's favour. His attenuated oral vaccine was deemed to have advantages over Salk's vaccine. It was found to confer longer-lasting immunity, so that repeated boosters were not necessary, and it acted quickly, immunity being achieved in a matter of days. Taken orally, on a sugar cube or in a drink, the vaccine was much easier to administer than the injected Salk vaccine. Also the Sabin vaccine offered the prospect of passive vaccination because it caused an active infection of the bowel resulting in the excretion of live attenuated virus. This could help to protect people who had not been vaccinated through exposure to faecal matter and sewage.

On 24 August 1960 when the surgeon-general recommended licensing Sabin's vaccine for domestic use, Salk continued to argue that even though it had been successful in the Soviet trial, the vaccine could actually cause cases of polio.[44] He would prove to be correct, but in developing countries the cheaper Sabin oral vaccine had far more appeal and the risk was minimal compared with the difference it made overall to child morbidity and to cases of paralysis. The advantages of the attenuated vaccine were soon recognised even in the developed world.

SALK'S REIGN ENDS, SUSPICION MOUNTS

The Sabin oral polio vaccine (OPV) was licensed in 1962 and gradually supplanted its rival and predecessor. The frightening polio epidemics which marred the first half of the twentieth century were gone. By 1968, Salk's vaccine was no longer being administered in the United States and US pharmaceutical companies had stopped producing it. By the 1970s the Sabin vaccine replaced the Salk vaccine in many parts of the world. However, some countries including the Netherlands continued to use only

Salk's vaccine even though the advantages of the live attenuated vaccine seemed clear-cut.

And the reason? As early as 1962, it was suspected that in a very small number of cases, mostly adults, the live vaccine could lead to paralytic poliomyelitis. In 1964, an advisory committee established by the US surgeon-general reviewed the incidence of polio between 1955 and 1961, a period when only the Salk vaccine was used, and between 1961 and 1964, when the Sabin vaccine predominated. It was the judgment of the committee that of the 87 cases of paralytic polio reported in the United States after 1961, 57 were compatible with having been caused by the attenuated poliovirus regaining its virulence. [45] It was exactly what Jonas Salk had warned might happen.

By the mid 1960s, health officials in the United States had to weigh the many benefits of Sabin's OPV against the small but definite risks that were now known to be associated with its use. Polio was rampant in many countries despite the inroads made and the aim was still global eradication. There were other factors to consider. Immunisation programs with the OPV and manufacturing facilities were already in place. The costs involved in switching back to the Salk vaccine and the risk of affecting public confidence were too great to risk. These anomalies, however, made it difficult for health authorities to establish immunisation standards and for a time a course of injections was given that included both vaccines. The tortoise and the hare were running side by side.

In an overall review of the vaccines, the Centers for Disease Control and Prevention in the United States found that between 1960 and 1983 of a total of 210 cases of polio, 99 may have been caused by the Sabin vaccine. Sabin, however, could not accept this assessment and hypothesised that other diseases which cause paralysis can mimic polio and his vaccine was not the cause. Salk accused Sabin of not believing the scientific evidence. [46] The animosity continued between the two scientists but Sabin's reputation in the medical world remained untarnished.

During the tug-of-war between the Salk and the Sabin vaccines, Jonas Salk had been aggressively marginalised by the medical community and perhaps permanently bruised by the attacks he had suffered. In 1963, when he founded the Salk Institute for Biological Sciences in La Jolla in California, his cynical comment that he could not possibly have become a member of this institute if he had not founded it himself reveals insight into his ostracism and the depth of the hurt.[47] To add insult to injury his own institute did not bring him the professional satisfaction he may have hoped for. Jonas Salk harboured the view that many of the great scientists who were attracted to work there were no different to those who had sneered at his work on polio, dismissing him as a mere technician. Great minds and great egos walk closely together.

When asked about scientists devoting their lives to humanity and the rivalries that often ensue, Salk's answer was reminiscent of words uttered by Howard Florey. Salk commented that it is not a bent to help humanity that drives scientists: 'The motivation to do what we do is different in each instance' and in some instances, he said, one does not understand what that is until 'you see the effect it has produced'.[48] He said there is a difference between a scientist dealing with nature in the laboratory and dealing with human nature outside it, which includes how colleagues or others will react — often not from altruistic motives. Jonas Salk's story is certainly proof of that.

Jonas Salk saw scientists falling into two categories, the 'evolvers' and the 'maintainers of the status quo'. According to Salk, when it comes to medical breakthroughs it is the evolvers who cause things to change while the maintainers do everything to stop things changing. The two are different in interpretation, temperament and personality and evolvers are, like Salk, a much rarer species.

When assessing Jonas Salk's career two things are certain. He won the race to find an effective vaccine against polio but received few honours for being the first to save generations of children not only from death but, in some cases, as the cliché goes, a fate worse than death. Jonas Salk was awarded a Congressional Medal of Honour in 1955 and the Presidential Medal of Freedom in 1977 but he was not elected to the National Academy of Sciences and did not win a Nobel Prize. Perhaps his standing amongst his peers never recovered but he won the adulation of a grateful world.

Jonas Salk continued to conduct research and publish books, some in collaboration with his sons who also became medical scientists. In his last years he joined the search for a vaccine for AIDS. Jonas Salk died of congestive heart failure on 23 June 1995, aged 80.

Basil O'Connor remained a steadfast supporter of Jonas Salk and summed up what he saw as a great injustice. Salk had 'showed the world how to eliminate paralytic polio', O'Connor said, 'and you'd think he had halitosis or had committed a felony'.[49] Nobel laureate Renato Dulbecco, in an obituary he wrote for Salk, expressed the same sentiments with the appropriate gravitas: 'The fact that a fundamental advance in human health could not be recognised as a scientific contribution raises the question of the role of science in our society.'[50]

It was Jonas Salk's firm belief that in the future science should be able to provide a greater understanding of how the mind works, and how we can use our minds to better advantage to improve health by enhancing the positive and reducing the negative. He shared Louis Pasteur's view of humankind that some people are constructive and others destructive and it is necessary to have enough of the former to overcome the problems of each age. Jonas Salk made a superhuman effort to reduce the negative in the world by finding a cure for polio, one of the greatest problems of his age.

Albert Sabin went on to play a significant role in the vaccination programs run by the Pan-American Union and the World Health Organization. Sabin was researching the role of viruses in cancer at the time of his death in 1993. He was 86 years old.

Authorities in various countries interpreted the risks and benefits of the killed and the attenuated vaccines differently, depending on how successful they had already been in reducing the incidence of polio. In the 1970s, because of its lower cost and long-term efficacy, the World Health Organization included the Sabin vaccine in the packet of subsidised vaccines it provided to poor countries under its immunisation program. In 1974 the WHO launched its Expanded Programme on Immunisation (EPI) because, worldwide, less than 5 per cent of children in the first year of life were immunised against six initial target diseases: diphtheria, tetanus, pertussis, measles, tuberculosis and polio. Extraordinary minds during a period of almost a century had developed vaccines for all of these diseases.

With approximately 350,000 cases of polio still occurring worldwide in 1988, the World Health Assembly launched the Global Polio Eradication Initiative. During a two-year period, 1995–96, approximately 400 million children under the age of five were immunised against polio, mostly with the Sabin vaccine. By 1998 more than 450 million children had been vaccinated under this scheme and the number of polio cases worldwide had fallen to approximately 7000 in 1999.

In the United States the oral vaccine is no longer administered particularly because of vaccine-induced paralytic polio. During the 1990s improved vaccines were introduced with variable results. The latest Inactivated Polio Vaccine (IPV) is known to be 90 per cent effective after two doses and 99 per cent effective after three doses. In Australia in 2005 this injectable IPV replaced the oral polio vaccine, again because of the very small risk of vaccine-induced polio. It is now recommended that children receive doses of IPV or IPV combined with the DTaP (diphtheria, tetanus and acellular pertussis).

The WHO is committed to the same goal as Jonas Salk: ridding the world of polio. The Western Pacific Region and European Region were certified polio free in 2002. By 2003 only 784 cases were reported worldwide. The number of countries where polio remained a chronic problem in 2004 had fallen from 125 to just six: Egypt, Niger, Nigeria, Afghanistan, India and

Pakistan.[51] In these countries the WHO works with governments and UNICEF to coordinate immunisation drives. Every six weeks thousands of local health workers and volunteers fan out through cities and villages, each worker carrying a thermos of vaccine vials, maps and clipboards. We are reminded of Franklin Delano Roosevelt's sentiments that anything can be achieved if everyone is willing to work together.

The cost of the polio vaccination campaigns is enormous and questions often arise regarding the economic value and sustainability. But in 2004 Dr Bruce Aylward, the coordinator of the WHO's polio eradication program, noted that the world is like a forest and one case of polio could start a wildfire that might take years to put out.[52]

On 12 April 2005, the 50th anniversary of Jonas Salk's vaccine was celebrated but the planet was still not polio free. Polio, like other diseases, could once again become common because the virus that causes it still exists. In fact the Global Polio Eradication Initiative faced an increase in global cases in 2006, the result of an ongoing outbreak in northern Nigeria and a new outbreak in western Uttar Pradesh, India.[53] Most of the cases occurred in Nigeria after immunisation was curtailed in 2002 due to rumours that the program was a Western plot to sterilise Muslim girls. An outbreak of polio in Somalia in July 2005 highlighted the difficulty of wiping out a stubborn global scourge. Two hundred Somali children were left paralysed by the outbreak and by then nineteen countries had been reinfected with polio because of the situation in Nigeria.

Yemen, Indonesia, Saudi Arabia, Sudan and Iraq have all been re-infected since 2004 causing a threat to the region. Because of the war in Iraq and the breakdown of services and infrastructure in November 2006, a national polio immunisation drive conducted by UNICEF, the second for the year, was launched by the Iraqi Ministry of Health despite security concerns. Iraq's last polio case was reported in 2000. During April and May 5400 mobile vaccinators travelled house to house across Iraq to immunise every child under the age of five, and over 96 per cent of the target population, almost 5 million children, were immunised.[54]

The recent global resurgence of the poliovirus has brought a renewed threat to the whole world, making routine immunisation campaigns critical to safeguard all children and ensure they do not suffer the fate that was once visited on so many. Jonas Salk made great personal sacrifices to save the children of his generation and his fervent hope was that children everywhere would be safe from polio forever.

POSTSCRIPT

The fearsome-looking iron lung that once filled hospital wards now has a marginal place in medical treatment. It is half a century since vaccination put an end to polio epidemics and modern, much smaller mechanical ventilators that push air into the airway with positive pressure have been developed. One victim of polio who still relies on an iron lung to keep her breathing is an Australian woman, June Middleton. June is something of an anomaly and in February 2007 she was presented with a certificate from the Guinness World Records for a record she would have preferred not to achieve: the longest time spent in an iron lung. At 80 years of age June Middleton has spent eighteen hours a day for the last 57 years of her life inside an artificial lung machine. June contracted polio in 1949 at the age of 23 and since that time two generations of children have been born and most would never have feared poliomyelitis nor would they have heard of an iron lung.

CHAPTER

10

TARGETING CHILDHOOD LEUKAEMIA

GERTRUDE ELION, GEORGE HITCHINGS AND RATIONAL DRUG DESIGN

I watched him go over a period of months in a very painful way, and it suddenly occurred to me that what I really needed to do was to become a scientist, and particularly a chemist, so that I would go out there and make a cure for cancer.[1]

Gertrude Elion

My greatest satisfaction has come from knowing that our efforts helped to save lives and relieve suffering. When I was baptised, my father held me up and dedicated my life to the service of mankind. I am very proud that, in some measure, I have been able to fulfill his hopes.[2]

Dr George Hitchings

When Gertrude Elion joined the Wellcome Research Laboratories in New York in 1944 as an assistant to Dr George Hitchings, she was a woman entering what was considered to be a man's world. Fate brought two brilliant and like minds together. Both had committed their lives to research in order to find cures for diseases such as cancer — diseases that had robbed them of loved ones and that caused great suffering in the world. Both were humanitarians determined to improve the lives of others. Together they developed a range of therapeutic and curative drugs, including the first cure for childhood leukaemia. Here were two dedicated scientists who worked together harmoniously and whose story, for once, is untainted by rivalry, intrigue or scandal; and the story is all the more exceptional because one of them was a woman.

The scope and importance of the work of Gertrude Elion and George Hitchings is nothing short of astonishing. Probably the greatest legacy resulting from their research was the development of 6-MP, a drug that has provided both treatment and cure for childhood leukaemia. The prospect was very bleak for leukaemia sufferers in the 1950s. Today, most children suffering from leukaemia who are treated with 6-MP, in combination with other drugs, become free of the disease and there is a strong likelihood that it will never recur. Most childhood leukaemias now have very high remission rates with some forms as high as 90 per cent. Because of Gertrude Elion and George Hitchings, for the majority of children suffering from childhood leukaemia today the prognosis is good and a cure is the most likely outcome.

Leukaemia, which occurs worldwide, is a form of cancer, specifically cancer of the white blood cells (also called leucocytes). Leukaemia represents just over 5 per cent of all types of cancers but for childhood cancers it is closer to 25 per cent.[3] When a child has leukaemia, large numbers of abnormal white blood cells are produced in their bone marrow, crowding it and flooding the bloodstream. As a result the white blood cells cannot perform their proper role of protecting the body against disease because they are defective. As leukaemia progresses, the cancer interferes with the body's production of other types of blood cells, including red blood cells and platelets and there is an increased risk of infection caused by the abnormalities in the white cells.

There are different types of childhood leukaemia, which can be classified as acute or chronic. In children, about 98 per cent of leukaemias are acute. This is where it becomes more complicated. Acute childhood leukaemias can then be divided into acute lymphocytic leukaemia (ALL) and acute myelogenous leukaemia (AML), depending on whether the specific white blood cells called lymphocytes are involved. Lymphocytes are critically important because they are linked to the body's immune defences. Approximately 60 per cent of children with leukaemia have ALL, and about 38 per cent have AML. Children may also have the slow-growing chronic myelogenous leukaemia (CML) but this is very rare.[4]

The symptoms that children suffer are very distressing. Because the infection-fighting white blood cells are defective, sufferers can experience episodes of fevers and infections and can also become anaemic because leukaemia affects the bone marrow's production of oxygen-carrying red blood cells. Consequently children with leukaemia become exceptionally vulnerable. They are tired, short of breath, have a poor appetite and they bruise and bleed very easily — leukaemia also destroys the bone marrow's ability to produce clot-forming platelets. There are a range of other symptoms as well: pain in the bones or joints, swollen lymph nodes in the neck, groin and other parts of the body; and with some leukaemias headaches, seizures, balance problems, abnormal vision and even problems with blood flow to and from the heart all occur.

As to the cause of leukaemia, the consensus is that a number of factors are involved. It is now known that childhood leukaemia results from abnormal gene function and that an inherited predisposition to leukaemia is a significant factor. The question of genetic susceptibility was studied by Frederick Gunz at Sydney Hospital in Australia in the 1970s. He concluded that evidence from family studies reinforced the theory of a genetic basis in some people, particularly for chronic lymphatic leukaemia. Twin studies have also established a genetic link and siblings of people who have the disease can have up to a four-fold increase in risk.

It is accepted that ionising radiation can also be a cause. Around three years after the atom bombs were dropped on Hiroshima and Nagasaki in 1945 there was a rise in the incidence of leukaemia. This peaked at around six years and returned to normal incidence twenty years after the bombings. Overall, however, relatively few people were affected compared with the number exposed to radiation, which raised the question of individual susceptibility. Concern about nuclear power causing leukaemia has been highlighted because of clusters of cases reported in areas surrounding nuclear power stations in various parts of the world. Childhood cases appear to be more prominent within these clusters. Again, because relatively small numbers of people are affected individual susceptibility seems a reasonable assumption.

A major study conducted by the Centre for Clinical Epidemiology at Leeds University in England began in 1984. The centre collects information from patients and their families. In order to understand the processes that can lead to leukaemia and related cancers, information on lifestyle patterns, environmental exposure and genetic make-up is being analysed. Research at the centre has already found that certain exposures can increase the likelihood of a person developing leukaemia. For example, there appears to be an association between smoking and acute leukaemia in adults. Also people with certain genes appear to be at greater risk of developing leukaemia if they are exposed to chemicals such as benzene. The study is ongoing and over time will collect data on millions of people.

NOT WOMEN'S WORK

The first great inroads into curing leukaemia were made by George Hitchings and Gertrude Elion, and both seemed destined from an early age to carry out their life-saving work. Gertrude Belle Elion, better known to colleagues, family and friends as Trudy, was born in New York City on 23 January 1918 at the end of World War I. Both of her parents were immigrants, her father having migrated to the United States from Lithuania when he was twelve years old and her mother from Poland at the age of fourteen.[5]

Gertrude's father became a successful dentist after graduating from the New York University School of Dentistry in 1914. The family lived in a large apartment in Manhattan adjoining Gertrude's father's dental office. Gertrude had one brother who was born when she was six and not long after his birth the family moved to the Bronx. There were open spaces where the children played and the Bronx Zoo was almost in their backyard. In many interviews, Elion spoke about her happy childhood.

The Elion children attended a public school within walking distance of their house and, even though class sizes were large, Gertrude believed that they received a good basic education. She was a child with an insatiable thirst for knowledge and she excelled at an early age. At twelve Gertrude was accelerated to a class two years ahead of her peers and her junior high school report card from 1930 reflects her abilities in a wide range of subjects. Her one consistently low grade was in Physical Education. Later when she was in college receiving As for all subjects there was still one exception: a C in Physical Education.

Gertrude was only fifteen when she enrolled at Hunter College. It was the 1930s, a time of economic hardship due to the Great Depression. Gertrude later wrote that she would not have been able to receive a higher education had it not been for good grades that she achieved in high school and the fact that Hunter College did not charge its students fees, which would have been a tragedy for such a gifted woman.

The death of Gertrude's grandfather from stomach cancer shortly before she began her studies at Hunter College had a profound and abiding effect on her. He had followed the family to America from his homeland and was a devoted grandfather, reading to his little granddaughter and taking her on walks. He contributed much to Gertrude's contented early years. As he lay dying Gertrude spent time with him in the hospital. She later recalled the sad time.

I watched him go over a period of months in a very painful way,
and it suddenly occurred to me that what I really needed to do was

to become a scientist, and particularly a chemist, so that I would go out there and make a cure for cancer.[6]

It was a defining moment in her life and at the young age of fifteen Gertrude Elion made the selfless decision to devote herself to medicine. As a first step she studied chemistry and by 1937 had completed her Bachelor's degree. Another tragic event in her young life led Gertrude to renew her commitment. She met and fell in love with a young man and they planned to marry. Not long after her fiancé graduated from university and started his career working for Merrill Lynch he became ill. Then soon after Gertrude's own graduation from Hunter College, her fiancé died of a bacterial infection, subacute bacterial endocarditis, an inflammation of the heart lining.[7] Two years later when penicillin was discovered, Gertrude realised that the man she loved could have been saved and this tragic event reinforced in her mind the importance of scientific discovery. Gertrude Elion said that it was never her intention not to marry after this loss but she did remain single for the rest of her life. She was not without close family, however, and remained very much a part of her brother's life even when they were living in different parts of the country. Gertrude was devoted to his children, her four nephews and two nieces.

Apart from the personal challenges, there were other hurdles to face. After college, Elion knew that she needed to have a PhD if she wanted to proceed with her ambition to do laboratory research but her family could not afford to send her to graduate school. Despite her excellent academic record she was unable to get either a graduate fellowship or assistantship, so she did what many women were forced to do at a time in history when the glass ceiling was barely above the floor, and that was to look for a job in which her talents would be squandered. Elion described the experience as hitting a brick wall. She said that nobody took her seriously: 'They wondered why in the world I wanted to be a chemist when no women were doing that. The world was not waiting for me.'[8] Things were doubly tough because jobs were scarce during the Depression and the few positions that existed in laboratories were not considered 'women's jobs'.

With little choice open to her Gertrude Elion embarked upon a more traditional career, but clung desperately to her goal. To get some practical skills she enrolled in a secretarial school and took on temporary work. She taught biochemistry to nurses in the New York Hospital School of Nursing for three months. Then by chance, she met a chemist who needed a laboratory assistant, and even though he was unable to pay any salary initially (not uncommon during the Depression), Elion stayed for a year and a half and gained valuable experience. Over this time she did begin to earn a wage and, using her meagre savings and some financial assistance from her parents, she was able to enter graduate school at New York University in 1939.

Gertrude Elion was a rarity, the only female in her chemistry class. Her recollection, however, is that she was accepted by her male classmates and did not feel out of place. Within a year Elion had completed the prerequisite courses to begin research for her Master's degree. But there were bills to pay while she was studying and for two years she worked as a substitute teacher in secondary schools in New York City teaching chemistry, physics and general science and she also had a part-time job as a doctor's receptionist. This left the evenings and weekends for research and study at New York University. Against the odds Gertrude Elion obtained her Master of Science degree in chemistry in 1941. World War II was ravaging Europe, and in December when Pearl Harbor was bombed by the Japanese, America joined the war. As the United States geared up for the war it entered a new era of economic prosperity and the Great Depression came to an end.

The war changed many things. Men were required in the armed services and suddenly there was a shortage of industrial chemists. Elion was finally able to get a job in a laboratory. It was not in research but it was in a lab. World War II made a difference to the thwarted aspirations of many women in countries like the United States, Britain and Australia. Unexpectedly women found themselves with careers that had previously not been an option for them. As more and more men enlisted, women filled the jobs that they vacated. Gertrude was hired as an analytical chemist for a major food company — a far cry from the groundbreaking medical work that she was destined to do. Her job included tasks such as measuring the acidity of pickles, testing the colour of mayonnaise and ensuring that the berries used in the manufacture of jam were not mouldy.[9] It's a job that someone had to do.

It is hardly surprising that after a year and a half Elion became restless with the repetitive nature of the work; the only compensations were that she was using some of her scientific skills and learning a lot about instrumentation, but she must have felt that her brain was atrophying. In the end, the job was simply too mind-numbing for a woman of Elion's intellectual capacity and she decided to make a move. Through an employment agency she applied successfully for a research job in pharmaceuticals at Johnson & Johnson in New Jersey, but even here the work was not all she had hoped for. Instead of synthesising medicines her time was mostly taken up with checking the strength of sutures.

In 1944, after Elion had been working in the laboratory for about six months it was disbanded. That was the bad news but the good news was that she was offered a number of positions in other research laboratories. The one which intrigued Elion most was a position as a biochemist assisting George Hitchings at the Burroughs Wellcome pharmaceutical company. The Wellcome Research Laboratories were located in Tuckahoe in New York. Elion suddenly found herself researching the metabolism of nucleic acids — the material that determines the genetic make-up of a cell and directs the process of protein synthesis — with a view to making substances that could attack diseases. This was a far cry from measuring the acidity of pickles.

In her autobiography, Gertrude Elion explained that she was not entirely sure what Hitchings was doing. She said that Hitchings 'talked about purines and pyrimidines, which I must confess I'd never even heard of up to that point, and it was really to attack a whole variety of diseases by interfering with DNA synthesis'.[10] This all sounded extraordinarily exciting to Gertrude Elion and accorded with her mission to use science to fight disease.

The lifelong professional relationship between Hitchings and Elion would prove to be profoundly productive and successful. Elion was eager to learn and Hitchings was prepared to give her more responsibility than she thought herself ready for. Hitchings was impressed with his new assistant. He found her intelligent, hard-working and ambitious, the perfect combination for the 'left-field' research he was determined to do. Gertrude Elion had a real career at last, a career that took her from organic chemistry into the realms of microbiology, pharmacology, immunology and virology. Gertrude Elion would spend the next 39 years at Burroughs Wellcome, reaching the position of head of the Department of Experimental Therapy in 1967.

These two great minds were able to carry out all of their iconic work at Burroughs Wellcome, a British pharmaceutical company now known as GlaxoSmithKline. Times had changed and medical and scientific research were no longer the preserve of universities. Throughout the twentieth century drug companies became more and more involved in research. Today billions of dollars are at stake.

When George Hitchings joined Burroughs Wellcome in 1942 as a biochemist, after working for nine years in temporary positions at the Harvard School of Public Health and other universities, he finally found an environment in which he could conduct the research he wanted to do and this was a rare privilege. In 1944 when Gertude Elion began working with Hitchings, the two had no idea that they were about to embark on a pioneering scientific journey that would lead to cures for many diseases.

MAKING FALSE DNA BUILDING BLOCKS

The death of a close family member, combined with an abiding passion for science, similarly led George Hitchings to a career in the medical and chemical sciences. Hitchings was born on the Olympic Peninsula in

Washington State in 1905. Because George's father was a shipbuilder the family moved often from one place to another along the coast during George's early years. Sadly, when George was only twelve his father died. It was a prolonged illness and this tragic experience turned the boy's thoughts towards medicine.

Hitchings was unequivocal about the direction his life should take. He later explained that his determination to help save lives was all-consuming, even shaping his selection of courses at Seattle's Franklin High School. Hitchings demonstrated his early resolve by focusing on science subjects and as salutatorian at his class graduation he chose the life of Pasteur as the subject for his oration.[11] The combination of Pasteur's basic research principles and using science to achieve practical results for the common good remained a goal for Hitchings throughout his career. Gertrude Elion had also been influenced by Pasteur. While at school she had read Paul DeKruif's *Microbe Hunters* and was fascinated by the achievements of Edward Jenner, Paul Ehrlich, Louis Pasteur and others in chemistry, physics and biology. She and Hitchings in their own way were to join the cohort of microbe hunters.

The next step for Hitchings was to enrol in a chemistry degree, which he did at the University of Washington in 1923. He followed this with a Master's degree, which he began in 1928, and a PhD in biochemistry at Harvard, which he finished in 1933. It was at Harvard that Hitchings became interested in research into the metabolism of nucleic acids, which we now know are the building blocks of DNA. His work centred on what to the lay person sounds arcane — the analytical methods used in physiological studies of purines, which are a class of compounds. In the same year that he was awarded his PhD, George Hitchings married Beverly Reimer, a woman he described as highly artistic, intelligent and empathetic but who was able to make accurate intuitive appraisals of people.

It is amazing to think that at the time Hitchings began his research into nucleic acids, the eventual discoverers of the DNA structure knew nothing about the subject. James Watson was three years old at the time and Francis Crick was a student at Mill Hill School in North London.[12] So in the 1930s nucleic acids were not considered to be a critical field in scientific research, ironically because not enough was known about them. This made it difficult for Hitchings to find a permanent appointment at an institution where he could indulge in this research. Hitchings was a little ahead of his time, and times were even tougher because the Great Depression had taken hold. Consequently George Hitchings wandered in the wilderness for the next nine years, going from one temporary position to another but wherever he went Beverly went with him. Hitchings worked at various universities including Western Reserve University (now Case Western Reserve) and the Harvard School of Public Health. When Hitchings joined Burroughs Wellcome in 1944 he too felt that at last his career had begun. He was able to concentrate his investigative energies on the metabolism of nucleic acids, the molecular carriers of genetic information.

Hitchings had been evolving the idea that it should be possible to make drug discovery more rational, less 'hit and miss'. Although he was not entirely sure at the time how it could be achieved, the recent development of sulfa drugs that could interfere with the metabolism of microbes led Hitchings to believe that other substances could do the same. It was in that year that Oswald Avery at the Rockefeller Institute published a paper suggesting cautiously that deoxyribonucleic acid, DNA, was genetic material.[13] It was another nine years after this that Watson and Crick at Cambridge University discovered the double-helix structure of DNA, revealing how genetic information might be copied during cell replication.

In their work together George Hitchings and Gertrude Elion devised something akin in its conception to Emil von Behring's Blood Serum Therapy and Paul Ehrlich's 'magic bullets'. Their brainchild was 'rational drug design', which meant doing things opposite to standard practice. Rational drug design was a controlled scientific process for creating new drugs by designing new molecules with specific molecular structures that would inhibit the replication of rapidly dividing cancer and bacteria cells in specific diseases rather than discovering new drugs and then trialling them against different diseases. Target the disease and design the drug accordingly.

Elion described the 'rational drug design' process as letting the drug lead the scientist to the answer that nature was trying to keep hidden.[14] This ingenious idea and the work that followed led to the development of the 'designer drug' 6-MP, their weapon against childhood leukaemia. Hitchings hypothesised that rapidly dividing cells like bacteria and cancer cells had to be making lots of nucleic acids, therefore it might be possible to stop the growth of these cells with 'antagonists' to the purine and pyrimidine bases, antagonists being the drugs that Elion and Hitchings would make through rational drug design.[15] The idea was that synthetic chemical compounds would be similar to the natural ones and would interfere with the body's DNA production. They would be similar enough to those in nucleic acids so that they could integrate themselves into natural metabolic pathways. Once there, these 'antimetabolites' would be different enough to shut things down by interfering with the metabolism of nucleic acids, in particular purines and pyrimidines. It is this sort of science that is inconceivable to the non-scientific mind. The antimetabolites would look like the real thing but would be fake, the art-world equivalent of copying a masterpiece and tricking even the experts. They would make false DNA building blocks.

George Hitchings began examining nucleic acids, which are now known as DNA and RNA. Gertrude Elion was assigned to investigate and synthesise a large number of purines, including adenine and guanine. To find out how to make compounds she would go to the library and look up scientific literature, work out how to do it and then make them.[16] The next job, because so little was known about DNA and therefore nucleic acid structure and function, was to find out if the compounds actually did anything. For Hitchings and Elion it was like feeling their way in the dark. What they soon discovered was that without the presence of certain purines bacterial cells could not produce nucleic acids. So work began on the antimetabolite compounds that locked up enzymes necessary for the incorporation of these purines into nucleic acids. Elion later explained that when a micro-organism like *Lactobacillus casei* was put in a defined medium, it was possible to tell if something was a real growth antagonist when it was added. Then it was necessary to analyse why it was an antagonist. 'We knew that this organism would grow and from that it could make DNA and folic acid,' she explained. She extrapolated:

> *You could make everything just from the amino acids, medium, and folic acid, and so on. We knew folic acid was essential, or if you could replace folic acid with a purine, it would grow ... It would make lactic acid. If the organisms didn't grow, we knew we had something and we might be antagonising folic acid or it might be antagonising the purine. So you could with that one organism really make an analysis of three different kinds. You could add purine or folic acid and reverse the antagonism.* [17]

While Gertrude Elion was immersing herself in microbiology and synthesising compounds her ambition to get a doctoral degree was reignited. She began studying at night at the Brooklyn Polytechnic Institute, but after several taxing years of commuting, studying and working, she was informed that if she wished to continue she would have to convert to a full-time program. Elion had come to a crossroads in her life and was forced into making a critical decision — stay with Hitchings and the job she found stimulating and fulfilling or commit entirely to the academic studies that meant so much to her. She stayed, and countless numbers of people have benefitted from what must have seemed an enormous sacrifice at the time.

In 1948 Hitchings and Elion found that a synthetic purine derivative, diaminopurine, inhibited the growth of bacteria. They tested it on the growth of mouse tumour cells and leukaemia cells in tissue culture and found that it did in fact inhibit growth.[18] The following year Joseph Burchenal at the Sloan Kettering Institute in New York used diaminopurine to treat four patients with chronic granulocytic leukaemia, two of whom went into remission, giving them and the researchers great hope. However, the other two patients improved initially but relapsed later and experienced severe bone marrow suppression. The results indicated that diaminopurine had toxic effects.

It was her disappointment over the failure of diaminopurine as a reliable cure for leukaemia that took Elion to the next phase of her research. The rigour she and Hitchings applied to their task is certainly reminiscent of Paul Ehrlich in his search for compound 606. By 1951 they had made and tested over 100 purine analogues, including diaminopurine and thioguanine. They found that the enzymes latched onto both of these analogues instead of adenine and guanine and both had activity against a wide variety of rodent cancers and leukaemias. It was in 1952 that Elion substituted an oxygen atom with a sulfur atom on a purine molecule and so created 6-mercaptopurine, a purine derivative also known as 6-MP.[19]

This new material, 6-MP, became the first purine antagonist to be useful in the treatment of acute lymphoblastic leukaemia in children. At that time children were treated with steroids and methotrexate but most survived only for a few months. Approximately 3 per cent survived for around a year. Children given the new drug went into complete remission. No abnormal cells could be detected in the bloodstream. The median survival time was extended to one year and a few patients actually stayed in remission for years afterwards.[20] In 1999 when discussing her reaction to seeing leukaemia patients in remission due to her drug, Gertrude Elion said, 'The first time that I went to the leukaemia clinic at Sloan Kettering, and saw the first children who had been treated with 6-mercaptopurine, who were in remission, I can remember then the feeling of, we've really done it, it really works.'[21]

The success of the drug 6-MP seemed miraculous and was reported in the press. Excitement about the designer drug was so great that within days the US Food and Drug Administration approved 6-MP for use late in 1953, only ten months after clinical trials began.[22] Sadly, though, there was a repetition of what had happened with diaminopurine and some children, after first improving, relapsed and died. What Elion had showed, however, by synthesising 6-MP, was that small changes in a compound that was essential to cell division could chemically 'fool' the malignant cells and thereby combat them. Elion decided to examine everything about 6-MP, devoting the next six years of her life to this research. As a result, by the 1980s an 80 per cent cure rate for childhood leukaemia was achieved using 6-MP in combination with one or more of about a dozen other drugs that act against leukaemia with a continuation of drug therapy during remission.[23] This method of treatment cures the majority of cases today, something that was beyond reach before Elion and Hitchings devised rational drug design.

The contemporary treatment for leukaemia is complex and is also specific for each type of childhood leukaemia, and usually involves chemotherapy carried out in different stages. Certain features of a child's leukaemia, such as the child's age and initial white blood cell count, are used in determining the intensity of treatment that is needed to achieve the best chance for cure. Often many chemotherapeutic drugs are employed in the regime, each directed at a certain aspect of the disease. The drug 6-MP is still used in combination therapy for patients with acute lymphoblastic leukaemia.

Treatment options can include bone marrow transplantation, another medical breakthrough, from other donors or other unaffected bone marrow sites that may be within the patient's body. In addition, blood products and antibiotics may also be administered to try to normalise abnormal blood component levels and reduce the risk of infection.[24] The goal is remission — no evidence of cancer cells in the body. Once remission has occurred, maintenance chemotherapy is usually used in cycles over a period of two to three years to keep the cancer from recurring.

The multiplicity of treatments is a testament to the cumulative work of innumerable researchers including Gertrude Elion and George Hitchings and theirs is one of the success stories in the anti-cancer crusade.

ELION AND HITCHINGS BROADEN THEIR FOCUS

Using the same principle that had made 6-MP possible, Elion and Hitchings began work on developing other drugs. During their research they discovered that another form of leukaemia could be treated with 6-thioguanine and that 6-MP had wider applications than they had first anticipated.[25] As the research led by Hitchings and Elion expanded at Burroughs Wellcome so did the number of scientists who were involved. Always quick to collaborate, Elion and Hitchings began working with Dr Joseph Murray, a transplant surgeon at the Peter Bent Brigham Hospital in Boston. They provided him with their compounds including 6-MP to see if they might have an effect on organ rejection.

Dr Roy Calne, a pioneer of transplantation surgery who had come from England to work with Joseph Murray at the laboratory at the Harvard Medical School, found a new use for 6-MP. Calne performed kidney transplants on dogs and found that 6-MP and its analogues prevented rejection of the new organ.[26] This showed that 6-MP could not only interfere with the multiplication of white blood cells, but could also suppress the immune system. Calne became a key figure in establishing life-saving transplantation as part of routine clinical practice through his work on drugs to suppress organ rejection. The understanding of immunological tolerance and rejection and the development of immuno-suppressant drugs is what has made organ transplantation successful. Organ transplantation can give decades of nearly normal life to people who would otherwise die.

Apparently Hitchings and Elion became frequent visitors to Murray's laboratory and were referred to fondly as the 'two chemists from Tuckahoe'. The story goes that they got to know most of the lab dogs by name. There is a photograph of Gertrude Elion on the front steps of the Harvard Medical School with Roy Calne, George Hitchings, Joseph Murray, two other doctors and the dogs Tweedledum, Tweedledee, Titus, and Lollipop, the last dog being the recipient of the first successful kidney transplant made possible by 6-MP.[27]

The discovery that 6-MP was an immunosuppressant led the Hitchings team to a new drug, azathioprine (Imuran), which although it was not effective against cancer cells advanced the field of organ transplantation for humans. Imuran suppresses the immune system by interfering with the growth of T-lymphocytes, the specialised white blood cells that are one of the main instigators of the rejection process, when the immune system reacts to the transplanted organ as if it were a harmful foreign invader.[28] This was, in fact, a great leap forward for medical science and suppression was to have huge implications for future developments in surgery. Imuran was one of the drugs Elion had synthesised while trying to improve upon 6-MP. Once again the prescient words of Pasteur are resurrected. In the case of Imuran chance did favour the prepared mind. Late in her career Elion pointed out that she had not on this occasion set out to rationally design a drug that would work as an immunosuppressant but, if ears and minds are open, then great advances can happen.

For the first time in history, patients could receive organ transplants without their bodies rejecting the new organs. The first successful kidney transplant had taken place between identical twins in Boston in 1954 but rejection thwarted all transplants other than those between twins. With Imuran, Joseph Murray performed the first kidney transplant between unrelated individuals in 1961 and it has remained an essential anti-rejection drug that people take after transplantation. Imuran is now used with prednisone and cyclosporine which all work in slightly different ways thus causing fewer side-effects.

Developments in drug design led to Roy Calne and his team pioneering the use of cyclosporine A, a drug so successful in preventing rejection that transplantation of hearts, livers and lungs became common. In 1990, when Joseph Murray was awarded a Nobel Prize, in his address he noted that more than 200,000 kidney transplants had been performed worldwide.[29]

In the 1960s Elion and Hitchings shifted their research to nucleic acid formation in lower animals and the differences between these processes in animals and in people. For the dynamic duo the swinging sixties became a roller-coaster of rational drug design. They determined that infectious diseases could be fought if drugs could be targeted to attack bacterial and viral DNA. This work resulted in pyramethamine, used to treat malaria, and trimethoprim (Septra) used to treat meningitis, septicaemia and bacterial infections of the urinary and respiratory tracts.[30] Allopurinal, another relative of 6-MP, was developed in Gertrude Elion's lab and apart from being a treatment for gout it also proved effective for use during chemotherapy.

As a result of these overwhelming successes Hitchings became Vice President of Research at Burroughs Wellcome in 1967, a promotion that effectively ended his hands-on participation in research. Elion was promoted as well, to head of the Department of Experimental Therapy. In this position she was a 'great minds magnet', attracting young and gifted scientists to Burroughs Wellcome who became known as a research 'dream team'.[31]

Despite her new responsibilities, Elion did continue her research work and was involved in the development of acyclovir, an antiviral drug effective against herpes. Originally acyclovir was synthesised by Dr Howard Schaeffer but Elion was instrumental in determining exactly how and why it worked. Acyclovir, marketed as the well-known Zovirax, interferes with the replication process of the herpes virus, but only the herpes virus, thus proving that drugs can be selective. It was the development of acyclovir that eventually led to the development of azidothymidine (AZT) by Elion's colleagues, one of the very few drugs that has any effect on AIDS.[32]

In 1970, the Wellcome laboratory moved to Research Triangle Park in North Carolina and both Gertrude Elion and George Hitchings moved too. In the 1970s George Hitchings made a life-changing decision when he resigned from his job as a scientific director at Burroughs where he had spent most of his long and productive career. He did stay on as a research scientist, back to the coalface in a way, but he now had more time to devote

to his own pursuits inside and outside the laboratory, particularly philan-
thropic work. Hitchings was committed to promoting research, and as one
of the leaders of the charitable Burroughs Wellcome Fund, he helped
support the medical research of other scientists. His concern for people
extended beyond their physical wellbeing and in 1983 Hitchings founded
the Triangle Community Foundation which not only provided healthcare to
the poor but assisted in protecting battered women and gave disadvantaged
children greater opportunities.[33]

Gertrude Elion retired in 1983, eight years after Hitchings, with the
status of scientist emeritus. For the next sixteen years she remained active
as an advisor to many professional organisations and as a consultant she
maintained her association with her former employer, Burroughs
Wellcome, while holding adjunct professorships at Duke University, the
University of North Carolina and Ohio State University. Indefatigable, she
served on advisory committees for the National Cancer Institute, the
American Cancer Society, the Leukemia Society of America and the tropical disease research division of the World Health Organization.[34] It could
all have been so different. Whatever project she worked on, Gertrude
Elion remained involved in the investigation of her old favourites, purines
and purine analogues as chemotherapeutic agents and she continued to
publish her findings throughout her life. Her first article had been published in 1939 and her last, in 1998, the year before her death. Elion
admitted that work had become her vocation and she never felt a need for
outside relaxation. But there were pastimes that she enjoyed — photogra-
phy, travel and music, especially Puccini, Verdi and Mozart operas.

There were so many synergies between Gertrude Elion and George
Hitchings. Like Hitchings, Elion was passionate about the importance of
research. Every year after her retirement she would share her knowledge
by mentoring a third-year medical student at Duke University. 'I think it's
a very valuable thing for a doctor to learn how to do research, to learn how
to approach research, something there isn't time to teach them in medical
school.'[35] When visiting academic institutions she often preferred spending

time with students rather than their teachers. Gertrude Elion and George Hitchings were cut from the same cloth. Both were devoted to improving the wellbeing of humankind and both were selfless in doing so.

ACCOLADES AND AWARDS

In 1988 Gertrude Elion and George Hitchings shared the Nobel Prize in Physiology or Medicine for their work on drug design with a third scientist, Sir James Black, who did seminal work which led to beta-blockers for cardiovascular disease and to H2-antagonists for peptic ulcers. The Nobel Committee noted that the prize was awarded for their discoveries of 'important principles for drug treatment, principles that have resulted in the development of a series of new drugs'. Jon Elion, one of Gertrude's nephews, recalled the Nobel festivities in Stockholm. All the laureates and officials, who were seated on the stage, were men and all were dressed in their formal black suits and ties and white shirts. Elion described fondly how his aunt stood out in what he called her 'Trudy blue chiffon dress'.[36]

Gertrude Elion expressed how she felt about receiving the Nobel Prize in a lecture she often gave afterwards to students. What thrilled her more, she said, was that her work led to the discovery of drugs that saved people who might otherwise have died from diseases such as leukaemia, kidney failure and herpes virus encephalitis. To Gertrude Elion, the Nobel Prize was only 'the icing on the cake'. She was often asked if the Nobel Prize was what she had aimed for in life. Her answer was that if getting an award was someone's goal in life and they did not achieve that goal, then their life would be negated. She never lost her original motivation, no matter how hard the road or how much success she achieved. What she and George Hitchings aimed for was to make people well, to save them from life-threatening diseases and that brought infinitely more satisfaction.

I think I'm most proud of the fact that so many of the drugs have really been useful in saving lives. I've run into people whose lives have been saved, and the kind of satisfaction that you get from

*having someone come up and say, 'My child had acute leukemia and
your drug saved him.' Or, 'My little girl had herpes encephalitis, and
she is now cured, she is back at school. She is doing very well. People
told me that she might be mentally affected, but she is not.' I run
into people who have had kidney transplants for twenty years who
are still taking the drug. And I don't think that anything else that
happens to you can match that type of satisfaction.*[37]

By all accounts Gertrude Elion did not trade on her celebrity. In the
customs hall, after flying back to America from the awards ceremony in
Stockholm, she was asked by a customs official if she had any jewellery to
declare. Jokingly she pulled out the Nobel Prize medallion.[38] This seems
totally in keeping with a woman who was described variously as direct in
manner, vigorous in debate, generous in crediting others for their achievements and wholly unpretentious. In fact there were many people with
whom she collaborated and who contributed to the evaluation of her
drugs, including Joseph Burchenal at Sloan Kettering Institute in New
York; Roy Calne, the English surgeon from Cambridge; Joseph Murray at
Harvard; and Dr Robert Schwartz and William Damashek at Tufts
University in Boston who pioneered the use of 6-MP with patients.

George Hitchings, for his part, was surprised when he won the Nobel
Prize. He had already received many other awards for his contribution to
humankind — devising rational drug design. At 83 years of age, however,
he thought he was too old to be considered for the Nobel although he was
still hard at work for science and philanthropy as president of the
Burroughs Wellcome Fund. Hitchings regretted that his wife of 52 years,
Beverly Reimer Hitchings, could not be by his side when he received the
award. Beverly had passed away in 1985.

In September 1988, shortly before the announcement of the Nobel
Prize, Hitchings met Joyce Shaver, who was 26 years his junior. They were
married in February 1989, after attending the award ceremonies in
Stockholm together with members of Hitchings' family and a man whose

cancer had been cured by a drug that Hitchings developed.[39] In an interview just before her husband died, Joyce Shaver gave some insight into what the Nobel Prize meant to Hitchings. On the day he was presented with the award Hitchings said that the real gift was not the prize itself but the individual people whom his medicines had helped. It would come as no surprise that Hitchings gave all of his prize money to the Triangle Community Foundation.

After winning the Nobel Prize, Hitchings continued to travel and lecture. During his lectures, apparently, he would always show his favourite slide of a beautiful young Pakistani woman in her wedding dress. He would then tell the story of how her life had been saved by a free sample of an antibiotic that Hitchings had developed and that a Burroughs Wellcome salesman had left with her doctor.[40] Every life was precious to Hitchings and he too had never lost sight of his goal to help humankind and cure disease. During his 30-year career Hitchings had developed and patented 85 different drugs.

The woman who had begun as George Hitchings' assistant and who became his respected colleague, Gertrude Elion, was the holder of 45 patents herself as a result of the discoveries she had made. Elion had synthesised and co-developed the first successful drugs for the treatment of leukaemia — thioguanine and mercaptopurine — as well as azathioprine (Imuran), which not only prevented the rejection of kidney transplants but was a treatment for rheumatoid arthritis; she had played a major role in the development of allopurinol, the treatment of gout, and acyclovir, the first effective treatment for herpes virus infections.

The first major award Elion won for this seminal work was the Garvan Medal in 1968 and she was thrilled to receive it.[41] The Garvan Medal, however, was the only American Chemical Society prize for which she could compete. Until 1980, women were ineligible for any other ACS awards. The Garvan Medal was established in 1936 to recognise outstanding US women chemists. Other awards did follow and in 1991 Gertrude Elion received a National Medal of Science, which was presented to her by the President of the United States. Elion did not rest in her retirement and continued her association with a plethora of academic societies and in 1991 she was elected to the Institute of Medicine.

Ironically, Gertrude Elion never completed her PhD. At the time that she had been forced to make the choice between her job and further study, Hitchings had assured her that she would not need the degree to do the work that she was doing with him at Burroughs Wellcome. And she didn't. In the 1950s when Hitchings successfully sponsored her before the American Society of Biological Chemists, he dismissed any objections to her election before they arose. He summed up the situation Elion often faced when, according to Elion he quipped, 'I know she has three strikes against her. She doesn't have a PhD, she is a woman, and she works for industry. Nevertheless, I am going to tell you about her.'[42] There was certainly a lot to tell and the society need not have worried about Elion's academic qualifications. During her career she was awarded 23 honorary degrees which included not just one, but three PhDs.

Both scientists, Gertrude Elion and George Hitchings, had long and distinguished careers spanning more than half a century and their work was prodigious. But fate dealt a cruel hand to George Hitchings in the end. He became blind and he developed Alzheimer's disease. Although he was well advanced in years, it is a tragedy for a great mind to be destroyed in this way. Today in laboratories throughout the world scientists like Hitchings are seeking a cure for Alzheimer's, which is becoming an increasing problem as more of us live longer thanks to the myriad medical advances that have been made since Edward Jenner produced the first vaccine. There is something very paradoxical about this.

George Hitchings died on 27 February 1998. Almost a year later on Sunday, 21 February 1999, Gertrude Elion collapsed while out on her daily walk. She was taken to the University of North Carolina Hospital and died at midnight. She was 81 years old. Unlike her dear colleague, Elion's mind was as sharp as ever. Only a week before her death she had participated in a project team meeting at GlaxoSmithKline discussing the development of a new cancer drug called Arranon.

Fifty-five years after she synthesised the first of her drugs and six years after her death, Elion's legacy was evident when Arranon was licensed in the United States in late 2005. It was the product of many hands and minds. The drug has a role in treating certain rare forms of leukaemia and lymphoma when patients have exhausted standard treatment options. In the early 1980s Elion knew that among the compounds her laboratory had synthesised over the years there might be other things that would work against leukaemia or lymphoma. She had given two glass vials with black tops to Joanne Kurtzberg, a specialist in paediatric oncology at Duke University Medical Center.[43] In one of the vials was a precursor of Arranon.

It was a long road for the drug, and Elion helped to fuel the research. Eventually, a group led by Thomas Krenitsky, who had been a colleague of Elion and who now has his own research company, worked through the chemistry to overcome the difficulties that had arisen with synthesis. His invention, known among his colleagues as 506U78, has become the injected cancer drug Arranon. An accumulation of the drug in T-cells inhibits DNA synthesis, stopping rampant cell replication. For some patients Arranon provides another treatment option, and in some cases provides sufficiently long remissions to allow bone marrow transplants to take place.[44] Arranon followed by transplant was the course of treatment for a boy who received the drug when he was four and at the age of ten he was still well and playing Little League baseball.

The fight to cure every case of childhood and adult leukaemia continues. Researchers have now turned their attention to stem cells. This is certainly the new frontier in medical science. In August 2006 researchers and their colleagues at the Dana-Farber Cancer Institute and Children's Hospital in Boston reported on having isolated rare cancer stem cells that cause leukaemia in a mouse model of the human disease.[45] The leukaemia stem cells that were isolated proved to be surprisingly different from normal blood stem cells, a finding that may be good news for developing a drug that selectively targets them.

The discovery provides answers to the longstanding questions of whether cancer stem cells must be similar to normal stem cells, and what type of cell first becomes abnormal in leukaemia. The research data supports the idea that leukaemia stem cells do not have to originate from normal blood stem cells, an important finding because it indicates that in the future it will be possible to specifically target leukaemia stem cells without killing normal stem cells.

The researchers at the Dana-Farber Cancer Institute were able to isolate leukaemia stem cells in mice and discovered a gene activity pattern which they called a 'signature' of self-renewal. [46] Next they must determine which genes among the several hundred that were particularly active or inactive are the most responsible for the cancer cell's behaviour. Using the Hitchings–Elion model, these genes might eventually become targets for new types of drugs. So far, researchers have not identified and isolated a pure population of leukaemia stem cells in humans with the disease. But the work which began with Hitchings and Elion continues.

The Hitchings–Elion partnership was a remarkable one. Gertrude Elion was determined to break down the gender barrier, George Hitchings aided her and medical science was the beneficiary. Professionally Hitchings and Elion were admired by a host of colleagues and students and are remembered for their devotion to science, their cutting edge work and their desire, rooted deep in personal loss, to find a cure for human disease. Devoid of ego, their enthusiasm for their work was contagious and apart from the panoply of weapons they aimed at disease and the drugs that they created through rational drug design, they lit the way for others. Their partnership was even more remarkable because although it took place within a drug corporation laboratory it was not product and reputation driven, but arose from pure altruism and the desire to discover new drugs that gave salvation through science.

POSTSCRIPT

In 1998, the company for which both Gertrude Elion and George Hitchings had provided loyal service and inspired research dedicated a new research centre to these two illustrious scientists and humanitarians. The building, which has a cubist-like façade, is called the Elion-Hitchings Building. Although the name of the company is now GlaxoSmithKline, many Hitchings and Elion stories are still told within the walls. The following one about Gertrude Elion may be apocryphal.

Towards the end of her life, Gertrude Elion pulled into a VIP parking space at GlaxoSmithKline, quite uncharacteristic for a woman who never expected privileges, but which probably had more to do with her age and mobility. She was unknown to the parking-lot guard who suggested as she walked towards the building that there were spaces elsewhere that were not reserved. With poise, the Nobel laureate asked if it would make a difference if her name was on the front of the building. Without hesitation and with great deference, the guard opened the door so that Gertrude Elion could enter her building.

GLOSSARY

acquired immunity: immunity which is not innate or natural. It is acquired via an infection or through vaccination. It can also be acquired through the transfer of antibodies or lymphocytes from an immune donor.

actinomycete: a group of fungus-like bacteria, most of which are harmless. Common in soil life, they play a role in the decomposition of organic matter. Selman Waksman discovered that they produce antinomycin, a natural antibiotic.

antibodies: a type of protein produced as an immune response by specialised B cells in the immune system to foreign substances (antigens) such as chemicals, viruses and bacteria which threaten the body. Each type of antibody is unique and defends the body against one specific type of antigen.

antigen: a foreign substance (protein, toxin, chemical, virus, bacterium) which when it enters an organism is capable of triggering an immune response.

antitoxin: an antibody produced by the immune system to counteract a toxin such as a bacterial toxin (exotoxin), an animal toxin (zootoxin) or plant toxin (phytotoxin). The antitoxin neutralises the effect of the toxin. Antitoxins produced within one type of organism can be injected into other organisms, including humans, to kill bacteria and other micro-organisms, as in Blood Serum Therapy. The procedure involves injecting an animal with a safe amount of a specific toxin, for example, diphtheria, allowing the animal to produce the antitoxin needed to neutralise the toxin. Later blood is withdrawn from the animal, the antitoxin is obtained and processed and then injected into a human or another animal to induce passive immunity.

avirulent: specifically, micro-organisms that are not able to cause disease.

Chamberland filter: a porcelain filter with small pores used in filtration sterilisation. It was devised by the French bacteriologist Charles-Édouard

Chamberland, who was a close associate of Louis Pasteur. His invention facilitated the discovery of microbial exotoxins and filterable viruses.

DNA sequence information: DNA sequence information is gained through biochemical methods. The DNA sequence is the order of DNA base pairs, nucleotide bases, in a fragment of DNA, a gene, a chromosome of an entire genome. The sequence of DNA comprises the inheritable genetic information for all living organisms.

exotoxin: a potent toxin (poison) which is a soluble protein formed and excreted by micro-organisms including bacteria, fungi, algae and protozoa. Exotoxins can destroy cells or disrupt normal cellular metabolism in a host. Most exotoxins can be destroyed by heating.

immunogenicity: the degree to which a substance possesses the ability to create immunity or provoke an immune response within an organism.

lymphocytes: a class of cells within the immune system that produce antibodies to attack infected and cancerous cells and which are also responsible for the body's rejection of foreign tissue. This includes B cells which when activated produce antibody and T cells which function in cellular immunity.

nucleic acid: an essential complex organic acid found in all living cells such as DNA and RNA, consisting of long chains of nucleotide units (composed of phosphoric acid, a carbohydrate and a base derived from purine and pyrimidine) that convey genetic information.

organic compounds: chemical substances which are organic i.e. their molecules contain carbon. Organic compounds can be found in nature or they can be synthesised in the laboratory.

pandemic: is an epidemic (a rapidly spreading disease which is more extensive than would normally be expected) which spreads over a vast geographical area or even worldwide and affects a large proportion of the population.

pathogen: an infectious agent which causes disease to attack its host. A pathogen is usually a biological agent, a micro-organism such as a bacterium, protozoa, virus or fungus.

pathogenic bacteria: infectious bacteria. Bacteria (singular, bacterium) are microscopic, unicellular organisms which are present in the air, in soil, on the skin. While many types cause disease others such as intestinal bacteria which help with the digestion of food, are useful to humans.

protozoa: a diverse family of single-celled animals most of which can only be seen under a microscope. Protozoa breathe, move and reproduce like multi-celled animals. They live mostly in water or in damp environments. Some can cause disease while others eat harmful bacteria.

recombinant: in molecular biology refers to genetic recombination, a new combination of genes in a cell or an individual, combinations which are not found in the 'parent'. These combinations can be genetically engineered in order to change the characteristics of an organism.

suppurated: discharging pus or festering.

toxin: poison produced by living organisms or a harmful substance which accumulates in the body. It frequently refers to a protein, highly toxic to other living organisms, that is produced by certain plants, animals and pathogenic bacteria.

virulent: extremely toxic, specifically in reference to micro-organisms that are markedly pathogenic (disease causing).

World Health Assembly: the decision-making forum through which the World Health Organization (WHO) is governed by its 193 member states. It meets each year in May in Geneva and is attended by health ministers from all member states. Its executive board is comprised of 34 members who are technically qualified in the field of health. The main tasks of the Assembly are to decide major policy and approve WHO programs and budgets.

NOTES

CHAPTER ONE

1.   Baron, John, 1827, *The Life of Edward Jenner*, Vol. I, Chapter 4, London, Henry Colburn, cited in Who Named It? <www.whonamedit.com>

2.   Strauss, Eugene W. and Strauss, Alex, 2006, *Medical Marvels: The 100 greatest advances in medicine*, Prometheus Books, New York, p. 78.

3.   Barquet, Nicolau and Domingo, Pere, 1997, *Smallpox: The triumph over the most terrible of the ministers of death*, Annals of Internal Medicine, Vol. 127, Issue 8 (Part 1), pp. 635-42.

4.   Who Named It?, *Edward Jenner*, <hhtp://www.whonamedit.com/doctor.cfm/1818html>

5.   Macauley, Thomas B., 1800, *The History of England from the Accession of James II*, Claxton, Remsen and Haffelfinger, Philadelphia, cited in LearnWell.org, Online Continuing Education in Health and Ethics, Nursing Continuing Education Institute, Smallpox Epidemic: Could you deal with it? 2006, <www.learnwell.org/smallpox.htm>

6.   Saunders, Vicki and Durrheim, David N., 2003, *Cuckoos, Cows and a Country Doctor: The pioneering work of a rural health professional in the development of public health*, Journal of Rural and Remote Environmental Health 2(2), <www.jcu.edu.au/jrtph/vol/v02saunders.pdf>

7.   *ZKEA Emerging Disease: Biological Warfare: Biological Terrorism*, Smallpox History, <www.zkea.com/archives/archive02001.html>

8.   Friedman, Meyer and Friedland, Gerald W., 1998, *Medicine's 10 Greatest Discoveries*, New Haven, Connecticut, Yale University Press, p. 67.

9.   The Jenner Museum, *Edward Jenner and Smallpox*, <www.jennermuseum.com/overview/index.shtml>

10. Strauss, Eugene W. and Strauss, Alex, 2006, op. cit., p. 104.

11. Barquet, Nicolau and Domingo, Pere, 1997, loc. cit.

12. Tucker, Jonathan B., 2001, *Smallpox: From eradicated disease to bioterrorist threat*, Center for Nonproliferation Studies, Monterey Institute of International Studies, Washington, <http://cns.miis.edu/research/cbw/smallpox.htm>

13. Strauss, Eugene W. and Strauss, Alex, 2006, op. cit., p. 77.

14. Barquet, Nicolau and Domingo, Pere, 1997, loc. cit.

15. Who Named It?, *Edward Jenner*, loc. cit.

16. ABC Radio National, 23 November 1997, *Ockham's Razor* transcript 23, 'Defending Edward Jenner', <www.abc.net.au/rn/science/ockham/or231197.htm>

17. Who Named It?, *Edward Jenner*, loc. cit.

18. Barquet, Nicolau and Domingo, Pere, 1997, loc. cit.

19. Parish, H.J., *Victory with Vaccines: The story of immunisation*, Edinburgh, E & S Livingstone, 1968, cited in Barquet, Nicolau and Domingo Pere, 1997, loc. cit.

20. Who Named It?, *Edward Jenner*, loc. cit.

21. Strauss, Eugene W. and Strauss, Alex, 2006, op. cit., p. 105.

22. Who Named It?, *Edward Jenner*, loc. cit.

23. Barquet, Nicolau and Domingo, Pere, 1997, loc. cit.

24. History Learning Site, 2000, *Edward Jenner*, <www.historylearningsite.co.uk/edward_jenner.htm>

25. Who Named It?, *Edward Jenner*, loc. cit.

26. ibid.

27. Barquet, Nicolau and Domingo, Pere, 1997, loc. cit.

28. Friedman, Meyer and Friedland, Gerald W., 1998, op. cit., p. 79.

29. Jenner, Edward, *An Inquiry Into the Causes and Effects of the Variolae Vaccinae*, Or Cow-Pox. 1798, The Harvard Classics: 1909–14, Great Books on Line, bartelby.com, <www.bartleby.com/38/4/1.html>

30. Friedman, Meyer and Friedland, Gerald W., 1998, op. cit., p. 83.

31. Who Named It?, *Edward Jenner*, loc. cit.

32. Friedman, Meyer and Friedland, Gerald W., 1998, op. cit., p. 82.

33. Barquet, Nicolau and Domingo, Pere, 1997, loc. cit.

34. Friedman, Meyer and Friedland, Gerald W., 1998, op. cit., p. 88.

35. Saunders, Vicki and Durrheim, David N., 2003, loc. cit.

36. Friedman, Meyer and Friedland, Gerald W., 1998, op. cit., p. 89.

37. Barquet, Nicolau and Domingo, Pere, 1997, loc. cit.

38. National Network for Immunization Information, *Vaccine Information: Smallpox*, <www.immunizationinfo.org/vaccineInfo/vaccine_detail.cfv?id=26>

39. Saunders, Vicki and Durrheim, David N., 2003, loc. cit.

40. The Jenner Museum, *Edward Jenner and Smallpox*, loc. cit.

41. Friedman, Meyer and Friedland, Gerald W., 1998, op. cit., p. 90.

42. ibid.

43. Saunders, Vicki and Durrheim, David N., 2003, loc. cit.

44. Friedman, Meyer and Friedland, Gerald W., 1998, op. cit., p. 92.

45. Jenner, Edward, 1801, *The Origin of the Vaccine Inoculation*, London, D.N. Shury, cited in Barquet, Nicolau and Domingo Pere, 1997, loc. cit.

46. PBS Online, Science Odyssey: People and Discoveries, *World Health Organization declares smallpox eradicated*, <www.pbs.org/wgbh/aso/databank/eventindex.html>

47. The Jenner Museum, *Edward Jenner and Smallpox*, loc. cit.

48. PBS Online, Science Odyssey: People and Discoveries, loc. cit.

49. Tucker, Jonathan B., 2001, *Smallpox: From eradicated disease to bioterrorist threat*, loc. cit.

50. The Jenner Museum, *Edward Jenner and Smallpox*, loc. cit.

51. Retroscreen Virology Ltd, *Twenty Five Years On: Smallpox revisited*, <www.retroscreen.com/?sec=23>

52. Organic Consumers Association, 2005, *International Campaign to Stop Genetic Engineering of Smallpox Virus Announced*, <http://www.smallpoxbiosafety.org/who/prenglish.html>

53. Tucker, Jonathan B., 2001, *Smallpox: From eradicated disease to bioterrorist threat*, loc. cit.

54. Organic Consumers Association, 2005, loc. cit.

55. Jefferson, Thomas, Letter, 14 May 1806, From Revolution to Reconstruction, 2006, *The Letters of Thomas Jefferson: 1743–1826, A Tribute of Gratitude*, <odur.let.rug.nl/~usa/P/tj3/writings/brf/jeflxx.htm>

CHAPTER TWO

1. Cited in Hawke, Caitlin, 2002, 'The Cutting Edge: Focus on Anthrax Then and Now', *Pasteur Perspective: The newsletter of the Pasteur Foundation devoted to the world of the Institut Pasteur*, No. 11, spring, New York, p. 1.

2. Scientists, *Pasteur*, <ambafrance-ca.org/HYPERLAB/PEOPLE/ _pasteur.html>

3. Coppedge, David, F., 2000, *Shining Through Material Darkness: Louis Pasteur*, World's Greatest Creation Scientists from Y1K to Y2K, <www.creationsafaris.com/wgcs_4.htm>

4. De Kruif, Paul, 1927, *Microbe Hunters*, Harcourt Brace, New York, reprinted San Diego, Harcourt Brace, 1996, p. 5.

5. Strauss, Eugene W. and Strauss, Alex, 2006, op. cit., p. 74.

6. Strauss, Eugene W. and Strauss, Alex, 2006, op. cit. p. 31.

7. Cohn, David V., *The Life and Times of Louis Pasteur*, 1999, LabExplorer, <www.labexplorer.com/louis_pasteur.htm>

8. ibid.

9. ibid.

10. Hellman, Hall, 2001, *Great Feuds in Medicine: Ten of the liveliest disputes ever*, John Wiley & Sons Inc., New York, p. 78.

11. Debré, Patrice, (trans: Elborg Forster), 1998, *Louis Pasteur*, Baltimore, Johns Hopkins Press, p. 103.

12. Hellman, Hall, 2001, op. cit. p. 79.

13. Cohn, David V., loc. cit.

14. Pasteur, Louis, Lecture at the Sorbonne in 1864, cited in Wilson, John L., *Stanford University School of Medicine and the Predecessor Schools: A historical perspective*, 1998, Chapter 5, 'Louis Pasteur (1822–1895)', Stanford School of Medicine History, <elane.stanford.edu/wilson/Text/5f.html>

15. Scientists, *Pasteur*, loc. cit.

16. Hellman, Hall, 2001, loc cit.

17. Coppege, David, F., *Shining Through Material Darkness: Louis Pasteur*, loc. cit.

18. Hellman, Hall, 2001, op. cit., p. 85.

19. Debré, Patrice, 1998, op. cit., p. 142.

20. Doctors Independent Network (DIN), *Louis Pasteur*, <www.dinweb.org/dinweb/DINMuseum/Louis%20Pasteur.asp>

21. Pasteur, Louis, Speech to the Academy of Medicine in Paris, cited in Cohn, David V., *The Life and Times of Louis Pasteur*, 1999, LabExplorer, <www.labexplorer.com/louis_pasteur.htm>

22. Pasteur, Louis, *Germ Theory And Its Applications to Medicine and Surgery: Read before the French Academy of Sciences*, 29 April 1878, Internet Modern History Sourcebook, 1998, <www.fordham.edu/halsall/mod/1878pasteur-germ.html>

23. Cohn, David V., *The Life and Times of Louis Pasteur*, 1999, loc.cit.

24. ibid.

25. ibid.

26. Mollaret, H.H., *Contribution to the knowledge of relations between Koch and Pasteur*, NTM-Schriftenr. Gesch. Naturwiss, Technik, Med, Leipzig 20 (1983)1, pp. 57–65. Translated by Cohn, E. T., Fasciotto-Dunn, B. H., Kuhn, U. and Cohn, D. V., Molleret, <pyramid.spd.louisville.edu/~eri/fos/Molleret.html>

27. ibid.

28. ibid.

29. Sanofi Pasteur Australia, *Rabies*, <www.sanofipasteur.com.au/avpi-australia/front/templates/vaccinations-travel-health-vaccine>

30. Coppedge, David, F., loc. cit.

31. Cohn, David V., loc. cit.

32. Pasteur, Louis, *'Method for Preventing Rabies after a Bite'*, report to the French Academy of Sciences in 1885, First Treatment of Rabies, Founders of Science, <www.foundersofscience.net/Rabies.htm>

33. ibid.

34. ibid.

35. ibid.

36. Koch, Robert, *Dr Robert Koch's Latest Estimate of Pasteur's Methods and Discoveries, and of the Present Position of the General Inoculation Problem*, editorial in *Boston Medical and Surgical Journal*, 18 January 1883, Vol. CVIII, No. 3, <www.foundersofscience.net/past_koc.htm>

37. DIN Doctors Independent Network, loc. cit.

38. Pasteur, Louis cited at Coppege, David, F., loc. cit.

39. Vallery-Radot, René, 1926, *The Life of Louis Pasteur*, Doubleday, Garden City, p. 195.

40. Hellman, Hall, 2001, op. cit., p. 88.

41. World Health Organization, *Human and Animal Rabies: A neglected disease*, <www.who.int/rabies/en>

42. World Health Organization, *Rabies Bulletin Europe, 1st Quarter, 2006*, <www.who-rabies-bulletin.org>

43. Watts, Jonathan, 'China Rabies Outbreak Triggers Second Dog Cull', *Guardian*, 4 August 2006.

CHAPTER THREE

1. Schatz, Albert, *My Experience in World War II, 1942*, Rutgers Oral History Archive of World War II, the Korean War, the Vietnam War and the Cold War, 2003, Rutgers University, <oralhistory.rutgers.edu/Docs/memoirs/schatz_albert/schatz_albert_memoir.html>

2. GlaxoSmithKline, 2007, *The White Plague*, <www.gsk.com/infocus/whiteplague.htm>

3. Who Named It? *Leon Charles Albert Calmette*, <http://www.whonamedit.com/doctor.cfm/2413.html>

4. Raymo, Chet, *Thus we Behold a Deadly Beauty*, Boston Globe Online, <www.boston.com/globe/seaarch/stories/health/science_musings/092898.htm>

5. Nobel Prize, *Robert Koch*, <http://nobelprize.org/nobel_prizes/medicine/laureates/1905/koch-bio.html>

6. Who Named It? *Heinrich Hermann Robert Koch*, <www.whonamedit.com/doctor.cfm/2987.html>

7. Nobel Prize, *Robert Koch*, loc. cit.

8. Who Named It? *Heinrich Hermann Robert Koch*, loc. cit.

9. History Learning Site, 2000, *Robert Koch*, <www.historylearningsite.co.uk/robert_koch.htm>

10. Strauss, Eugene W. and Strauss, Alex, 2006, op. cit., p. 192.

11. Who Named It? *Heinrich Hermann Robert Koch*, loc. cit.

12. Institute for Animal Health, *Robert Koch: Advancing the field of bacteriology*, <www.iah.bbsrc.ac.uk/schools/scientists/KOCH.htm>

13. History Learning Site, 2007, Robert Koch, <www.historylearningsite.co.uk/robert_koch.htm>

14. Who Named It? *Heinrich Hermann Robert Koch*, loc. cit.

15. Nobel Prize, *Robert Koch*, <http://nobelprize.org/nobel_prizes/medicine/laureates/1905/koch-bio.html>

16. Strauss, Eugene W. and Strauss, Alex, 2006, op. cit., p. 192.

17. Nobel Prize, *Robert Koch*, loc. cit.

18. Strauss, Eugene W. and Strauss, Alex, 2006, op. cit., p. 193.

19. History Learning Site, *Robert Koch*, loc. cit.

20. Robert Koch Institute, *Robert Koch and the Institute*,
    <www.rki.de/cln_006/nn_231644/EN/Content/Institute/History/history__node__en.ht
    ml__nnn=true>

21. Who Named It? *Heinrich Hermann Robert Koch*, loc. cit.

22. Who Named It? *Leon Charles Albert Calmette*,
    <http://www.whonamedit.com/doctor.cfm/2413.html>

23. Hoslink, *Pioneers in Medical Laboratory Science — Albert Calmette*,
    <http://www.hoslink.com/pioneers.htm>

24. ibid.

25. Who Named It? *Leon Charles Albert Calmette*, loc. cit.

26. ibid.

27. Hubbard, John P (ed.), *Trends:WHO reports first results of mass vaccination with BCG*, Pediatrics,
    Vol. 6 No. 3, September 1950,
    <pediatrics.aappublications.org/cgi/content/abstract/6/3/481>

28. Doherty, Mark T. and Rook, Graham, 'Progress and Hindrances in Tuberculosis Vaccine
    Development', *The Lancet*, 17 March 2006, 367(9514): pp. 947–9.

29. Friedman, Meyer and Friedland, Gerald W., 1998, op. cit., p. 190.

30. Simmons, John Galbraith, 2002, *Doctors and Discoveries: Lives that created today's Medicine*,
    Boston, Houghton Mifflin Company, New York, p. 257.

31. Nobel Prize, *Selman A. Waksman — Nobel Lecture*,
    <nobelprize.org/nobel_prizes/medicine.laureates/1952/waksman-lecture.html>

32. Schatz, Albert, *My Experience in World War II, 1942*, loc. cit.

33. Simmons, John Galbraith, op. cit., p. 259.

34. Simmons, John Galbraith, loc. cit.

35. ibid.

36. Strauss, Eugene W. and Strauss, Alex, 2006, op. cit., p. 256.

37. Simmons, John Galbraith, op. cit., ibid.

38. Pollard, Ruth, 'TB's Extreme New Face', *Sydney Morning Herald*, 21 September 2006, p. 18.

39. Pellerin, Cheryl, *Progress Challenges Highlighted on World Tuberculosis Day 2006*, Washington File,
    <http://usembassy-australia.state.gov/hyper/2006/0323/epf410.htm>

40. GlaxoSmithKline, 2007, *The White Plague*, loc. cit.

CHAPTER FOUR

1. Quote cited in The Black Death 1347–1350 Culprit: Oriental rat flea, *Quotes from the Plague*,
   <www.insecta-inspecta.com/fleas/bdeath/Quotes.html>

2. Twoop Timelines, *Bubonic Plague – A Historical Timeline*,
   <www.twoop.com/medicine/archives/2005/10/bubonic_plague.html>

3. Kiple, Kenneth F. (ed.), 1993, *The Cambridge World History of Human Diseases*, Cambridge
   University Press, Cambridge, p. 612.

4. Twoop Timelines, *Bubonic Plague – A historical timeline*, loc. cit.

5. Kruszelnicki, Karl S., 2006, *Arrow Up Yours & Plague 2*, ABC Great Moments in History,
   <www.abc.net.au/science/k2/moments/s662193.htm>

6. World Health Organization, *Plague Fact Sheet*, <www.who.int/topics/plabue/en/.>

7. Wood, James, *Black Death and Plague not Linked*, 12 April 2002, BBC News,
   <news.bbc.co.uk/1/hi/health/1925513.stm>

8. ibid.

9. History Learning Site, *Medieval England — The Black Death*
    <www.historylearningsite.co.uk/black_death_of_1348>

10. Channel 4, 2007, *Plague*,
    <www.channel4.com/history/microsites/H/history/plague/plague.html>

11. Twoop Timelines, *Bubonic Plague – A historical timeline*, loc. cit.

12. Who Named It? *Alexandre-Émil-Jean Yersin*,
    <www.whonamedit.com/doctor.cfm/2454.html>

13. Hoslink Pioneers in Med Lab Science, *Alexandre Yersin*, <www.hoslink.com/pioneers.htm>

14. Burns, William, MRC National Institute for Medical Research, *NIMR: Mill Hill Essays 2003: Alexandre Yersin and his adventures*, <www.nimr.mrc.ac.uk/millhillessays/2003/yersin>

15. Who Named It? *Alexandre-Émil-Jean Yersin*, loc. cit.

16. Hoslink, Pioneers in Med Lab Science, *Alexandre Yersin*, loc. cit.

17. Kitasato's Drama Without a Script, *Act I: Before Unravelling the Enigma*,
    <www.microbes.jp/hiwa/English/dorama/report1.html>

18. Channel 4, 2007, *Plague*, loc. cit.

19. Canadian Medical Association Journal, 2007, *The Late Baron Shibasaburo Kitasato*,
    <www.pubmedcentral.nih.gov/articlerender.fcgi?artid=382621>

20. Who Named It? *Alexandre-Émil-Jean Yersin*, loc. cit.

21. ibid.

22. Jewish Encyclopedia, *Waldemar Mordecai Wolff Haffkine*,
    <www.jewishencyclopedia.com/directory.jsp?letter=H&partition=1&pageNum=5>

23. Friedman, (Rabbi Mark), *Great Scientist, Great Jew*, Canadian Jewish News, 4 August 2005,
    <www.cjnews.com>

24. ibid.

25. Indian Post, *Dr Waldemar Mordecai Wolff Haffkine*,
    <www.indianpost.com/viewstamp.php/Alpha/D/DR.%20WALDEMAR%20MORDECAI%20HAFFKINE>

26. ibid.

27. Jewish Encyclopedia, *Waldemar Mordecai Wolff Haffkine*, loc. cit.

28. ibid.

29. Hawgood, Barbara J, 2005, *Waldemar Mordecai Haffkine, CIE (1860-1930): Prophylactic vaccination against cholera and bubonic plague in British India*, Journal of Medical Biography,
    <www.hawgood.co.uk/barbara/Haffkine.htm>

30. Jewish Encyclopedia, *Waldemar Mordecai Wolff Haffkine*. loc. cit.

31. Indian Post, *Dr Waldemar Mordecai Wolff Haffkine*, loc. cit.

32. Jewish Encyclopedia, *Waldemar Mordecai Wolff Haffkine*, loc. cit.

33. PBS Online, Science Odyssey: People and Discoveries, *Bubonic Plague hits San Francisco*,
    <www.pbs.org/wgbh/aso/databank/medhealth.html>

34. ibid.

35. Twoop Timelines, *Bubonic Plague – A historical timeline*, loc. cit.

36. World Health Organization, Epidemic and Pandemic Alert and Response, *2002 Plague in India*, <www.who.int/entity/csr/don/2002_02_20/en/indes.html>

37. World Health Organization, Epidemic and Pandemic Alert and Response, *2002 Plague in Algeria*, <www.who.int/entity/csr/don/2003_06_24a/en/>

38. World Health Organization, Epidemic and Pandemic Alert and Response, *Suspected Plague in the Democratic Republic of Congo* <www.who.int/csr/don/2006_11_07/en/index.html>

39. Buzzle, *Bubonic Plague: Case confirmed in Los Angeles*, <www.buzzle.com/editorials/4-19-2006-93918.asp>

40. World Health Organization, Epidemic and Pandemic Alert and Response, <www.who.int/csr/en>

41. Titus, Nicole, *Plague-infected Mice Escape from Jersey Lab*, 20 September 2005, Avion, <www.avionnewspaper.com/media/paper798/news/2005/09/20/Science/PlagueInfected.Mice.Escape.F>

42. Khamsi, Roxanne, *Lab Loses Trio of Plague Mice*, news@nature.com, 2005, MacMillan Publishers Ltd. <cmbi.bjmu.edu.cn/news/0509/78.htm>

43. Channel 4, 2007, *Plague*, loc. cit.

44. Khamsi, Roxanne, loc. cit.

CHAPTER FIVE

1. Walker, Benjamin Edward, *Unpublished Memoirs: The rain must fall*, <www.westmidlands.com/millennium/1900/1900-1924/1907.html>

2. Kitasato's Drama Without a Script, *Act I: Before Unravelling the Enigma*, loc. cit.

3. CDC Centres for Disease Control and Prevention, Department of Health and Human Services, *Tetanus Chapter (Pink Book)*, <www.cdc.gov/vaccine/pubs/pinkbook/downloads/tetanus.pdf>

4. ibid.

5. Sanofi Pasteur, *Welcome to sanofi pasteur in Japan: Tetanus*, <www.sanofipasteur.jp/sanofi-pasteur/front/index.jsp?codePage=VP_PD_Tetanus&codeRubrique=19....>

6. Healthline, *Tetanus Health Article*, <www.healthline.com/adamcontent/tetanus>

7. E-notes World of Microbiology and Immunology, *Emil von Behring*, <science.enotes.com/microbiology-encyclopedia/?start=60>

8. Todar's Online Textbook of Bacteriology, 2002, *Diphtheria*, <textbookofbacteriology.net/diphtheria.html>

9. Answers.com, *Diphtheria*, <www.answers.com/topic/diphtheria>

10. RDS Understanding Animal Research in Medicine, *Diphtheria Vaccine*, <www.rds_net.org.uk/pages/page.asp?i_ToolbarID=PageID=66>

11. Encyclopedia of Children's Health, *Diphtheria*, <www.healthofchildren.com/D/Diphtheria.html>

12. Grundman, Kornelia, 2001, *Emil von Behring: The founder of serum therapy*, Nobel Prize, <nobelprize.org/nobel_prizes/medicine/articles/behring/index.html>

13. Hoslink, *Pioneers in Medical Laboratory Science — Alexandre Yersin*, <http://www.hoslink.com/pioneers.htm>

14. Encyclopedia of Children's Health, *Diphtheria*, loc. cit.

15. Nobel Prize, *Emil von Behring: The Nobel Prize in Physiology and Medicine 1901, Biography*, <http://nobelprize.org/nobel_prizes/medicine/laureates/1901/behring-bio.html>

16. Hoslink, *Pioneers in Medical Laboratory Science — Emil von Behring*, <http://www.hoslink.com/pioneers.htm>

17. E-notes World of Microbiology and Immunology, *Emil von Behring*, loc. cit.

18. Grundman, Kornelia, 2001, loc. cit.

19. ibid.

20. A Traveller's Guide to the History of Biology and Medicine, *Chapter 3: Clausthal-Zellerfeld*, <www.historyofbiologyandmedicine.com/westgermany.htm>

21. Grundman, Kornelia, 2001, loc. cit.
22. ibid.
23. RDS Understanding Animal Research in Medicine, *Diphtheria Vaccine*, <www.rds_net.org.uk/pages/page.asp?i_ToolbarID=PageID=66>
24. Grundman, Kornelia, 2001, loc. cit.
25. A Traveller's Guide to the History of Biology and Medicine, *Chapter 3: Clausthal-Zellerfeld*, loc. cit.
26. Grundman, Kornelia, 2001, loc. cit.
27. ibid.
28. Internet FAQ Archives, *Emil von Behring Biography (1854–1917)*, Encyclopedia of Health, <www.faqs.org/health/bios/23/Emil-von-Behring.html>
29. ibid.
30. Grundman, Kornelia, 2001, loc.cit.
31. Answers.com, *Diphtheria*, <www.answers.com/topic/diphtheria> loc.cit
32. Grundman, Kornelia, 2001, loc. cit.
33. Encyclopedia of Children's Health, *Diphtheria*, loc. cit.
34. Nobel Prize, *Emil von Behring: The Nobel Prize in Physiology and Medicine 1901, Biography*, loc. cit.
35. Internet FAQ Archives, *Emil von Behring Biography (1854–1917)*, loc. cit.
36. Todar's Online Textbook of Bacteriology, 2002, *Diphtheria*, <textbookofbacteriology.net/diphtheria.html>
37. RDS Understanding Animal Research in Medicine, *Diphtheria Vaccine*, loc. cit.
38. Immunizations, *In Depth Reports: Diphtheria, tetanus and pertussis*, <162.1.2.78/ADAM/doc/In-DepthReports/10/000090.htm>
39. Encyclopedia of Children's Health, *Diphtheria*, loc. cit.
40. ibid.
41. World Health Organization, *Diphtheria in Afghanistan*, <www.who.int/csr/don/archive/country/afg>
42. CDC Centres for Disease Control and Prevention, Department of Health and Human Services, *Tetanus Chapter (Pink Book)*, loc. cit.
43. Sanofi Pasteur, *Welcome to Sanofi Pasteur in Japan: Tetanus*, loc. cit.
44. ibid.
45. Ehrlich, Paul, *Croonian Lecture — On Immunity with Special Reference to Cell Life, 13 March 1900*, Theoretical Immunology, <post.queensu.ca/~forsdyke/theorimm.htm>

CHAPTER SIX

1. Gide, André, cited in Strauss, Eugene W. and Strauss, Alex, 2006, op. cit., p. 101.
2. Crosby, Alfred W. Jr., 2003, *The Columbian Exchange: Biological and Cultural Consequences of 1492*, Westport Connecticut, Praeger, p. 126.
3. Kiple, Kenneth F. (ed.), 1993, *The Cambridge World History of Human Diseases*, Cambridge University Press, Cambridge, p. 1025
4. Impact of Sieges, *Siege Warfare 1494–1648*, <www.renaissancesoldier.com/features/siege/effects/disease.html>
5. Strauss, Eugene W. and Strauss, Alex, 2006, op. cit., p.102.
6. STD Helper.com, *History Advice*, Syphilis, <www.stdhelper.com/syphilis-history.html>
7. Poynter Centre, *Syphilis in History*, <wisdomtools.com/pointer/syphilis.html>

8. STD Helper.com, *History Advice*, loc. cit.

9. Thumbnails, *39 — Ehrlich: Chemotherapy is launched*, <dodd.cmcvellore.ac.in/hom/39%20-%20Ehrlich%20Chemo.html>

10. Kiple, Kenneth F. (ed.), 1993, *The Cambridge World History of Human Diseases*, Cambridge University Press, Cambridge, p.1032.

11. Poynter Centre, *Syphilis in History*, loc. cit.

12. Nobel Prize, *Paul Ehrlich — Nobel lecture*, <nobelprize.org/nobel_prizes/medicine/laureates/1908/ehrlich-lecture.html>

13. Thumbnails, *39 — Ehrlich: Chemotherapy is launched*, loc. cit.

14. Magner, Lois N., 2002, *A History of the Life Sciences*, CRC Press, p. 189.

15. Bowden, Mary Ellen, 2003, *Paul Ehrlich: Pharmaceutical achiever*, The Chemical Heritage Foundation, <www.chemheritage.org/EducationalServices/pharm/chemo/readings/ehrlich/pabio/htm>

16. Thumbnails, *39 — Ehrlich: Chemotherapy is launched*, loc. cit.

17. Nobel Prize, *Paul Ehrlich — Nobel lecture*, loc. cit.

18. A Traveller's Guide to the History of Biology and Medicine, *Chapter 3: Clausthal-Zellerfeld*, <www.historyofbiologyandmedicine.com/westgermany.htm>

19. Nobel Prize, Paul Ehrlich — Nobel Lecture, loc. cit.

20. Thumbnails, *39 — Ehrlich: Chemotherapy is launched*, loc. cit.

21. Bowden, Mary Ellen, 2003, *Paul Ehrlich: Pharmaceutical achiever*, loc. cit.

22. A Traveller's Guide to the History of Biology and Medicine, *Chapter 3: Clausthal-Zellerfeld*, loc. cit.

23. Thumbnails, *39 — Ehrlich: Chemotherapy is launched*, loc. cit.

24. ibid.

25. Bowden, Mary Ellen, 2003, *Paul Ehrlich: Pharmaceutical achiever*, loc. cit.

26. Ehrlich, Paul, *Croonian Lecture — On immunity with special reference to cell life*, 13 March 1900, Theoretical Immunology, <post.queensu.ca/~forsdyke/theorimm.htm>

27. ibid.

28. ibid.

29. Nobel Prize, *The Immune System Pioneers: Ilya Mechnikov and the phagocyte cells*, <nobelprize.org/educational_games/medicine/immunity/immune-pioneers.html>

30. The Chemical Heritage Foundation, 2001, Magic Bullets: Chemistry vs Cancer — Pharmaceutical achievers, *Paul Ehrlich*, <www.chemheritage.org/EducationalServices/pharm/chemo/home.htm>

31. Moss, Ralph W., 1995, *Questioning Chemotherapy*, Equinox Press, New York, p. 11.

32. The Chemical Heritage Foundation, 2001, Magic Bullets: Chemistry vs Cancer — Pharmaceutical achievers, *Paul Ehrlich*, loc. cit.

33. Nobel Prize, *Paul Ehrlich — Nobel lecture*, loc. cit.

34. Bowden, Mary Ellen, 2003, *Paul Ehrlich: Pharmaceutical achiever*, loc. cit.

35. Thumbnails, *39 — Ehrlich: Chemotherapy is launched*, loc. cit.

36. ibid.

37. Nobel Prize, *The Immune System Pioneers: Ilya Mechnikov and the phagocyte cells*, loc. cit.

38. Nobel Prize, *Paul Ehrlich — Nobel lecture*, loc. cit.

39. PBS Online, Science Odyssey: People and Discoveries, *Ehrlich Finds Cure for Syphilis*, <www.pbs.org/wgbh/aso/databank/medhealth.html>

40. PBS Online, Science Odyssey: People and Discoveries, *Fleming Discovers Penicillin*, <www.pbs.org/wgbh/aso/databank/medhealth.html>

41. Thumbnails, *39 — Ehrlich: Chemotherapy is launched*, loc. cit.

42. Poynter Centre, *Syphilis in History*, <wisdomtools.com/pointer/syphilis.html>

43. Nobel Prize, *Paul Ehrlich — Nobel lecture*, loc. cit.

44. Poynter Centre, *Syphilis in History*, loc. cit.

45. ibid.

46. Thumbnails, *39 — Ehrlich: Chemotherapy is launched*, loc. cit.

47. PBS Online, Science Odyssey: People and Discoveries, *Fleming Discovers Penicillin*, loc. cit.

48. Britannica Online Encyclopedia, *Paul Ehrlich: Syphilis studies*, <www.britannica.com/eb/article-2054/Paul-Ehrlich>

49. Look Smart Find Articles, *A Portrait of History: Paul Ehrlich archives of pathology*, <findarticles.com/p/articles/mi_qa3725/is_200106/ain9003500/pg_2>

50. Strauss, Eugene W. and Strauss, Alex, 2006, op. cit., p. 103.

51. Moss, Ralph W., 1995, loc. cit.

52. World Health Organization, Media Center, *Global Cancer Rates Could Increase by 50% to 15 million by 2020*, <www.who.int.mediacentre/2003/pr27/en/>

53. Thumbnails, *39 — Ehrlich: Chemotherapy is launched*, <dodd.cmcvellore.ac.in/hom/39%20-%20Ehrlich%20Chemo.html>

54. The Chemical Heritage Foundation, 2001, Magic Bullets: Chemistry vs Cancer — Pharmaceutical achievers, *Paul Ehrlich*, loc.cit.

55. Moss, Ralph W., 1995, loc. cit.

56. World Health Organization, *Women's Health News: New vaccines against HPV could save hundreds of thousands of lives if delivered effectively*, 12 December 2006.

57. Richwine, Lisa., *Gene therapy used to treat skin cancer*, 1 September 2006, News In Science, <http://www.abc.Net.au/science/news/stories/s1730700.htm>

CHAPTER SEVEN

1. Banting, Frederick G., *Nobel Lecture*, Nobel Lectures, Physiology or Medicine 1922–1941, <nobelprize.org/nobel_prizes/medicine/laureates/1923/banting-lecture.html>

2. The Association of the British Pharmaceutical Industry, *Target Diabetes*, <www.abpi.org.uk/publications/publication_details/targetDiabetes/default.asp>

3. Hite, Pamela F., Barnes, Ann M. and Johnston, Philip E., 2006, *Exuberance Over Exubera*, Clinical Diabetes 24:110-114, American Diabetes Association, <clinical.diabetesjournals.org/cgi/content/full/24/3/110>

4. Alberti, George, 2001, *Lessons from the History of Insulin*, Diabetes Voice, Vol. 46, December, No. 4, <www.diabetesvoice.org>

5. Simmons, John Galbraith, 2002, *Doctors and Discoveries: Lives that created today's medicine*, Houghton Mifflin Company, Boston, p. 206.

6. Alberti, George, 2001, loc. cit.

7. Hoogerdijk, Derek, *The Discovery of Insulin*, Quasar, University of Alberta, <www.quasar.ualberta.ca/edse456/apt/vignettes/insulin.htm>

8. Madehow.com, *How Insulin is Made*, <www.madehow.com/Volume-7/Insulin.html>

9. Simmons, John Galbraith, 2002, loc. cit.

10. Madehow.com, *How Insulin is Made*, loc. cit.

11. ibid.

12. International Diabetes Institute, 2006, *Diabetes Explained*, <www.diabetes.com.au>

13. World Health Organization Media Center, *Diabetes:What is diabetes*, Fact Sheet No 312, September 2006, <www.who.int/mediacentre/factsheets/fs312/en>.

14. Simmons, John Galbraith, 2002, op. cit., p. 205.

15. ibid.

16. Canadian Diabetes Association, 2007, *Captain Banting:War hero*,
    <www.diabetes.ca/Section_About/BantingIndex.asp>

17. Canadian Diabetes Association, 2007, *Co-discoverer of Insulin*,
    <www.diabetes.ca/Section_About/BantingIndex.asp>

18. After the discovery of insulin and years after he had been living in Canada, Charles Best, who
    was experiencing resentment amongst the scientific fraternity because he was seen as an out-
    sider, had to prove his claim to Canadian citizenship. Herbert Best signed an affidavit in 1924
    asserting that even though they had lived in the United States he had never given up his
    Canadian citizenship. *See* Best, Henry Bruce Macleod, *Speech to:The Academy of Medicine,Toronto,
    24 April 1996*, Discovery of Insulin, <http://www.discoveryofinsulin.com/Home.htm>

19. Shampo, Marc and Kyle, Robert A., 2004, *Charles Best–Codiscoverer of Insulin*, Mayo Clinic
    Proceedings, 79(12):p. 1546, <www.mayoclinicproceed-
    ings/com/pdf%2F7912%2F7912sv.pdf >

20. Best, Henry Bruce Macleod, *Speech to:The Academy of Medicine,Toronto, 24 April 1996*, loc. cit.

21. Simmons, John Galbraith, 2002, op. cit., p. 207.

22. Best, Charles, cited in Best, Henry Bruce Macleod, *Speech to:The Academy of Medicine,Toronto,
    24 April 1996*, loc. cit.

23. Alumni Association, University of Alberta, *In the Footsteps of Pioneers*,
    <www.ualberta.ca/ALUMNI/history/founding/88sprfootsteps.htm>

24. ibid.

25. Bliss, Michael, 1982, *The Discovery of Insulin*, Chicago, University of Chicago Press, Chapter
    Four, XI.

26. During the period 1910 to 1920 Dr Frederick Madison Allen became a leading diabetes spe-
    cialist in the United States and after an exhaustive study of 100 diabetic patients published
    Studies Concerning Glycosuria and Diabetes in 1913 followed by *Total Dietary Regulation in
    the Treatment of Diabetes*. Allen recommended that diabetics eat only a low-calorie diet, an
    approach which extended life for some people for a brief period. *See* Canadian Diabetes
    Association, 2007, *The History of Diabetes*, <www.diabetes.ca/Section_About/timeline.asp>

27. Bliss, Michael, 1982, op. cit., Chapter Five, III.

28. Hite, Pamela F., Barnes, Ann M. and Johnston, Philip E., 2006, *Exuberance Over Exubera*, loc.
    cit.

29. Bliss, Michael, 1982, loc. cit.

30. ibid.

31. Simmons, John Galbraith, 2002, loc. cit.

32. Best, Henry Bruce Macleod, *Speech to:The Academy of Medicine,Toronto, 24 April 1996*, loc. cit.

33. ibid.

34. ibid.

35. ibid.

36. Best, Charles, cited in Best, Henry Bruce Macleod, *Speech to:The Academy of Medicine,Toronto,
    24 April 1996*, loc. cit.

37. Discovery of Insulin, Sir Frederick Banting Educational Committee, *The Discovery of Insulin:A
    Canadian medical miracle of the 20th century*, James Bertram Collip
    <http://www.discoveryofinsulin.com/Home.htm>

38. Best, Charles, cited in Best, Henry Bruce Macleod, *Speech to:The Academy of Medicine,Toronto,
    24 April 1996*, loc. cit.

39. Banting, Frederick, cited in Best, Henry Bruce Macleod, *Speech to: The Academy of Medicine, Toronto, 24 April 1996*, Discovery of Insulin, <http://www.discoveryofinsulin.com/Home.htm>

40. Williams, Michael, 2007, John James Rickard Macleod, Diabetologia, <www.diabetologia-journal.org/past%20masters/macleod.htm>

41. Best, Henry Bruce Macleod, *Speech to: The Academy of Medicine, Toronto, 24 April 1996*, loc. cit.

42. Discovery of Insulin, Sir Frederick Banting Educational Committee, *The Discovery of Insulin: A Canadian medical miracle of the 20th century*, Charles Herbert Best, <http://www.discoveryofinsulin.com/Home.htm>

43. Shampo, Marc & Kyle, Robert A., 'Charles Best–Codiscoverer of Insulin', *Mayo Clinic Proceedings*, December 2004 ;79(12):1546.

44. Best, Henry Bruce Macleod, *Speech to: The Academy of Medicine, Toronto, 24 April 1996*, loc. cit.

45. ibid.

46. Canadian Diabetes Association, 2007, *The History of Diabetes*, loc. cit.

47. Endocrine Web's Diabetes Centre, *What is Insulin?*, <www.endocrineweb.com./diabetes/2insulin.html>

48. Madehow.com, *How Insulin is Made*, loc.cit.

49. Endocrine Web's Diabetes Centre, *What is Insulin*, loc. cit.

50. Madehow.com, *How Insulin is Made*, loc.cit.

51. Doble, Claire, 'Unexpected Directions, Diabetes', *Sydney Morning Herald*, Health and Fitness, 23 February 2006. <www.sciencedaily.com/releases/2007/04/070410162659.htm>

52. World Health Organization Media Center, '*Diabetes: What is diabetes*, Fact Sheet No 312, September 2006, <www.who.int/mediacentre/factsheets/fs312/en>

53. University of Michigan Transplant Centre, 2007, *Islet Transplantation Program*, <www.med.umich.edu/trans/public/islet/>

54. Junior Diabetes Research Foundation, 2004, *Fact Sheet: The Edmondton Protocol*, <www.jdrf.org.au/publications/factsheets/the_edmondton_protocol.pdf>

55. CNN, *Islet Cell Transplant: Experimental treatment for type 1 diabetes*, 3 October 2006, <www.cnn.com/HEALTH/library/DA/00046.html>

56. ScienceDaily, *Emory to Develop Islet Transplant Technology*, 26 March 2007, <www.sciencedaily.com/releases/2007/03/070319175919.htm>

57. Cairney, Richard, *Edmondton Protocol Takes Giant Lead Forward*, ExpressNews, University of Alberta, 3 February 2005, <www.expressnews.ualberta.ca/article.cfm?id=6354>

58. Junior Diabetes Research Foundation, 2004, loc.cit.

59. ScienceDaily, *Stem Cell Transplant Resets Immune System in Type I Diabetes Patients*, 11 April 2007, <www.sciencedaily.com/releases/2007/04/070410162659.htm>

CHAPTER EIGHT

1. Chain, Ernst, cited in Wong, George, 2003, *Penicillin: The wonder drug*, University of Hawaii, <www.botany.hawaii.edu/faculty/wong/BOT135/Lect21b.htm>

2. Lax, Eric, 2007, *Feature — Norman who?*, Popular Science, <www.popularscience.co.uk/features/feat12.htm>

3. ibid.

4. PBS Online, Science Odyssey: People and Discoveries, *Fleming Discovers Penicillin*, loc. cit.

5. PBS Online, Science Odyssey: People and Discoveries, *Alexander Fleming 1881–1955*, <www.pbs.org/wgbh/aso/databank/medhealth.html>

6. Torok, Simon, *Howard Florey — Maker of the miracle mould*, The Helix, <www.abc.net.au/science/slab/florey/story.htm>

7. Ho, David, *Alexander Fleming*, The Time 100: Scientists and Thinkers, 29 March 1999, <jcgi.pathfinder.com/time/time100/scientist/profile/fleming.html>

8. Swan, Norman, *Howard Florey: Part 2*, 21 September 1998, Radio National Health Report, ABC Online, <http://www.abc.net.au/science/slab/florey/story.htm>

9. Ho, David, *Alexander Fleming*, loc. cit.

10. PBS Online, Science Odyssey: People and Discoveries, *Fleming Discovers Penicillin*, loc. cit.

11. Ho, David, *Alexander Fleming*, loc. cit.

12. Torok, Simon, *Howard Florey — Maker of the miracle mould*, loc. cit.

13. Jayaram Paniker, C.K. (ed), 2006, *Textbook of Microbiology*, Orient Longman, New Delhi, p. 466.

14. Torok, Simon, *Howard Florey — Maker of the miracle mould*, loc. cit.

15. Swan, Norman, *Howard Florey: Part 1*, 14 September 1998, Radio National Health Report, ABC Online, <http://www.abc.net.au/science/slab/florey/story.htm>

16. Florey, Howard, cited in Swan, Norman, *Howard Florey: Part 1, 14 September 1998, loc. cit.*

17. The Tall Poppies Campaign, Australian Institute of Policy and Science, 2007, *The Oxford Team: Mary Ethel Hayter Reed — Lady Florey*, <www.tallpoppies.net.au/florey/researcher/theperson/main-content.html>

18. ibid.

19. Swan, Norman, *Howard Florey: Part 1*, loc. cit.

20. York, Barry, *Howard Florey and the Development of Penicillin*, NLA News, September 2001, Vol. XI, No. 12, National Library of Australia, <www.nla.gov.au/pub/nlanews/2001/sep01/sep01news.html>

21. Swan, Norman, *Howard Florey: Part 1,* loc. cit.

22. ibid.

23. Florey, Howard, cited in Swan, Norman, *Howard Florey: Part 2*, 21 September 1998, Radio National Health Report, ABC Online, <http://www.abc.net.au/science/slab/florey/story.htm>

24. SBS Australia, *Penicillin: The magic bullet*, Arcimedia, 3 August 2006.

25. ibid.

26. Torok, Simon, *Howard Florey — Maker of the miracle mould*, loc. cit.

27. Science Watch Website, *Making Penicillin Possible: Norman Heatley remembers*, <www.sciencewatch.com/interviews/norman_heatly.htm>

28. ibid.

29. York, Barry, *Howard Florey and the Development of Penicillin*, loc. cit.

30. Science Watch Website, *Making Penicillin Possible: Norman Heatley remembers*, loc. cit.

31. Lax, Eric, *Feature — Norman who?*, loc. cit.

32. ibid. In the 1980s, Heatley was asked to build a replica by the Science Museum in London which he said cost a lot more than the £5 he spent on the original. 'The rubbish dumps aren't what they were in the 1940s,' he commented.

33. ibid.

34. Florey, Howard, cited in Swan, Norman, *Howard Florey: Part 2*, loc. cit.

35. SBS Australia, *Penicillin: The magic bullet*, Arcimedia, 3 August 2006.

36. Science Watch Website, *Making Penicillin Possible: Norman Heatley remembers*, loc. cit.

37. SBS Australia, *Penicillin: The magic bullet*, Arcimedia, 3 August 2006.

38. Science Watch Website, *Making Penicillin Possible: Norman Heatley remembers*, loc. cit.

39. Torok, Simon, *Howard Florey — Maker of the miracle mould*, loc. cit.

40. SBS Australia, *Penicillin: The magic bullet*, Arcimedia, 3 August 2006.

41. ibid.

42. Science Watch Website, *Making Penicillin Possible: Norman Heatley remembers*, loc. cit.

43. SBS Australia, *Penicillin: The magic bullet*, Arcimedia, 3 August 2006.

44. Science Watch Website, *Making Penicillin Possible: Norman Heatley remembers*, loc. cit.

45. Florey, Howard, cited in Swan, Norman, *Howard Florey: Part 2*, loc. cit.

46. ibid

47. Science Watch Website, *Making Penicillin Possible: Norman Heatley remembers*, loc. cit.

48. Swan, Norman, *Howard Florey: Part 2*, loc. cit.

49. ibid.

50. SBS Australia, *Penicillin: The magic bullet*, Arcimedia, 3 August 2006.

51. Lax, Eric, 2007, *Feature — Norman who?*, loc. cit.

52. PBS Online, Science Odyssey: People and Discoveries, *Fleming Discovers Penicillin*, loc. cit.

53. SBS Australia, *Penicillin: The magic bullet*, Arcimedia, 3 August 2006.

54. Swan, Norman, *Howard Florey: Part 2*, loc. cit.

55. Torok, Simon, *Howard Florey — Maker of the miracle mould*, loc. cit.

56. Nobel Prize, *Ernst B. Chain — Biography*,
    <nobelprize.org/nobel_prizes/medicien/laureates/1945/chain-bio.html>

57. Nobel Prize, *Sir Alexander Fleming: The Nobel Prize in Physiology or Medicine*,
    <nobelprize.org/nobel_prizes/medicine/laureates/1945/fleming_docu.html>

58. PBS Online, Science Odyssey: People and Discoveries, *Alexander Fleming 1881–1955*, loc. cit.

59. Florey, Howard, Oral History Interview, 1967, cited in York, Barry, 'Howard Florey and the Development of Penicillin', *National Library of Australia News*, Vol. XI, No. 12, September 2001.

60. Hole, Jackson, 2005, *Barry Marshall — Nobel Prize in Medicine*, Academy of Achievement,
    <www.achievement.org/autodoc.printmember/mar1int-1>

61. Swan, Norman, *Howard Florey: Part 1*, loc. cit.

62. Torok, Simon, *Howard Florey — Maker of the miracle mould*, loc. cit.

63. The Tall Poppies Campaign, Australian Institute of Policy and Science, 2007, *The Person — Marriage: Mary Etherl Hayter Reed*,
    <www.tallpoppies.net.au/florey/researcher/theperson/main-content.html>

64. Swan, Norman, *Howard Florey: Part 2, loc. cit.*

65. Heatley, Norman, cited in The Tall Poppy Campaign, Australian Institute of Policy and Science, 2007, *The Oxford Team: Norman Heatley*,
    <www.tallpoppies.net.au/florey/researcher/working/main-content.htm>.

66. Swan, Norman, Howard Florey: Part 2, loc. cit.

67. Torok, Simon, *Howard Florey — Maker of the miracle mould*, loc. cit.

68. Strauss, Eugene W. and Strauss, Alex, 2006, op. cit., p. 263.

CHAPTER NINE

1. Academy of Achievement, 2005, *Interview: Jonas Salk M. D.*, 16 May 1991,
   <www.achievement.com/autodoc/page/sal0int-1>

2. Lapiana, Joseph J. and Winkowski, Robert B., 'Poliomyelitis: The era of fear', *Innovative Curriculum Series*, The Wright Centre for Science Education, Tufts University, Massachusettes, p. 20.

3. Who Named it? *Heine-Medin Disease*, <www.whonamedit.com/synd.cfm/544.html>
4. Sass, Edmund, 2001, *Poliomyelitis: A brief history*, from Sass, Edmund, *Polio's Legacy: An oral history*, University Press of America, 1996, <www.cloudnet.com/edrbsass/polio.htm>
5. ibid.
6. Who Named it? *Heine-Medin Disease*, loc. cit.
7. Bayly, Beddow M., 1956, *The Story of the Salk Antipoliomyelitis Vaccine*, Whale, <www.whale.to/vaccine/bayly.html>
8. Answers.com, *Poliomyelitis*, <www.answers.com/topic/poliomyelitis>
9. Sass, Edmund, 2001, *Poliomyelitis: A Brief History*, loc. cit.
10. Roosevelt, Franklin Delano, cited in Lapiana, Joseph J. and Winkowski, Robert B., 'Poliomyelitis: The era of fear', op. cit., p. 21.
11. Academy of Achievement, 2005, *Interview: Jonas Salk M. D.*, loc. cit.
12. Sass, Edmund, 2001, *Poliomyelitis: A brief history*, loc. cit.
13. Academy of Achievement, 2005, *Interview: Jonas Salk M. D.*, loc. cit.
14. Hellman, Hall, 2001, op. cit., p. 131.
15. Sheed, Wilfrid, 'Jonas Salk', *Time*, Vol. 153, No. 12, 29 March 1999, pp. 168–70.
16. Sass, Edmund, 2001, *Poliomyelitis: A brief history*, loc. cit.
17. Hellman, Hall, 2001, op. cit., p. 129.
18. Notable Biographies, *Albert Sabin: Biography*, <www.notablebiographies.com/Ro-Sc/Sabin-Albert.html>
19. Hellman Hall, 2001, op. cit., p 132.
20. PBS Online, Science Odyssey: People and Discoveries, *Salk Produces Polio Vaccine*, <www.pbs.org/wgbh/aso/databank/medhealth.html>
21. Nobel Prize, *Medicine 1954*, <nobelprize.org/nobel_prizes/medicine/laureates/1954/>
22. Hellman, Hall, 2001, op. cit., p. 131.
23. Salk, Jonas, cited in Hellman, Hall, 2001, op. cit., p. 132.
24. Sheed, Wilfrid, 'Jonas Salk', *Time*, Vol. 153, No. 12, 29 March 1999, pp. 168–70.
25. PBS Online, Science Odyssey: People and Discoveries, *Salk Produces Polio Vaccine*, loc. cit.
26. Academy of Achievement, 2005, *Interview: Jonas Salk M. D.*, loc. cit.
27. ibid.
28. Oransky, Ivan., *Medical Nihilism and the HPV Vaccine*, Boston Globe Online, 4 March 2007, <www.boston.com/yourlife/health/diseases/articles/2007/03/04/medical_nihilism_and_the_hpv_vaccine/->
29. Hellman, Hall, 2001, op. cit., p. 137.
30. Lindner, Ulrike and Blume, Stuart S., *Vaccine Innovation and Adoption: Polio Vaccine in the UK, the Netherlands and West German, 1955–1965*, PubMed Central, <www.pubmedcentral.nih.gov/articlerender.fcgi?artid=1592614>
31. *Lancet*, 2 April 1955, p. 702 cited at Bayly, Beddow M., 1956, loc. cit.
32. Sass, Edmund, 2001, loc. cit.
33. Bayly, Beddow M, 1956, loc. cit.
34. ibid.
35. Time Magazine Archives, *Closing in on Polio*, 29 March 1954, <www.time.com/time/magazine/article/0,9171,819686,00.html>
36. Bayly, Beddow M., 1956, loc. cit.
37. Hellman, Hall, 2001, op. cit., p. 138.
38. Academy of Achievement, 2005, *Interview: Jonas Salk M. D.*, loc. cit.

39. Sanofi Pasteur SA, *Conquering Polio: Competition to develop an oral vaccine*, <www.polio.info/polio-eradication/front/templates/index.jsp?siteCode=POLIO&codeRubrique=2>

40. PBS Online, Science Odyssey: People and Discoveries, *Salk Produces Polio Vaccine*, loc. cit.

41. Unfortunately for Koprowski the results of his trials have remained controversial. One theory for the origin of the global AIDS pandemic is that it developed from contaminated vaccines used in the trials of Koprowski's polio vaccine, which was given to over 1 million people. It is suggested that AIDS originated as a result of the inadvertent vaccination of trial participants with an HIV-like virus present in the monkey kidney cell cultures used to prepare the vaccine. Counterarguments were that Koprowski's vaccine was also tested on thousands of people in Poland, but there was no evidence of early HIV infection there. Many hypotheses regarding the origin of AIDS have been proposed. In 2006, 25 years after the first AIDS cases emerged, scientists from the University of Alabama in the United States, led by Dr Beatrice Hahn, confirmed that the HIV virus plaguing humans originated in wild chimpanzees in a remote part of Cameroon. Genetic analysis identified chimp communities whose viral strains were most closely related to the human strain of the AIDS virus, HIV-1. Results of the study were published in *Science* magazine on 25 May 2006. *See* Hahn, Beatrice H. et al., *Chimpanzee Reservoirs of Pandemic and Nonpandemic HIV-1*, 26 May 2006, Science magazine, <www.sciencemag.org/cgi/content/abstract/1126531v1>

42. Bayly, Beddow M., 1956, loc. cit.

43. Sanofi Pasteur SA, *Conquering Polio: Competition to develop an oral vaccine*, loc.cit.

44. Hellman, Hall, 2001, op. cit., p. 138.

45. Blume, Stuart and Geesink, Ingrid, Essay on Science and Society: *A Brief History of Polio*, Science, 2 June 2000, Vol 288, no.5471, pp.1593 – 1594.

46. Hellman, Hall, 2001, op. cit., p. 139.

47. PBS Online, Science Odyssey: People and Discoveries, *Jonas Salk 1914–1995*, <www.pbs.org/wgbh/aso/databank/medhealth.html>

48. Academy of Achievement, 2005, *Interview: Jonas Salk M. D.*, loc. cit.

49. Hellman, Hall, 2001, op. cit., p.141.

50. ibid.

51. Baker, Aryn, 'One Child at a Time: A new outbreak of polio in Africa underscores the difficulty of wiping out a stubborn global scourge', *Time*, 12 July 2004 / No. 27, p. 48.

52. ibid.

53. UNICEF, *Despite Difficulties, Polio Immunisation Drive Underway in Iraq*, 15 November, 2006, <www.unicef.ie/news110.htm>

54. ibid.

CHAPTER TEN

1. Elion, Gertrude B., 2007, *Autobiography*, Les Prix Nobel, <nobelprize.org/nobel_prizes/medicine/laureates/1988/elion-autobio.html>

2. Hitchings, George, cited in The Chemical Heritage Foundation, 2001 *George Hitchings: Pharmaceutical achiever*, <http//www.chemheritag.org/educationalservices/pharm/chemo/home.html>

3. National Cancer Institute — US National Institutes of Health, 2007, *Childhood Acute Lymphoblastic Leukemias*, <www.cancer.gov/cancer_information/doc_pdq.aspx?...>

4. Leukaemia Foundation, *About the Diseases: Leukemias*, <www.leukaemia.org.au/web/aboutdiseases/living_childhood.php>

5. Avery, Mary Ellen, *Gertrude B. Elion, January 23, 1918–February 21, 1999*, Biographical Memoirs, National Academy of Sciences, <www.nap.edu/html/biomems/gelion.html>

6. Elion, Gertrude, cited in Avery, Mary Ellen, loc. cit.

7. Chemical Heritage Foundation, 2001, *Gertrude Belle Elion — A lifeline*, <www.chemheritage.org/EducationalServices/pharm/chemo/readings/lifeline.htm>

8. Elion, Gertrude, cited in Avery, Mary Ellen, loc. cit.

9. Academy of Achievement, 2005, *Interview: Gertrude Elion Nobel Prize in Medicine, 6 March 1991*, <www.achievement.org/autodoc/printmember/eli0int-1>

10. Elion Gertrude, cited in Avery, Mary Ellen, loc. cit.

11. Bowden, Mary Ellen, 2002, *George Hitchings (1905–1998) and Gertrude Elion (1918–1999)*, The Chemical Heritage Foundation, <chemheritage.org/.../pharm/chemo/readings/hitch/pabio.htm>

12. The Chemical Heritage Foundation, 2001, *George Hitchings: Pharmaceutical achiever*, loc. cit.

13. GlaxoSmithKline, 2007, *The Legacy of Great Science: The work of Nobel Laureate Gertrude Elion lives on*, 16 March 2007, GSK in focus, <www.gsk.com/infocus/gertrude_elion.htm>

14. ibid.

15. Strauss, Eugene W. and Strauss, Alex, 2006, op. cit., p. 266.

16. Academy of Achievement, 2005, *Interview: Gertrude Elion Nobel Prize in Medicine, 6 March 1991*, loc. cit.

17. Avery, Mary Ellen, *Gertrude B. Elion, January 23, 1918–February 21, 1999*, loc. cit.

18. Strauss, Eugene W. and Strauss, Alex, 2006, *Medical Marvels: The 100 greatest advances in medicine*, op. cit., p. 266.

19. Bowden, Mary Ellen, 2002, *George Hitchings (1905–1998) and Gertrude Elion (1918–1999)*, loc. cit.

20. Strauss, Eugene W. and Strauss, Alex, 2006, op. cit., p. 267

21. Academy of Achievement, 2005, *Interview: Gertrude Elion Nobel Prize in Medicine, 6 March 1991*, loc. cit.

22. Avery, Mary Ellen, *Gertrude B. Elion, January 23, 1918–February 21, 1999*, loc. cit.

23. ibid.

24. virtualmedicalcentre.com, *Childhood Leukaemia*, <www.virtualbloodcentre.com/diseases.asp?did=698>

25. Bowden, Mary Ellen, 2002, *George Hitchings (1905–1998) and Gertrude Elion (1918–1999)*, loc. cit.

26. Chemical Heritage Foundation, 2001, *Gertrude Belle Elion — A lifeline*, <www.chemheritage.org/EducationalServices/pharm/chemo/readings/lifeline.htm>

27. GlaxoSmithKline, 2007, *The Legacy of Great Science: The work of Nobel Laureate Gertrude Elion lives on*, loc. cit.

28. Transweb.org, *Imuran: another miracle drug*, <www.transweb.org/reference/articles/drugs/imuran.html>

29. GlaxoSmithKline, 2007, *The Legacy of Great Science: The work of Nobel Laureate Gertrude Elion lives on*, loc. cit.

30. Bowden, Mary Ellen, 2002, *George Hitchings (1905–1998) and Gertrude Elion (1918–1999)*, loc. cit.

31. Elion, Gertrude, cited in Avery, Mary Ellen, *Gertrude B. Elion, January 23, 1918–February 21, 1999*, loc. cit.

32. ibid

33. Nobel Prize, George H. Hitchings, *The Nobel Prize in Physiology or Medicine, 1988: Autobiography*, <nobelprize.org/nobel_prizes/medicine/laueates/1988/hitchings-autobio.html>

34. Elion, Gertrude B., 2007, *Autobiography*, Les Prix Nobel, <nobel-prize.org/nobel_prizes/medicine/laureates/1988/elion-autobio.html>

35. Elion, Gertrude, cited in Avery, Mary Ellen, *Gertrude B. Elion, January 23, 1918–February 21, 1999*, loc. cit.

36. Avery, Mary Ellen, *Gertrude B. Elion, January 23, 1918 – February 21, 1999*, loc. cit.

37. Academy of Achievement, 2005, *Interview: Gertrude Elion Nobel Prize in Medicine*, 6 March 1991, <www.achievement.org/autodoc/printmember/eli0int-1>

38. GlaxoSmithKline, 2007, *The Legacy of Great science: The work of Nobel Laureate Gertrude Elion lives on*, loc. cit.

39. The Chemical Heritage Foundation, 2001, *George Hitchings: Pharmaceutical achiever*, loc. cit.

40. ibid.

41. Jewish Women's Archive, 2003, *Article from Burroughs Wellcome Newsletter Announcing Gertrude Elion's Receipt of the American Chemical Society's Garvan Medal 1968*, <www.jwa.org/archive/jsp/presInfo-print.jsp?resID=679>

42. GlaxoSmithKline, 2007, The Legacy of Great Science: The work of Nobel Laureate Gertrude Elion lives on, loc. cit.

43. ibid.

44. ibid.

45. Dana-Farber Cancer Institute and Children's Hospital Boston, 2007, *Press Release: Scientists isolate leukemia stem cells in a model of human leukemia*, 1 August 2006, <www.dana-farber.org/abo/news/press/default.html>

46. ibid.

BIBLIOGRAPHY

BOOKS

Adler, Robert E., *Medical Firsts from Hippocrates to the Human Genome*, John Wiley & Sons Inc., Hoboken, N.J., 2004.

Bickel, Lennard, *Florey: The man who made penicillin,* Melbourne University Press, Melbourne, 1995.

Bliss, Michael, *The Discovery of Insulin*, University of Chicago Press, Chicago, 1982.

Boccaccio, Giovanni (trans. G.H.McWilliam), *The Decameron,* Penguin Classics, 2003.

Clark, Ronand W., *The Life of Ernst Chain: Penicillin and beyond,* St Martin's Press, New York, 1985.

Crosby, Alfred W. Jr., *The Columbian Exchange: Biological and cultural consequences of 1492*, Praeger, Westport Connecticut, 2003.

Daniel, Thomas M. & Robbins, Frederick C. (ed.), *Polio,* University of Rochester Press, Rochester, 1997.

De Kruif, Paul, *Microbe Hunters*, New York, Harcourt Brace, 1927, reprinted Harcourt Brace, San Diego, 1996.

Debré, Patrice, (trans. Elborg Forster), *Louis Pasteur*, Johns Hopkins University Press, Baltimore, 1998.

Dubos, René and Dubos, Jean, *The White Plague,* Rutgers University Press, New Brunswick, 1998.

Friedman, Meyer and Friedland, Gerald W., *Medicine's 10 Greatest Discoveries,* Yale University Press, New Haven, 1998.

Glynn, Ian & Glynn, Jennifer, *The Life and Death of Smallpox,* Profile Books, London, 2004.

Gould, Tony, *A Summer Plague: Polio and its survivors,* Yale University Press, New Haven, 2005.

Hargittai, István, *Candid Science: Conversations with famous chemists,* Imperial College Press, London, 2000.

Hays, J.N., *Epidemics and Pandemics: Their impacts on human history*, California, ABC-CLIO, Santa Barbara, 2005.

Hellman, Hall, *Great Feuds in Medicine: Ten of the liveliest disputes ever,* John Wiley & Sons Inc., New York, 2001.

Hopkins, D.R., *Princes and Peasants: Smallpox in history,* University of Chicago Press, Chicago, 1983.

Jayaram Paniker, C.K. (ed.), *Textbook of Microbiology*, Orient Longman, New Delhi, 2006.

Kelly, John, *The Great Mortality: An intimate history of the Black Death*, Fourth Estate, London, 2005.

Kiple, Kenneth F. (ed.), *The Cambridge World History of Human Diseases*, Cambridge University Press, Cambridge, 1993.

Klein, Aaron E., *Trial by Fury: The polio vaccine controversy,* Charles Scribner's Sons, New York, 1972.

Kluger, Jeffrey, *Splendid Solution: Jonas Salk and the conquest of polio*, G.P. Putnam's Sons, New York, 2004.

Lapiana, Joseph J. and Winkowski, Robert B., 'Poliomyelitis: The era of fear', *Innovative Curriculum Series,* The Wright Centre for Science Education, Tufts University, Massachusetts.

Laszlo, John, *The Cure of Childhood Leukemia: Into the age of miracles*, Rutgers University Press, New Brunswick, 1995.

Lax, Eric, *The Mould in Dr Florey's Coat,* Henry Holt and Co, New York, 2000.

Lyons, Gerald, *Breakthroughs: An exploration of some of the amazing advances in Science, Medicine and*

Technology, William Collins Pty Ltd, Sydney, 1984.

Macauley, Thomas Babington, *The History of England from the Accession of James the Second,* Longman, Brown, Green and Longman, London, 1852.

Macfarlane, Gwyn, *Howard Florey: The making of a great scientist*, Oxford University Press, Oxford, 1979.

Marriott, Edward, *Plague: A story of science, rivalry and the scourge that won't go away*, Metropolitan Books, New York, 2003.

Miller, Genevieve (ed.), Letters of Edward Jenner and Other Documents Concerning the Early History of Vaccination, Johns Hopkins University Press, Baltimore, 1983.

Morton, Leslie T. & Moore, Robert J., *A Chronology of Medicine and Related Sciences,* Scholar Press, Aldershot, 1997.

Moss, Ralph W, *Questioning Chemotherapy,* Equinox Press, New York, 1995.

Oldstone, Michael B.A., *Viruses, Plagues and History,* New York, Oxford University Press, Oxford, 1998.

Paul, John R., *A History of Poliomyelitis,* Yale University Press, New Haven, 2005.

Reynolds, Moira Davidson, *American Women Scientists: 23 inspiring biographies 1900–2000*, McFarland & Company, Jefferson N.C., 1999.

Scott, Susan and Duncan, Christopher, *Return of the Black Death: The world's greatest serial killer*, John Wiley & Sons, Chichester, 2004.

Shell, Marc, *Polio and its aftermath: The paralysis of culture*, Cambridge MA, Harvard University Press, 2005.

Simmons, John Galbraith, *Doctors and Discoveries: Lives that created today's medicine*, Boston, Houghton Mifflin Company, 2002.

Smith, J. R., *The Speckled Monster: Smallpox in England 1670–1970,* Whitley Press, Chelmsford, 1987.

Strauss, Eugene W. and Strauss, Alex, *Medical Marvels: The 100 greatest advances in medicine*, Prometheus Books, New York, 2006.

Tucker, Jonathan B., *Scourge: The once and future threat of smallpox*, Atlantic Monthly Press, New York, 2001.

Twigg, Graham, *The Black Death: A biological reappraisal*, B.T. Batsford Ltd., London, 1984.

Vallery-Radot, René, *The Life of Louis Pasteur,* Doubleday, Garden City N.Y, 1926.

Warrell, David A., Cox, Timothy M. and Firth, John D. (eds), *Oxford Textbook of Medicine*, Oxford University Press, Oxford, 2003.

JOURNAL, PERIODICAL AND NEWSPAPER ARTICLES

Baker, Aryn, 'One Child at a Time: A new outbreak of polio in Africa underscores the difficulty of wiping out a stubborn global scourge', *Time*, No. 27, 12 July 2004.

Barquet, Nicolau and Domingo, Pere, 'Smallpox: The triumph over the most terrible of the ministers of death', *Annals of Internal Medicine,* 127, 1997.

Doble, Claire, 'Unexpected Directions, Diabetes', *Sydney Morning Herald*, Health and Fitness supplement, February 23, 2006.

Doherty, T. Mark and Rook, Graham, 'Progress and Hindrances in Tuberculosis Vaccine Development', *Lancet*, 17 March 2006, 367 (9514).

Farley, John and Geison, Gerald L., 'Science, Politics and Spontaneous Generation in Nineteenth Century France: The Pasteur–Pouchet debate', *Bulletin of the History of Medicine*, Vol. 48, No. 2, summer 1974.

Friedman, (Rabbi) Mark, 'Great Scientist, Great Jew', *Canadian Jewish News,* 4 August 2005.

Hawke, Caitlin, 'The Cutting Edge: Focus on anthrax then and now', *Pasteur Perspective: The newsletter of the Pasteur Foundation devoted to the world of the Institit Pasteur,* No. 11, spring 2002.

Jenkins, Scott and Perrone, Joseph, 'The Need for Biodefense Standards', *The Scientist: Magazine of the life sciences,* 1 August 2006.

Murtagh, John E., 'Diabetes Mellitus: The general practitioner's perspective', *Clinical and Experimental Optometry,* 82.2–3 March–June 1999.

Pollard, Ruth, 'TB's Extreme New Face', *Sydney Morning Herald*, 21 September 2006.

Shampo, Marc and Kyle, Robert A., 'Charles Best — Codiscoverer of Insulin', *Mayo Clinic Proceedings,* December 2004; 79(12):1546.

Sheed, Wilfrid, 'Jonas Salk', *Time,* Vol. 153, No. 12, 29 March 1999.

Watts, Jonathan, 'China Rabies Outbreak Triggers Second Dog Cull', *Guardian,* 4 August 2006.

WEBSITES

A Traveller's Guide to the History of Biology and Medicine, Chapter 3: Clausthal-Zellerfeld,
    <www.historyofbiologyandmedicine.com/westgermany.htm>

ABC Radio National, 23 November 1997, *Ockham's Razor* transcript 23, 'Defending Edward Jenner', <www.abc.net.au/rn/science/ockham/or231197.htm>

——Swan, Norman, *Health Report,* Howard Florey: Parts 1 & 2,' 14 & 21 September 1998,
    <http://www.abc.net.au/science/slab/florey/story.htm>

Academy of Achievement, 2005, *Biography: Jonas Salk M.D. — Developer of polio vaccine,*
    <http://.org/autodoc/printmember/sal0int-1>

——*Interview: Gertrude Elion Nobel Prize in Medicine,* 6 March 1991,
    <www.achievement.org/autodoc/printmember/eli0int-1>

——*Interview: Jonas Salk M.D.,* 16 May 1991, <www.achievement.com/autodoc/page/sal0int-1>

——Hole, Jackson, *Barry Marshall — Nobel Prize in Medicine,*
    <www.achievement.org/autodoc.printmember/mar1int-1>

The Age online, 7 October 2005, Cervical cancer vaccine breakthrough,
    <www.theage.com.au/news/National/Cervical-cancer-vaccine-break-through/2005/10/07/1128562982238.html>

Alberti, George, *Lessons from the History of Insulin,* Diabetes Voice, Vol. 46, No. 4/2001,
    <www.diabetesvoice.org>

Answers.com, *Diphtheria,* <www.answers.com/topic/diphtheria>

——*Poliomyelitis,* <www.answers.com/topic/poliomyelitis>

——*Tetanus,* <www.answers.com/topic/tetanus>

Association of the British Pharmaceutical Industry, *Target Diabetes,*
    <www.abpi.org.uk/publications/publication_details/targetDiabetes/default.asp>

Avery, M.E., *Gertrude B Elion,* Hunter: Department of Physics and Astronomy,
    <www.ph.hunter.cuny.edu/scientists/Elion.html>

——*Gertrude B. Elion,* Biographical Memoirs, National Academy of Sciences,
    <www.nap.edu/html/biomems/gelion.html>

Banting, Frederick G., *Nobel Lecture,* Nobel Lectures, Physiology or Medicine 1922–1941,
    <nobelprize.org/nobel_prizes/medicine/laureates/1923/banting-lecture.htm>

Bayly, Beddow M., *The Story of the Salk Antipoliomyelitis Vaccine,* Whale,
    <www.whale.to/vaccine/bayly.html>

Berman, Jessica, 25 September 2005, *Researchers Improve Tuberculosis Vaccine,*
    <www.voanews.com/english/2005-09-25-voa31.cfm>

Best, Henry Bruce Macleod, 24 April 1996, *Speech to: The Academy of Medicine, Toronto,* Discovery of
    Insulin, <http://www.discoveryofinsulin.com/Home.htm>

BioCycle World, Albert Schatz: Educator, microbiologist, streptomycin discoverer,
    <www.jgpress.com/archives_free/00375.html>

Bowden, Mary Ellen, *George Hitchings (1905–1998) and Gertrude Elion (1918–1999),* Chemical
    Heritage Foundation, 2002, <http://www.chemheritage.org/educationalservices/ph-
    arm/chemo/readings/hitch/pabio.htm>

——2003, *Paul Ehrlich: Pharmaceutical achiever,*
    <www.chemheritage.org/educationalservices/pharm/chemo/readings/ehrlich.htm>

——The Chemical Heritage Foundation, 2001, Magic Bullets: Chemistry vs Cancer —
    Pharmaceutical Achievers, *Paul Ehrlich,*
    <www.chemheritage.org/educationalservices/pharm/chemo/home.htm>

Britannica Online Encyclopedia, *Paul Ehrlich: Syphilis studies,*
    <www.britannica.com/eb/article-2054/Paul -Ehrlich>

Burns, William, MRC National Institute for Medical Research, *NIMR: Mill Hill Essays 2003:*
    Alexandre Yersin and his adventures, <www.nimr.mrc.ac.uk/millhillessays/2003/yersin>

Buzzle, *Bubonic Plague: Case confirmed in Los Angeles,*
    <www.buzzle.com/editorials/4-19-2006-93918.asp>

Cairney, Richard, *Edmondton Protocol takes giant leap forward,* ExpressNews, University of Alberta,
    3 February, 2005, <www.expressnews.ualberta.ca/article.cfm?id=6354>

California: History 135F Plagues and Contagion, 2005,
    <e3.uci.edu/clients/bjbecker/PlaguesandPeople/week6f.html>

Canadian Diabetes Association, 2007, *The History of Diabetes,*
    <www.diabetes.ca/Section_About/timeline.asp>

——*Banting House National Historic Site: Frederick Banting,*
    <www.diabetes.ca/Section_About/BantingIndex.asp>

Canadian Lung Association, 2007, *An History of the Fight against TB in Canada: Prevention of TB —*
    BCG Vaccine, <http://www.lung.ca/tb/tbhistory/prevention/vaccine.html>

Canadian Medical Association Journal, 2007, *The Late Baron Shibasaburo Kitasato,*
    <www.pubmedcentral.nih.gov/articlerender.fcgi?artid=382621>

CDC Centres for Disease Control and Prevention, Department of Health and Human Services,
    Tetanus Chapter (Pink Book),
    <www.cdc.gov/vaccine/pubs/pinkbook/downloads/tetanus.pdf>

Cells alive!, *Bacteriophage: When E. coli has a Virus,* <http://www.cellsalive.com/phage.htm>

Channel 4, 2007, (Britain), *Plague,*
    <www.channel4.com/history/microsites/H/history/plague/plague.html>

Chemical Heritage Foundation, 2001, *Gertrude Belle Elion — A lifeline,*
    <www.chemheritage.org/EducationalServices/pharm/chemo/readings/lifeline.htm>

——*George Hitchings: Pharmaceutical achiever,*
    <http//www.chemheritag.org/educationalservices/pharm/chemo/home.html>

CNN, *Islet Cell Transplant: Experimental treatment for type 1 diabetes,* 3 October 2006,
    <www.cnn.com/HEALTH/library/DA/00046.html>

Cohn, David V., *Pasteur Koch Controversy on Anthrax Inoculation,* Founders of Biological and Medical
    Sciences, <www.foundersofscience.net>

——*The Life and Times of Louis Pasteur,* 1999, LabExplorer,

<www.labexplorer.com/louis_pasteur.htm>

Coppedge, David, F., *Shining Through Material Darkness: Louis Pasteur*, 2000, World's Greatest Creation Scientists from Y1K to Y2K, <www.creationsafaris.com/wgcs_4.htm>

Dana-Farber Cancer Institute and Children's Hospital Boston, 1 August 2006, *Press Release: Scientists isolate leukemia stem cells in a model of human leukemia*, <www.dana-farber.org/abo/news/press/default.html>

Department for Environmental Food and Rural Affairs UK (DEFRA), *Disease Fact Sheet: Rabies*, <www.defra.gov.uk/animalh/diseases/notifiable/ rabies/index.htm>

Discovery of Insulin, Sir Frederick Banting Educational Committee, *The Discovery of Insulin: A Canadian medical miracle of the 20th century*, James Bertram Collip, <www.discoveryofinsulin.com/Home.htm>

DoctorConnect, *2006 Australian of the Year — Professor Ian Frazer*, <www.doctorconnect.gov.au/internet/otd/publishing.nsf/Content/work-australian-of-the-year>

Doctors Independent Network (DIN), *Louis Pasteur,* <www.dinweb.org/dinweb/DINMuseum/Louis%20Pasteur.asp>

Edward Jenner Institute for Vaccine Research, <www.jenner.ac.uk>

Ehrlich, Paul, 13 March 1900, *Croonian Lecture — On Immunity with Special Reference to Cell Life,* Theoretical Immunology, <post.queensu.ca/~forsdyke/theorimm.htm>

Elion, Gertrude B., 2007, *Autobiography,* Les Prix Nobel, 2007, <nobel-prize.org/nobel_prizes/medicine/laureates/1988/elion-autobio.html>

Encyclopedia of Children's Health, *Diphtheria,* <www.healthofchildren.com/D/Diphtheria.html>

Endocrine Web's Diabetes Centre, 2007, *What is Insulin?,* <www.endocrineweb.com./diabetes/2insulin.html>

E-notes World of Microbiology and Immunology, *Emil von Behring,* <science.enotes.com/microbiology-encyclopedia/?start=60>

Florey Medical Research Fund, 2007, *About Howard Florey,* <www.florey.adelaide.edu.au/aboutflo.html>

Founders of Biological and Medical Sciences, *Dr Robert Koch's Latest Estimate of Pasteur's Methods and Discoveries ... from the Boston Medical and Surgical Journal,* 18 January, 1883, Vol. CVIII, No. 3, <www.foundersofscience.net/past_koc.htm>

——*Pasteur's Reply to Koch from the Boston Medical and Surgical Journal,* 1 March, 1883, Vol. CVIII, No. 9, <www.foundersofscience.net/past_koc.htm>

Gardner, Amanda, 10 April 2007, *Stem Cell Therapy May Combat Type I Diabetes,* MedicineNet.com, <www.medicinenet.com/script/main/art.asp?articlekey=80402>

GlaxoSmithKline, 16 March 2007, *The Legacy of Great Science,* <www.gsk.com/infocus/gertrude_elion.htm>

——*The White Plague,* <www.gsk.com/infocus/whiteplague.htm>

Grundman, Kornelia, 2001, *Emil von Behring: The founder of Serum Therapy,* <nobel-prize.org/nobel_prizes/medicine/articles/behring/index.html>

Hahn, Beatrice H. et al., 26 May 2006, *Chimpanzee Reservoirs of Pandemic and Nonpandemic HIV-1,* Science magazine, <www.sciencemag.org/cgi/content/abstract/1126531v1>

Hammond, Edward and Ching, Lim Li, 30 May 2006, *WHA Delays Decision on Smallpox Virus Stocks,* Report from the 59th World Health Assembly, <www.smallpoxbiosafety.org>

Hawgood, Barbara J, 2005, *Waldemar Mordecai Haffkine, CIE (1860–1930): prophylactic vaccination against cholera and bubonic plague in British India*, Journal of Medical Biography, <www.hawgood.co.uk/barbara/Haffkine.htm>

Healthline, *Tetanus Health Article*, <www.healthline.com/adamcontent/tetanus>

History Learning Site, 2000, *Robert Koch*, <www.historylearningsite.co.uk/robert_koch.htm>

Hite, Pamela F., Barnes, Ann M. and Johnston, Philip E., 2006, *Exuberance Over Exubera*, Clinical Diabetes 24:110-114, American Diabetes Association, <clinical.diabetesjournals.org/cgi/content/full/24/3/110>

Ho, David, 29 March 1999, *Alexander Fleming*, The Time 100: Scientists and Thinkers, <jcgi.pathfinder.com/time/time100/scientist/profile/fleming.html>

Hoogerdijk, Derek, *The Discovery of Insulin*, Quasar: University of Alberta, <www.quasar.ualberta.ca/edse456/apt/vignettes/insulin.htm>

Hoslink, *Pioneers in Medical Laboratory Science — Albert Calmette*, <www.hoslink.com/pioneers.htm>

——*Pioneers in Medical Laboratory Science — Alexandre Yersin*, <www.hoslink.com/pioneers.htm>

——*Pioneers in Medical Laboratory Science — Emil von Behring*, <www.hoslink.com/pioneers.htm>

Hubbard, John P (ed.), *Trends: WHO reports first results of mass vaccination with BCG*, iPediatrics, Vol. 6 No. 3, September 1950, <pediatrics.aappublications.org/cgi/content/abstract/6/3/481>

Images of Poliomyelitis: A critique of scientific literature, 2004, *The Salk Vaccine*, <www.geocities.com/harpub/salkvacc.htm>

Immunizations, *In-Depth Reports: Diphtheria, tetanus and pertussis*, <162.1.2.78/ADAM/doc/In-DepthReports/10/000090.htm>

Indian Post online, *Dr Waldemar Mordecai Wolff Haffkine*, <www.indianpost.com/viewstamp.php/Alpha/D/DR.%20WALDEMAR%20MORDECAI%20HAFFKINE>

Innovator Awards 2005 Website, *Albert Schatz*, <www.njinvent.org/2005/schatz.htlm>

Institute for Animal Health, *Robert Koch: Advancing the Field of Bacteriology*, <www.iah.bbsrc.ac.uk/schools/scientists/KOCH.htm>

International Diabetes Institute, 2006, *Diabetes Explained*, <www.diabetes.com.au>

International Travel Vaccination Centre, *Global Status of Polio*, <www.travelvaccines.com.au>

Internet FAQ Archives, *Emil von Behring Biography (1854–1917)*, Encyclopedia of Health, <www.faqs.org/health/bios/23/Emil-von-Behring.html>

Jenner, Edward, *An Inquiry into the Causes and Effects of the Variolae Vaccinae, a Disease Discovered in Some of the Western Counties of England, Particularly Gloucestershire, and Known by the Name of the Cow Pox (1798)*, 'The Three Original Publications on Vaccination Against Smallpox', The Harvard Classics: 1909–14, Great Books on Line, bartelby.com, <www.bartleby.com/38/4/1.html>

Jenner Museum, *Edward Jenner and Smallpox*, <www.jennermuseum.com/overview/index.shtml>

Jewish Encyclopedia, *Waldemar Mordecai Wolff Haffkine*, <www.jewishencyclopedia.com/directory.jsp?letter=H&partition=1&pageNum=5>

Jewish Womens Archive, 2003, *Article from Burroughs Wellcome newsletter announcing Gertrude Elion's receipt of the American Chemical Society's Garvan Medal 1968*, <www.jwa.org/archive/jsp/presInfo-print.jsp?resID=679>

Junior Diabetes Research Foundation, 2004, *Fact Sheet: The Edmondton Protocol*, <www.jdrf.org.au/publications/factsheets/the_edmondton_protocol.pdf>

Khamsi, Roxanne, *Lab loses trio of plague mice*, news@nature.com, 2005, MacMillan Publishers Ltd., <cmbi.bjmu.edu.cn/news/0509/78.htm>

Kitasato's Drama Without a Script, *Act I: Before Unravelling the Enigma,*
<www.microbes.jp/hiwa/English/dorama/report1.html>

Koch, Robert, 18 January 1883, *Dr Robert Koch's Latest Estimate of Pasteur's Methods and Discoveries, and of the Present Position of the General Inoculation Problem,* Boston Medical and Surgical Journal, Vol. CVIII, No. 3, Pasteur Koch Controversy,
<www.foundersofscience.net/past_koc.htm>

Kruszelnicki, Karl S., *Arrow Up Yours & Plague 2,* ABC Great Moments in History, 2006,
<www.abc.net.au/science/k2/moments/s662193.htm>

Lax, Eric, 2007, *Feature — Norman Who?,* Popular Science,
<www.popularscience.co.uk/features/feat12.htm>

Leukaemia Foundation, *About the Diseases: Leukaemias,*
<www.leukaemia.org.au/web/aboutdiseases/living_childhood.php>

Library and Archives Canada, 2007, *Famous Canadian Physicians: Frederick Banting,*
<www.collectionscanada.ca/physicians/002032-200-e.html>

Lindner, Ulrike and Blume, Stuart S., *Vaccine Innovation and Adoption: Polio vaccine in the UK, the Netherlands and West Germany, 1955–1965,* PubMed Central,
<www.pubmedcentral.nih.gov/articlerender.fcgi?artid=1592614>

Look Smart Find Articles, *A Portrait of History: Paul Ehrlich archives of pathology,* <findarticles.com/p/articles/mi_qa3725/is_200106/ain9003500/pg_2>

Madehow.com, *How Insulin is Made,* <www.madehow.com/Volume-7/Insulin.html>

Medical Discoveries, 2007, *Emil von Behring,* <www.discoveriesinmedicine.com/General-Information-and-Biographies/index.html>

MedlinePlus: US National Library of Medicine and the National Institutes of Health, *Rabies,*
<www.nlm.nih.gov/medlineplus/rabies.html>

Mollaret, H.H., *Contribution to the knowledge of relations between Koch and Pasteur,* NTM-Schriftenr. Gesch. Naturwiss, Technik, Med, Leipzig 20 (1983)1, pp 57–65, translated by Cohn, E.T., Fasciotto-Dunn, B.H., Kuhn, U. and Cohn, D.V., Molleret,
<pyramid.spd.louisville.edu/~eri/fos/Molleret.html>

National Network for Immunization Information, *Vaccine Information: Smallpox,*
<www.immunizationinfo.org/vaccineInfo/vaccine_detail.cfv?id=26>

New-Medical.Net, *It's 2006 and Two Hundred Children are Crippled by Polio in Somalia,* 27 March 2006, <http://www.news-medical.net/print_article.asp?id=16902>

nobelprize.org, *Ernst B. Chain — Biography,*
<nobelprize.org/nobel_prizes/medicine/laureates/1945/chain-bio.html>

——*Emil von Behring: The Nobel Prize in Physiology and Medicine 1901, Biography,* <nobelprize.org/nobel_prizes/medicine/laureates/1901/behring-bio.html>

——*George H. Hitchings, The Nobel Prize in Physiology or Medicine, 1988: Autobiography,* <nobelprize.org/nobel_prizes/medicine/laueates/1988/hitchings-autobio.html>

——*Medicine 1954,* <nobelprize.org/nobel_prizes/medicine/laureates/1954/html>

——*Paul Ehrlich — Nobel Lecture,*
<nobelprize.org/nobel_prizes/medicine/laureates/1908/ehrlich-lecture.html>

——*Robert Koch — Biography,*
<http://nobelprize.org/nobel_prizes/medicine/laureates/1905/koch-bio.html>

——*Selman A. Waksman — Nobel Lecture,*
<nobelprize.org/nobel_prizes/medicine.laureates/1952/waksman-lecture.html>

——*Sir Alexander Fleming: The Nobel Prize in Physiology or Medicine,* <nobelprize.org/nobel_prizes/medicine/laureates/1945/fleming_docu.html>

——*The Immune System Pioneers: Ilya Mechnikov and the phagocyte cells*,
   <nobelprize.org/educational_games/medicine/immunity/immune-pioneers.html>

Notable Biographies, *Albert Sabin: Biography*,
   <www.notablebiographies.com/Ro-Sc/Sabin-Albert.html>

Oransky, Ivan., 4 March 2007, *Medical Nihilism and the HPV Vaccine*, Boston Globe online,
   <www.boston.com/yourlife/health/diseases/articles/2007/03/04/medical_nihilism_and_
   the_hpv_vaccine/->

Organic Consumers Association, 2005, *International Campaign to Stop Genetic Engineering of Smallpox
   Virus Announced*, <http://www.smallpoxbiosafety.org/who/prenglish.html>

Owen, James, 25 May 2006, *AIDS Origin Traced to Chimp Group in Cameroon*, National Geographic
   News, <news.nationalgeographic.com/news/2006/05/060525-aids-chimps.html>

PapScreen Victoria, 16 March 2005, *Cervical Cancer Vaccine no Replacement for Pap Tests*,
   <www.cancervic.org.au/cancer1/whatsnew/mediareleases/2005/20050316.htm>

Paul Ehrlich Symposium 2004, *Welcome Address*, <www.paul-ehrlich-symposium-2004.de>

PBS Online, Science Odyssey: People and Discoveries, *Alexander Fleming*,
   <www.pbs.org/wgbh/aso/databank/medhealth.html>

——*Bubonic plague hits San Francisco*, <www.pbs.org/wgbh/aso/databank/medhealth.html>

——*Ehrlich finds cure for syphilis*, <www.pbs.org/wgbh/aso/databank/medhealth.html>

——*Fleming discovers penicillin*, <www.pbs.org/wgbh/aso/databank/medhealth.html>

——*Salk produces polio vaccine*, <www.pbs.org/wgbh/aso/databank/medhealth.html>

——*World Health Organization declares smallpox eradicated*,
   <www.pbs.org/wgbh/aso/databank/eventindex.html>

Pellerin, Cheryl, *Progress Challenges Highlighted on World Tuberculosis Day 2006*, Washington File,
   <http://usembassy-australia.state.gov/hyper/2006/0323/epf410.htm>

polyscience.org, 3 October 2005, *Nobel Prize for medicine awarded to discoverers of H. pylori*,
   <http://polyscience.org/2005/10/nobel-prize-heliobacter-pylori>

Poynter Centre, *Syphilis in History*, <wisdomtools.com/pointer/syphilis.html>

Raymo, Chet, *Thus we Behold a Deadly Beauty*, Boston Globe online,
   <www.boston.com/globe/seaarch/stories/health/science_musings/092898.htm>

RDS Understanding Animal Research in Medicine, *Diphtheria Vaccine*,
   <www.rds_net.org.uk/pages/page.asp?i_ToolbarID=PageID=66>

Retroscreen Virology Ltd, *Twenty Five Years On: Smallpox revisited*,
   <www.retroscreen.com/?sec=23>

Richwine, Lisa, 1 September 2006, *Gene therapy used to treat skin cancer*, News in Science,
   <www.abc.net.au/science/news/stories/s173077.htm>

Robert Koch Institute, *Robert Koch and the Institute*,
   <www.rki.de/cln_006/nn_231644/EN/Content/Institute/History/history__node__en.ht
   ml__nnn=true>

Rutgers University, 2003, *Albert Schatz: My Experience in World War II, 1942*, Rutgers Oral History
   Archive of World War II, the Korean War, the Vietnam War and the Cold War, <oralhis-
   tory.rutgers.edu/Docs/memoirs/schatz_albert/schatz_albert_memoir.html>

Sanofi Pasteur, *Welcome to Sanofi Pasteur in Japan: Tetanus*, <www.sanofipasteur.jp/sanofi-
   pasteur/front/index.jsp?codePage=VP_PD_Tetanus&codeRubrique=19...>

Sanofi Pasteur Australia, *Rabies*, <www.sanofipasteur.com.au/ avpi-aus-
   tralia/front/templates/vaccinations-travel-health-vaccine>

Sanofi Pasteur SA, *Conquering Polio: Competition to develop an oral vaccine*, <www.polio.info/polio-
   eradication/front/templates/index.jsp?siteCode=POLIO&codeRubrique=2>

Sass, Edmund, 2001, *Poliomyelitis: A Brief History*, from Sass, Edmund, *Polio's Legacy: An oral history*,
<www.cloudnet.com/edrbsass/polio.htm>

Saunders, Vicki and Durrheim, David N., 2003, *Cuckoos, Cows and a Country Doctor: The pioneering
work of a rural health professional in the development of public health*, Journal of Rural and
Remote Environmental Health, 2(2), <www.jcu.edu.au/jrtph/vol/v02saunders.pdf>

ScienceDaily, 26 March 2007, *Emory to Develop Islet Transplant Technology*,
<www.sciencedaily.com/releases/2007/03/070319175919.htm>

——11 April 2007, *Stem Cell Transplant Resets Immune System in Type I Diabetes Patients*,
<www.sciencedaily.com/releases/2007/04/070410162659.htm>

Science in Africa, *Spotting the Culprits — New tests for TB, May 2003*,
<www.scienceinafrica.co.za/2003/may/tb.htm>

Science Watch, *Making Penicillin Possible: Norman Heatley remembers*,
<www.sciencewatch.com/interviews/norman_heatly.htm>

Scientists, *Pasteur*, <ambafrance-ca.org/HYPERLAB/PEOPLE/_pasteur.html>

Scott, Patrick, *Edward Jenner and the Discovery of Vaccination*, Department of Rare Books and Special
Collections: University of South Carolina, <www.sc.edu/library/spcoll/nathist/jenner1.html>

Sizemore, Christine F., Laughon, Barbara E. and Fauci, Anthony S., *World TB Day, 24 March, 2006*,
National Institute of Allergy and Infectious Diseases & National Institutes of Health,
<www3.niaid.nih.gov>

Smith, Ryan, 3 February 2005, *World-first Living Donor Islet Cell Transplant a Success*, Eureka Alert,
<www.eurekalert.org/pub_releases/2005-02/uoa-wld020305.php>

Smithsonian National Museum of American History, 2006, Whatever Happened to Polio?
Exhibition information, *How Polio Changed Us: The March of Dimes*, <americanhis-
tory.si.edu/exhibitions/exhibition.cfm?key=38&exkey=352>

——Whatever Happened to Polio? Exhibition information, *Polio: The iron lung and other equipment*,
<americanhistory.si.edu/polio/howpolio/ironlung.htm>

Sydney Morning Herald online, 1 February 2007, *Victorian woman chalks up record for iron lung*,
<www.smh.com.au/news/National/Vic-woman-chalks-up-record-for-iron-
lung/2007/02/01/116991947>

Tall Poppies Campaign, Australian Institute of Policy and Science, 2007, *The Oxford Team: Ernst
Chain*, <www.tallpoppies.net.au/florey/researcher/theperson/main-content.html>

——*The Oxford Team: M.A. Jennings*,
<www.tallpoppies.net.au/florey/researcher/theperson/main-content.html>

——*The Oxford Team: Mary Ethel Hayter Reed — Lady Florey*,
<www.tallpoppies.net.au/florey/researcher/theperson/main-content.html>

——*The Oxford Team: Norman Heatley*,
<www.tallpoppies.net.au/florey/researcher/working/main-content.html>

Thumbnails, 39 — *Ehrlich: Chemotherapy is launched*,
<dodd.cmcvellore.ac.in/hom/39%20-%20Ehrlich%20Chemo.html>

Time Magazine Archives, 29 March 1954, *Closing in on Polio*,
<www.time.com/time/magazine/article/0,9171,819686,00.html>

Titus, Nicole, 20 September 2005, *Plague-infected Mice Escape from Jersey Lab Avion*,
<www.avionnewspaper.com/media/paper798/news/2005/09/20/Science/PlagueInfected.
Mice.Escape.F>

Todar's Online Textbook of Bacteriology, 2002, *Diphtheria*,
<http://textbookofbacteriology.net/diphtheria.html>

Torok, Simon, *Howard Florey — Maker of the miracle mould*, Helix,
    <www.abc.net.au/science/slab/florey/story.htm>

Transweb.org, *Imuran: another miracle drug,*
    <www.transweb.org/reference/articles/drugs/imuran.html>

Travelers Vaccines Website, 2006, *Disease Fact Sheet: Tetanus, diphtheria and poliomyelitis*,
    <www.travelersvaccines.com/En/Before_Leaving/Fact_Sheets11.cfm>

Trueman, Chris, 2007, *Edward Jenner*, History Learning Site,
    <www.historylearningsite.co.uk/edward_jenner.htm>

Tucker, Jonathan B., 2001, *Smallpox: From eradicated disease to bioterrorist threat,* Centre for
    Nonproliferation Studies, Monterey Institute of International Studies,
    <cns.miis.edu/research/cbw/smallpox.htm>

Twoop Timelines, *Bubonic Plague — A historical timeline,*
    <www.twoop.com/medicine/archives/2005/10/bubonic_plague.html>

UNICEF, 15 November 2006, *Despite Difficulties, Polio Immunisation Drive Underway in Iraq*,
    <www.unicef.ie/news110.htm>

University of Michigan Transplant Centre, 2007, 'Islet Transplantation Program',
    <www.med.umich.edu/trans/public/islet/>

Vaccine Place: Sanofi Pasteur Inc, 2006, *Polio Disease — 50ᵗʰ anniversary of the polio vaccine*,
    <www.vaccineplace.com>

virtualmedicalcentre.com, *Childhood Leukaemia*, <www.virtualbloodcen-
    tre.com/diseases.asp?did=698>

Walker, Benjamin Edward, *Unpublished Memoirs: The rain must fall,* Millenium, 'Our Century
    1900–1924 Diphtheria Strikes Staffordshire',
    <www.westmidlands.com/millennium/1900/1900-1924/1907.html>

Who Named It?, *Alexandre-Émil-Jean Yersin*, <www.whonamedit.com/doctor.cfm/2454.html>
——*Edward Jenner*, <http://www.whonamedit.com/doctor.cfm/1818.html>
——*Heine-Medin Disease*, <www.whonamedit.com/synd.cfm/544.html>
——*Heinrich Hermann Robert Koch*, <www.whonamedit.com/doctor.cfm/2987.html>
——*Leon Charles Albert Calmette*, <www.whonamedit.com/doctor.cfm/2413.html>

Williams, Michael, 2007, *John James Rickard Macleod*, Diabetologia, <www.diabetologia-
    journal.org/past%20masters/macleod.htm>

Wilson, John L., 1998, *Stanford University School of Medicine and the Predecessor Schools: A historical
    perspective,* Stanford School of Medicine History,
    <http://elane.stanford.edu/wilson/Text/5f.html - 32k>

Wong, George, 2003, *Penicillin: The wonder drug*, University of Hawaii, Botany,
    <www.botany.hawaii.edu/faculty/wong/BOT135/Lect21b.htm>

Wood, James, 12 April 2002, *Black Death and Plague not Linked,* BBC News,
    <news.bbc.co.uk/1/hi/health/1925513.stm>

World Health Organization International, *Diphtheria in Afghanistan*,
    <www.who.int/csr/don/archive/country/afg>
——*Epidemic and Pandemic Alert and Response*, <www.who.int/csr/en>
——*Epidemic and Pandemic Alert and Response, Suspected Plague in the Democratic Republic of Congo*
    <www.who.int/csr/don/2006_11_07/en/index.html>
——*Expanded Programme on Immunization*, <www.worldbank.org/HDNet/HDdocs.nsf/0/6...>
——*Human and Animal Rabies: A neglected disease*, <www.who.int/rabies/en>
——*Plague Fact Sheet*, <www.who.int/topics/plabue/en/>
——*Rabies Bulletin Europe, 1ˢᵗ Quarter, 2006*, <www.who-rabies-bulletin.org>

——*Smallpox*, <www.who.int/topics/smallpox/en/>

——*Smallpox Fact Sheet*, <www.who.int/csr/disease/smallpox/>

——12 December 2006, *Women's Health News: New vaccines against HPV could save hundreds of thousands of lives if delivered effectively*,
<www.who.int/entity/mediacentre/news/releases/2006/pr73/en/index.html>

World Health Organization Media Centre, September 2006, *Diabetes:What is diabetes*, Fact Sheet 312, <www.who.int.mediacentre/factsheets/fs312/en>

——*Global Cancer Rates Could Increase by 50% to 15 Million by 2020*,
<www.who.int.mediacentre/2003/pr27/en/>

——12 December 2006, New Vaccines Against Cervical Cancer Major Opportunity for Developing World, <www.who.int/entity/mediacentre/news/releases/2006/pr73/en/index.html>

York, Barry, September 2001, Howard Florey and the Development of Penicillin, NLA News, Vol. XI, No. 12, National Library of Australia,
<www.nla.gov.au/pub/nlanews/2001/sep01/sep01news.html>

VISUAL MEDIA

SBS Australia, *Penicillin:The magic bullet*, Arcimedia, 3 August 2006.

INDEX